D1551662

The CRC Press MODERN NUTRITION *Series*

The Mediterranean Diet: *Constituents and Health Promotion*

CRC SERIES IN MODERN NUTRITION
Edited by Ira Wolinsky and James F. Hickson, Jr.

Published Titles

Manganese in Health and Disease, Dorothy J. Klimis-Tavantzis

Nutrition and AIDS: Effects and Treatments, Ronald R. Watson

Nutrition Care for HIV-Positive Persons: A Manual for Individuals and Their Caregivers, Saroj M. Bahl and James F. Hickson, Jr.

Calcium and Phosphorus in Health and Disease, John J.B. Anderson and Sanford C. Garner

Edited by Ira Wolinsky

Published Titles

Practical Handbook of Nutrition in Clinical Practice, Donald F. Kirby and Stanley J. Dudrick

Handbook of Dairy Foods and Nutrition, Gregory D. Miller, Judith K. Jarvis, and Lois D. McBean

Advanced Nutrition: Macronutrients, Carolyn D. Berdanier

Childhood Nutrition, Fima Lifschitz

Nutrition and Health: Topics and Controversies, Felix Bronner

Nutrition and Cancer Prevention, Ronald R. Watson and Siraj I. Mufti

Nutritional Concerns of Women, Ira Wolinsky and Dorothy J. Klimis-Tavantzis

Nutrients and Gene Expression: Clinical Aspects, Carolyn D. Berdanier

Antioxidants and Disease Prevention, Harinda S. Garewal

Advanced Nutrition: Micronutrients, Carolyn D. Berdanier

Nutrition and Women's Cancers, Barbara Pence and Dale M. Dunn

Nutrients and Foods in AIDS, Ronald R. Watson

Nutrition: Chemistry and Biology, Second Edition, Julian E. Spallholz, L. Mallory Boylan, and Judy A. Driskell

Melatonin in the Promotion of Health, Ronald R. Watson

Nutritional and Environmental Influences on the Eye, Allen Taylor

Laboratory Tests for the Assessment of Nutritional Status, Second Edition, H.E. Sauberlich

Advanced Human Nutrition, Robert E.C. Wildman and Denis M. Medeiros

Handbook of Dairy Foods and Nutrition, Second Edition, Gregory D. Miller, Judith K. Jarvis, and Lois D. McBean

Nutrition in Space Flight and Weightlessness Models, Helen W. Lane and Dale A. Schoeller

Forthcoming Titles

The CRC Press MODERN NUTRITION *Series*

The Mediterranean Diet: Constituents and Health Promotion

Edited by
Antonia-Leda Matalas
Antonis Zampelas
Vassilis Stavrinos
Ira Wolinsky

CRC Press
Boca Raton   London   New York   Washington, D.C.

Library of Congress Cataloging-in-Publication Data

The Mediterranean diet / edited by Antonia L. Matalas ...[et al.]
   p. cm. (Modern nutrition)
Includes bibliographical references and index.
ISBN 0-8493-0110-6 (alk. paper)
1. Nutrition. 2. Diet--Mediterranean Region. I. Matalas, Antonia L. II. Modern
nutrition (Boca Raton, Fla.)
QP141 .M347 2000
613.2′0918′2—dc21

00-046818
CIP

© 2001 by CRC Press LLC

No claim to original U.S. Government works
International Standard Book Number 0-8493-0110-6
Library of Congress Card Number 00-046818
Printed in the United States of America 1 2 3 4 5 6 7 8 9 0
Printed on acid-free paper

SERIES PREFACE FOR MODERN NUTRITION

The CRC Series in Modern Nutrition is dedicated to providing the widest possible coverage of topics in nutrition. Nutrition is an interdisciplinary, interprofessional field par excellence. It is noted by its broad range and diversity. We trust the titles and authorship in this series will reflect that range and diversity.

Published for a scholarly audience, the volumes in the CRC Series in Modern Nutrition are designed to explain, review, and explore present knowledge and recent trends, developments, and advances in nutrition. As such, they will also appeal to the educated general reader. The format for the series will vary with the needs of the author and the topic, including, but not limited to, edited volumes, monographs, handbooks, and texts.

Contributors from any bona fide area of nutrition, including the controversial, are welcome.

We welcome this important and timely contribution to this series. This book will be useful to a broad spectrum of nutritionists and life scientists of all walks.

Ira Wolinsky, Ph.D.
University of Houston
Series Editor

Preface

We, the nutrition and dietetics faculty at Harokopio University, together with our co-workers, collaborators, and colleagues, are pleased to have assembled a volume on the very timely topic of the Mediterranean Diet. Harokopio University, the newest higher education institution in Greece, encompassed two departments at the time this book was written —the Department of Nutrition and Dietetics and the Department of Home Economics. The faculty in Harokopio University comprises a unique concentration of nutrition specializations and expertise. As such, we were in a singular position to produce this book.

This volume explores the relationships among the Mediterranean Diet, nutritional status, and disease, and evaluates nutritional practices intended to minimize or retard the incidence and progress of major diseases. Interest in changing dietary patterns is a recognition of the importance of the link between diet and health. Food-consumption patterns are closely tied to incidence and severity of major chronic debilitating diseases. In this sense, "You are what you eat."

The basic observation underlying current interest in the Mediterranean Diet is that adults living in certain olive-growing areas of the Mediterranean basin display high life expectancies and rates of chronic disease, including coronary heart disease, that are among the lowest in the world. These benefits are achieved despite socio-economic indicators that are often much lower than those of more industrialized nations in North America and Europe. Attention has focused on diet as the key factor. In the Mediterranean Diet, olive oil provides more calories than any other individual food; it is the principal source of dietary fat. The Mediterranean Diet is largely plant-food based and is characterized by consumption of large amounts of fruits and vegetables, legumes and grains, and small amounts of meat. The Mediterranean Diet, typified most by a traditional Greek diet with its recognized culinary qualities and nutritional adequacy, is the subject of ongoing studies as a cultural model for dietary improvement and health promotion in the USA and all of Europe. It may be a prototype of a healthy diet for all of us.

The volume is divided into three parts. The first begins with the classical antecedents of the Mediterranean Diet and then goes on to define what it is, and to describe its characteristics, patterns, and epidemiological aspects. The next section deals with specific food components and commodities constituting the diet, and addresses supply, production, usage, availability, consumption, choices, patterns, and contributions to the diet. The third section deals with health promotion and disease prevention and includes discussion of life expectancy, coronary heart disease, diabetes, cancer, and hypertension. The entire volume is pulled together by chapters giving dietary recommendations based on our understanding of the Mediterranean Diet, suggested future research, and applications.

The first chapter deals with the diet of the classical Greeks and Romans. Food patterns of both poor and elite Classical Hellenistic Greeks and Republican Empire

Romans were based on cereals, legumes, and a wide range of fruits, nuts, seeds, and vegetables, with relatively limited meat intake. The second chapter treats the modern historical background and dietary patterns in pre-World War II Greece, comparing these with contemporary European patterns. It concludes that the Greek version of the Mediterranean Diet, based on the diet followed by rural Cretan populations in the 1960s, represents a transition pattern, and not one that had persisted over time in the region. The last chapter in the background section of the book, a key chapter defining the modern Mediterranean Diet, discusses epidemiological aspects and current patterns. Evidence of the role of the Mediterranean Diet in longevity is discussed. Current guidelines based on the traditional Mediterranean Diet are given, with the example of guidelines for adults in Greece.

The next section of the book discusses the constituents of the Mediterranean Diet. Included are discussions of fats and oils; fruits, vegetables, legumes and grains; milk and dairy products; meat and meat products —their consumption, nutrient value, safety issues, and contribution to the Diet.

In the last section, Chapter 9 discusses longevity, and the authors present biochemical and nutritional evidence that the reported longevity and reduced mortality rates of Mediterranean populations are attributed, at least in part, to their dietary habits. Chapter 10 deals with diabetes mellitus, obesity, and the Mediterranean Diet, and Chapter 11 discusses the Mediterranean Diet and coronary heart disease. Epidemiological data indicate low morbidity and mortality rates for coronary heart disease rates for the Cretan population compared with other populations. The effects of significant components of the Mediterranean Diet on the development of coronary heart disease are also elaborated here. Chapter 12 deals with the important topic of the cancer-protective properties of the Mediterranean Diet. It focuses on cancer and dietary epidemiological evidence for southern European Mediterranean countries. The upward trend in total cancer mortality in the Mediterranean is paralleled by features of nutritional transition and westernization of the diet. In Chapter 13, we benefit from discussion of the Cyprus experience. For centuries, Cypriots have traditionally been nourished on a diet that resembles the Mediterranean Diet model. However, it was found recently that the majority of children in modern Cyprus have moved away from the traditional pattern, and now consume a western-type diet, with its attendant problems and challenges. The last chapter deals with nutrition policy aspects, such as food-supply issues, nutrient-supply issues, and nutrient risk-factor issues. Future research needs are discussed, with an emphasis on monounsaturated fatty acids.

To create this book, we put together a roster of individuals uniquely suited to the task. We feel honored to share in its creation with them. We hope that it will be useful to the scientific and consumer communities in evaluating the literature, and will facilitate the recommendation and adoption of dietary allowances and appropriate food choices.

Antonia-Leda Matalas, Ph.D.

Antonis Zampelas, Ph.D.

Vassilis Stavrinos, Ph.D.

Ira Wolinsky, Ph.D.

About the Editors

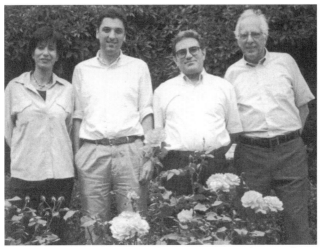

The editors: (left to right) Antonia-Leda Matalas, Antonis Zampelas, Vassilis Stavrinos, and Ira Wolinsky.

Antonia-Leda Matalas, Ph.D., is a member of the faculty of the Department of Nutrition and Dietetics, Harokopio University, Athens. Her undergraduate training was in the Aristotelian University of Thessaloniki and she received her Ph.D. in Nutrition from the Department of Nutrition, University of California at Davis. Her applied research interests include dietary assessment, eating disorders, nutritional policy, ecology of nutrition, and the Mediterranean Diet.

Antonis Zampelas, Ph.D., is on the faculty of the Department of Nutrition and Dietetics, Harokopio University, Athens. He received his B.S. in Food Science and Technology, Agricultural University of Athens, his M.Sc. in Food Science at the University of Reading, U.K. , and his Ph.D. in Nutrition at the University of Surrey, U.K. His research interests include nutritional aspects of lipid metabolism, nutrition and chronic diseases, and the Mediterranean Diet.

Vassilis Stavrinos, Ph.D., is Vice Rector of Harokopio University and a member of the Department of Nutrition and Dietetics. His undergraduate training was in Athens and his graduate degrees obtained at the University of London and University of Athens. He has further served as research fellow at the University of Louvain and Princeton University. His research interests include consumer issues.

Ira Wolinsky, Ph.D., is a nutrition scientist at the University of Houston. He received his B.S. degree in Chemistry from the City College of New York and his M.S. and Ph.D. degrees in Biochemistry from Kansas University. He has served in nutrition research and teaching positions at The Hebrew University, The University of Missouri, and Pennsylvania State University. He has published numerous nutrition papers in the open literature. Dr. Wolinsky has co-authored a book on the history of the science of nutrition, *Nutrition and Nutritional Diseases: The Evolution of Concepts*, and co-edited several CRC Press volumes, including *Nutritional Applications in Exercise and Sport*; *Nutritional Concerns of Women*; *Sports Nutrition, Vitamins and Trace Elements*; *Energy-Yielding Macronutrients*; and *Energy Metabolism in Sports Nutrition*.

Contributors

Spyros A. Georgakis, Ph.D.
Department of Food Hygiene
School of Veterinary Medicine
University of Thessaloniki
Thessaloniki, Greece
SpyrosG@vet.auth.gr

Dimitrios G. Gerasopoulos, Ph.D.
National Agricultural Research
  Foundation
Thermi, Thessaloniki
Greece
D-gerasopoulis@usq.net

Michael J. Gibney, Ph.D.
Department of Clinical Medicine
St. James Hospital
Dublin, Ireland
Iefs@indigo.ie

Louis E. Grivetti, Ph.D.
Department of Nutrition
University of California at Davis
Davis, CA
LEGrivetti@UCDavis.Edu

Gharalambos Hadjigeorgiou, M.D.
Healthy Children Program
Ministries of Health and Education
Strovolos, Cyprus

Michael Hourdakis, B.S.
Department of Nutrition and Dietetics
Harokopio University
Athens, Greece
MHourdakis@.yahoo.com

Anthony Kafatos, M.D., Ph.D.
Department of Social Medicine,
  Preventive Medicine and Nutrition
Medical School
University of Crete
Iraklion, Crete
Greece

Nicholas L. Katsilambros, M.D., Ph.D.
Department of Propaedeutic Medicine
Medical School
University of Athens
Athens, Greece
laennec@techlink.gr

Apostolos K. Kiritsakis, Ph.D.
Department of Foods
School of Food Technology and
  Nutrition
TEI of Thessaloniki
Sindos, Thessaloniki
Greece
Kiritsaka@aetos.it.teithe.gr

Yiannis A. Kourides, M.D.
Healthy Children Program
Ministries of Health and Education
Paphos, Cyprus

Konstantinos Kyritsakis, B.S.
Department of Food Science
University of Thessaloniki
Thessaloniki, Greece

Pagona Lagiou, M.D., Ph.D.
Department of Hygiene and
  Epidemiology
Medical School
University of Athens
Athens, Greece
nit@nut.uoa.gr

George Mamalakis, M.S.
Department of Social Medicine,
  Preventive Medicine and Nutrition
Medical School
University of Crete
Iraklion, Crete
Greece

Antonios J. Mantis, Ph.D.
Department of Food Hygiene
School of Veterinary Medicine
University of Thessaloniki
Thessaloniki, Greece
AMantis@vet.auth.gr

Antonia-Leda Matalas, Ph.D.
Department of Nutrition and Dietetics
Harokopio University
Athens, Greece
AMatala@hua.gr

Maria-Nectaria Mavroudi, Dipl.
Department of Foods
School of Food Technology and
  Nutrition
TEI of Thessaloniki
Sindos, Thessaloniki
Greece

George D. Nanos, Ph.D.
Department of Agriculture
University of Thessaly
Volos, Greece
Gnanos@UTH.gr

**Constantina Papoutsakis-Tsarouhas,
M.S., R.D.**
Department of Nutrition and Dietetics
Harokopio University
Athens, Greece
Tina.Papoutsakis@hua.gr

Helen M. Roche, Ph.D.
Department of Clinical Medicine
St. James Hospital
Dublin, Ireland

Savvas C. Savva, M.D.
Healthy Children Program
Ministries of Health and Education
Nicosia, Cyprus

Maria Shamounki, M.D.
Healthy Children Program
Ministries of Health and Education
Nicosia, Cyprus

Vassilis Stavrinos, Ph.D.
Department of Nutrition and Dietetics
Harokopio University
Athens, Greece
vstavrinos@hua.gr

Michael Tornaritis, Ph.D.
Healthy Children Program
Ministries of Health and Education
Strovolos, Cyprus
Iochrist@cylink.com.cy

Antonia Trichopoulou, M.D., Ph.D.
Department of Hygiene and
  Epidemiology
Medical School
University of Athens
Athens, Greece
Antonia@nut.uoa.gr

Tonia Vassilakou, Ph.D.
Department of Nutrition and
  Biochemistry
National School of Public Health
Athens, Greece

Ira Wolinsky, Ph.D.
Department of Human Development
University of Houston
Houston, TX
IWolinsky@UH.Edu

Mary Yannakoulia, M.S.
Department of Nutrition and Dietetics
Harokopio University
Athens, Greece
MYiannak@hua.gr

Nikos Yiannakouris, Ph.D.
Department of Home Economics
Harokopio University
Athens, Greece
NYiannak@hua.gr

Antonis Zampelas, Ph.D.
Department of Nutrition and Dietetics
Harokopio University
Athens, Greece
AZampelas@hua.gr

Acknowledgments

Our thanks to those who contributed to the production of this volume, either directly or indirectly, particularly Irini Granika. Also, special thanks to Sylvia Wood and Dawn Boyd, CRC Press, for their efforts in the production of this book.

Dedication

To the memory of Professor Costas Balis,
who made seminal contributions to the development of
Harokopio University

Contents

Part I

Background

1 Mediterranean Food Patterns: The View From Antiquity, Ancient Greeks and Romans

Louis E. Grivetti

CONTENTS

0-8493-0110-6/01/$0.00+$.50

I. INTRODUCTION AND SOURCES

The archaeological richness of Mediterranean societies is unrivaled elsewhere. Domestication of plants and animals occurred at several centers in southwestern Asia, writing was first invented in the region more than 5,000 years ago, and medical and dietary systems that evolved here are still practiced. The Mediterranean basin has been the cradle of several great civilizations, with economic-military-political centers located at Athens, Byblos, Carthage, Knossos, Memphis, Mycenae, Rome, Thebes, Troy, and elsewhere.

Food-related evidence from ancient Mediterranean cultures is diversified and vast. Carbonized seeds that date to the 10th millennium B.C.E. reveal hunting and gathering economies. Domestication of plants and animals in the region was followed by herding and settled agriculture. Stone technologies of the Paleolithic, Mesolithic, and Neolithic periods gave way to smelting of copper, bronze, and iron. Iron Age settlements ultimately evolved into sophisticated urban centers exemplified by ancient Athens and Rome.

The study of food in antiquity requires specialists from many disciplines, especially archaeology, botany, chemistry, classics, dietetics and nutrition, food science and technology, geography, history, linguistics, and zoology. Forensic scientists have lent their approaches to the study of excavated ancient human bones; mummy autopsies have provided information on "last meals" through analysis of stomach and intestinal contents; analysis of bone, hair, nails, and teeth has revealed data on energy-protein intake and the presence or absence of mineral and vitamin deficiencies or toxicities; coprolites and preserved excreta from public latrines have provided selected insights on diet and confirmed the presence of parasitic diseases. Household and temple frescoes, as well as tomb art and burial artifacts, have revealed food-related information: foods and meals presented to the dead, agricultural and animal husbandry activities, and food-production and cooking tools and containers. Pollen analysis of mud bricks, study of ancient religious texts, and perusal of ancient travel accounts permits the reconstruction of ancient food patterns. Public and private art from ancient Mediterranean societies has revealed extensive food-related information such as dining objects and artistic renderings of malnutrition and disease, while analyses of chemical residues have differentiated between objects that once held wine from those that contained anchovy pastes. Available, too, are actual cooked foods — ready to eat — almost in a state of suspended animation — preserved during the explosive eruption of Mt. Vesuvius in Italy.

Great civilizations leave written texts. Throughout the eastern Mediterranean, archaeologists and linguists have pored over and deciphered Egyptian hieroglyphs and the Phoenician alphabet, and have traced food-related terms from earliest Greek to Classical and Hellenistic periods, and earliest Latin to Republican and Empire texts, and ultimately into Byzantine and ecclesiastical Latin expressions. An impressive body of literature has survived from antiquity that documents agricultural practices, food storage, cooking, and dietary patterns.

A. Primary

Primary sources include archaeological reports of flora and fauna at excavated sites, for example, at the prehistoric site of Sitagroi in northeastern Greece;[1] at Minoan localities of Gournia, Hagia Triada, Knossos on Crete;[2] and at Herculaneum and Pompeii in Italy.[3–4] Vase paintings studied for food and dining context have revealed breads and various meats, while surveys of mosaics, relief-murals, and statuary have determined the roles of domesticated and wild animals in both Greek and Roman everyday life and diet.[5–7]

Most valuable, however, are original texts that contain observations and descriptions of foods and their preparation in everyday or festival contexts. While the ancient Greeks left only fragmented recipes, the important cookbook by Apicius of Rome, *De Re Coquinaria* (The Art of Cooking), written in the 1st century CE, can be perused nearly 2,000 years later for insights on the culinary habits of wealthy Romans.[8]

B. Secondary: Reviews and Compilations

Study of Mediterranean foods, especially those of the ancient Greeks and Romans, has attracted scholars for nearly a century.[9–14] Numerous food-related monographs and articles based on archaeological or literary data focus on specific items consumed by the Greeks and Romans. A sampling of this rich literature would include information on: apple,[15] barley cakes,[16] birds in general,[17] bread,[18] carrot,[19] celery,[20] cheese,[21] chicken,[22] fig,[23] fish in general,[24–27] honey,[28] lovage,[29] lupine,[30] marjoram,[31] meat in general,[32] medlar (loquat),[33] melon,[34] milk,[35] mint,[36] mushroom,[37] mustard,[38] olive,[39] oyster,[40] parsnip,[41] pepper,[42] poppy seed,[43] sesame,[44] spinach/orach,[45] thyme,[36] tracta/dry biscuit/crackers,[46–47] turnip,[41] and wheat/wheat cakes.[48]

Both ancient and contemporary authors have identified the fauna and flora of Greece,[49–53] and those of the Italian peninsula.[54–55] Additional reviews have identified Greek birds, edible and inedible;[17,56] fish names used by ancient Greek writers living in Egypt;[57] Greek and Roman hunting techniques;[58–59] even Greek and Roman dietary-medical uses of insects. Both marine and terrestrial invertebrates have been catalogued.[60–61]

II. GREEK FOODS

A. Most Ancient Greeks

Foods of the most ancient Greeks can be identified from flora and fauna remains excavated at late Paleolithic-, Neolithic-, Copper-, Bronze-, and Iron-Age sites. Oldest remains of seeds, dated to 11,000–7,300 BCE, pre-date plant domestication and agriculture but reveal use of such wild foods as barley, lentils, oats, and peas. The earliest evidence for domestication and agriculture in Greece dates to ca. 6,200–5,300 BCE, where the following crops were grown: barley, millet, oats, wheat; lentils, peas, and vetch. Gathered foods that also accompanied these domesticated crops included acorn, almond, cherry, grapes, olive, pistachio, plum, and pear.[62–63]

Excavations at Copper-, Bronze-, and early Iron-Age sites in Greece also have revealed dietary use of both wild and domesticated fruits and nuts, among them acorn, almond, anise, apple, blackberry, blackthorn/sloe, caper, cherry, coriander, cowberry, cucumber, elderberry, fig, grape, hawthorn, white mustard, olive, pear, plum/bullace, pomegranate, poppy, raspberry, rose hip, strawberry, strawberry tree, and water chestnut.[64]

Excavations at Sitagroi, a prehistoric village in northeastern Greece, revealed the presence of domesticated cattle, goats, pigs, and sheep, while additional remains — aurochs (wild progenitor of common cattle), badger, brown bear, beaver, bustard, wild cat, chamois, red deer, fallow deer, roe deer, duck, fox, geese, hare, hedgehog, marten, wild pig, quail, turtle, and various fish bones — showed the importance of hunting.[1]

Excavations at Dimini, Nemea, Olynthus, Orchomenos, Pylos, Sparta, Thebes, and Vardaroftsa yielded acorn, almond, barley, fava bean, beef/cattle, elk, fig, fish, geese/eggs, goat, grapes and wine-making equipment, lentils, millet, fresh water mussel, olive, pear, pea, pork/pig, pinna shells, scallop/pecten, lamb/sheep, tortoise, venison/deer, and wheat.[65-66] Although olive pits or stones have been excavated at most ancient Greek sites, pollen evidence suggests that olive use was rare in Greece until ca. 1300 BCE, and cultivated olive trees were uncommon until ca. 900–700 BCE.[66]

Turning to Crete, the late Stone Age or Neolithic levels at Knossos, dated to ca. 6000 BCE, revealed the presence of domesticated goats and sheep (75% of bones excavated), pigs (18% of the bones), and bovines (7%). Excavations at post-Neolithic sites at Gournia, Hagia Triada, and Knossos unearthed almond, barley, bean, beef/cattle, chick-pea, fig, fish, goat, olive, pea, pork/pig, lamb/sheep, venison/deer, wheat, and various types of edible marine hard-shelled mollusks.[2, 67]

Iron-Age Mycenaeans had a cereal-based diet, where barley and wheat were commonly prepared as porridge or bread. Although bones of cattle, goats, pigs, and sheep have been excavated at Mycenaean sites, presumably little meat was consumed and beans and lentils would have been the primary protein resources. Still, forensic analysis of Mycenaean-era skeletons has suggested that diets were low in protein, energy, and iron, since adult females (n = 154) averaged 160 cm in height, and adult males (n = 191) 167 cm. Further, average age at death was 32 for adult females, 39 for adult males.[68] On the other hand, the Mycenaean diet may have been superior to that of the early Classical Greek Period, given evidence of even shorter average stature: 153–154 cm for adult females, 162–163 cm for adult males.[69]

The ancient Achaeans, who occupied Mycenae, Pylos, and Sparta, were extolled by Homer of Chios. Earliest literary mention of Greek foods and culinary practices, in fact, are found within Homer's *Iliad*[70] and *Odyssey*,[71] where typical food patterns of the heroes who besieged Troy were characterized as bread, meat, and wine, but not fish and fowl. Some scholars have argued, however, that food-related descriptions that appear in Homer's texts reflect ritual/religious practices, and were not characteristic of everyday meal-time traditions even among the elite.[78]

B. CLASSICAL AND HELLENISTIC PERIODS

1. Dining Patterns

According to Athenaeus of Naucratis, the word *dais* signified a meal, and was derived from the verb, *daiesthai*, "to divide" or "to distribute equally," and he wrote that men who roasted meat were called *diatros*, or "dividers," because they provided equal portions of meat.[73] Athenaeus cited Philemon of Syracuse, who wrote that the Greeks ate four meals daily: *akratisma*, *ariston*, *hesperisma*, and *deipnon*. The first, *akratisma*, was equivalent to "breaking the fast," and from this word evolved *akratos*, or "bread sopped in unmixed wine," typically eaten as a breakfast food.[74]

Philemon's explanation not withstanding, considerable confusion reigned regarding Greek dining terminology. According to Athenaeus, in Homeric times breakfast was called *ariston* or *embroma*, and the fourfold terminology of Philemon changed through Greek history and became *akratisma* (breaking the fast), *deipnon* (midday meal), *dorpestos* (early evening meal), and *epidorpis* (later dinner). Athenaeus also wrote that meal-time terminology was so confused that Aeschylus of Eleusis had to teach his supervisors to distinguish among meals. Still others, according to Athenaeus, held that the words *ariston*, *deipnon*, or *epidorpis* signified the midday meal, while the evening meal was variously called *dorpestos* or *hesperisma*. Ultimately, the early-morning meal of the Heroic Era, *ariston*, became the midday meal; *akratisma,* or breakfast, remained in position, while *deipnon* shifted to the evening meal.[75]

Among both poor and elite, breakfast commonly consisted of barley or wheat bread dipped in undiluted wine, sometimes eaten with figs or olives.[76-77] Athenaeus also remarked that the word *amaristeton* applied to persons who skipped breakfast.[78]

The midday ariston was informal, commonly eaten outside the home, usually was light, and consisted of various warm foods.[76]

In contrast, the evening deipnon was heavy and consumed at home. Among wealthy Greeks, it consisted of elaborate cooking where guests could be entertained. A simple dinner–drinking party was called *potos,* while an elaborate dinner with several food courses and entertainment was a *symposium*. Three components characterized the Greek evening meal: *sitos*, *opson*, and *oinos*. Staple foods, collectively called *sitos*, were served first and included barley, lentils, and wheat. Complementing the sitos were relishes, or *opson,* such as cakes, cheese, eels, eggs, fish and shellfish, lettuce, mullet, oysters, shrimps, broiled tunny (tuna), and perhaps thrushes. Different meat courses commonly followed, maybe goat, mutton, and pork, sometimes sausage and lesser cuts such as feet and pig's snout, kid's head, and sometimes domesticated fowl. During the third component, *oinos*, which concluded dinner, wines were served with *tragemata*, or collectively, sweet cakes, various confections, curdled cream, dried and fresh fruits, honey, and nuts.[76, 79-81]

Athenaeus wrote that the banquets of the wealthy started with appetizers or *propoma*, among them small birds, sliced eggs, sometimes combination dishes that included salad leaves, Egyptian perfume, myrrh, pepper, and sedge. He cited Phaenias of Eresus, who wrote that common dessert foods were soft tender beans and chickpeas. Athenaeus also commented that, at the conclusion of Greek banquets, the tongues of animals served were cut out to signal that the feast was over and that guests should depart.[82]

Body position while eating varied by custom and era. Athenaeus observed that Homer's heroes sat upright while dining, and also cited Hegesander of Delphi, who wrote that Macedonian men were not permitted to recline at dinner until they had speared a wild boar without using a hunting net.[83] Scholars have assumed that most families ate at home, that adult women, slaves, and children ate independently of men, that adult women ate together, and that "respectable women" did not dine outside the house in the evening.[76,81]

2. Common Foods

What constituted suitable food to the Classical Greeks, whether in the Greek "heartland" or throughout Mediterranean lands? Athenaeus preserved the comment by Eubulus of Athens that "real food" consisted of items that promoted health and physical strength, especially beef boiled in huge quantities — with generous portions of foot and snout — and slices of young pork sprinkled with salt.[84] Still, a broad range of foods available to Greeks throughout the Mediterranean can be identified (Table 1).

Common meats during Classical and Hellenistic periods included beef, mutton, goat, and pork. Wild game augmented meals, specifically wild boar, deer, hare, and numerous varieties of domesticated and wild birds including beccafico (songbirds), blackbird, bustard, chicken, coot, crane, cuckoo, dove, duck, francolin (partridge), goose, grebe, guinea-fowl, jay, lark, nightingale, ostrich, owl, peacock/peahen, pelican, pheasant, pigeon, quail, starling, swan, thrush, and wagtail.[85-89]

Out in the "lands," away from the urban centers, farmers and wealthy absentee landowners regularly consumed goat, mutton, pork, and wild game. In contrast, urban Greeks probably consumed more fish than meat, since the term *opson*, which originally signified "relish," gradually shifted in meaning to "fish," a linguistic transition that suggested that bread and fish were common foods of the majority of urban Greeks. Fresh fish and seafoods would have included anchovy, carp, conger eels, eels from Lake Copais, gudgeon, halibut, mackerel, mullet, octopus, shark, sole, squid, tunny, and turbot, as well as various echinoderms, mussels, oysters, and snails.[85-88]

Milk was rarely was drunk (except in a medicinal context); most was converted to cheese. Butter was considered fit only for barbarians, and most was used medicinally to soothe wounds. Olive and sesame were the primary dietary fats/oils.[11, 87]

Barley and wheat were the most commonly grown cereals, while minor grains included millet and rye. Proper wheat bread, *artos*, was baked in the form of round loaves and consumed on festival days. Rural and urban poor did not regularly consume wheat bread but ate barley cakes or *maza,* similar to modern American-style pancakes or griddle cakes. These were sodden with water and eaten as porridge. Women bread vendors, *artopolides*, were recognized in urban centers.[85-88]

While many vegetables and legumes were common fare in rural Greece, fresh varieties probably would have been scarce in urban centers. Beans and lentils were

TABLE 1
Greek-Roman Regional Foods: Selections from *the Deipnosophists* by Athenaeus[161]

Foods of Animal Origin:
Mammal:
Beef: Troy (1:8:F)
Beef ribs: Thessaly (1:27:E)
Cheese: Gallipoli (9:370:D)
Deer: General (2:41:D)
Entrails: General (1:23:F)
Goat: Melos (1:4:C)
Hare: Astypalaea (9:400:D)
Lard: General (1:25:D)
Pig: Argive region (7:288:F)
Sausage: General (2:57:A)
Sheep/Lamb: Troy (1:9:C)
Spleen: General (2:49:F)
Sweetbreads: General (2:49:F)

Fish:
Anchovy; Phaleron (7:293:E)
Bream: Eretria (7:295:D)
Chromis: Pella (7:328:A)
Eel: Lake Copais (4:135:C-D)
Glaucus: Megara (7:295:B-C)
Mackerel; Hellespont (1:27:E)
Mullet: Abdera (7:307:B)
Plaice: Eleusis (7:330:A-B)
Ray: Syracuse (7:286:E)
Sardine: Chalcedon (7:329:A)
Sea Bream: Delos (7:327:D)
Shark (Dog Fish): Rhodes (7:295:A)
Sprat: Carystia (7:295:C)
Sturgeon: Bosporos (3:116:A-B)
Swordfish: Sicily (7:314:F)
Tunny: Samos (7:301:F)

Fowl:
Blackbird: General (2:65:D)
Chicken: General (2:65:E)
Dove: General (1:32:A-B)
Duck: General (2:65:E)
Eggs: Chicken (2:58:B)
Eggs: Goose (2:58:B)
Eggs: Peacock (2:58:B)
Finch: General (2:65:C)
Francolin: Boeotia (9:388:B)

Foods of Animal Origin (continued):
Fowl (continued):
Geese: Egypt (9:384:A)
Gold Finch: General (2:65:E)
Kestrel: General (2:65:E)
Parrot: General (2:65:E)
Partridge: Athens (9:390:A)
Pheasant: Phasia (9:386:E)
Pigeon: Sicily (9:395:C)
Quail: General (9:92:A-F)
Ring Dove: Egypt (9:394:C)
Sparrow: General (2:65:E)
Starling: General (2:65:E)
Thrush: Syracuse (2:64:F)

Invertebrates:
Barnacle: Egypt (3:91:A)
Crab: Parium (3:92:D)
Crayfish: Mt. Athos (3:105:D)
Honey: Attica (3:101:D-E)
Honey comb: General (2:56:E)
Locust: General (2:63:C)
Lobster: Thasos (3:105:D)
Mussel (fresh water): Ephesus (3:90:D)
Mussel (marine): Alexandria (3:87:F)
Oyster: Calchedon (3:92:E)
Prawn: Smyrna (1:7:B)
Scallop: Mitylene (3:86:E)
Sea Urchin: Sicily (3:91:A-B
Shrimp: Ambracian gulf (3:105:E)
Snail (terrestrial): General (2:64:E)
Squid: Abdera (7:324:B)
Whelk: Strait of Messene (3:92:D)

Foods of Plant Origin:
Bread and Grains:
Barley: Thebes (3:112:A)
Barley Cakes: Eretria (4:160:A)
Bread: Alexandrian (3:111:B)
Bread: Athens (3:112:C-D)
Bread: Macedonian (3:114:B)
Bread: Thessalian (3:114:B)
Millet: General (2:58:D)

TABLE 1 (CONTINUED)
Greek-Roman Regional Foods: Selections from *the Deipnosophists* by Athenaeus[161]

Foods of Plant Origin (continued):

Bread and Grains (continued):
Wheat: Athens (3:112:B)
Wheat: Lusitania (8:331:A)
Wheat flour: Phoenicia (1:28:A)

Condiments-Flavoring Agents:
Bay leaf: Cnidia (2:66:D)
Caper: General (2:63:A)
Chicory: General (2:71:A)
Coriander: General (2:70:A)
Cumin: Aethiopian (2:68:B)
Fennel: Marathon (2:56:C)
Marjoram: Tenedos (1:28:D)
Mint: General (2:49:E)
Mustard: Cyprus (1:28:D)
Myrrh: General (2:66:D)
Pennyroyal: General (2:63:A)
Pepper: Libyan (2:66:D)
Poppy: General (2:68:E)
Rue: General (2:63:A)
Safflower: General (2:71:A)
Sage: General (2:63:A)
Silphium: Cyrene (1:27:E)
Sorrel: General (2:71:A)
Thyme: Attica (2:43:C)
Truffles: Cyrene (2:62:A)
Vinegar: Pontic (9:366:C)

Fruits:
Apple: Delphi (3:80:D
Cherry: Milesia (2:51:B)
Date: Phoenicia (1:28:A)
Fig: Chios (3:80:C)
Grape: Lesbos (3:92:E)
Medlar: General (2:50:D)
Melon: General (2:68:E)
Mulberry: Alexandria (2:51:B)
Pear: Euboea (1:27:F)
Plum: Damascus (2:49:D)
Pomegranate: General (1:25:A)
Pumpkin: General (2:59:B)
Quince: General (2:59:B-C)

Foods of Plant Origin (continued):

Fruits (continued):
Raisins: Rhodes (1:27:F)
Sycamore Fig: Egypt (2:50:B-C)

Legumes-Nuts:
Acorn: Elis (1:28:A)
Almond: Lacedaemon/Sparta (2:52:C)
Bean: Lemnos (9:366:C)
Chestnut: Sardis (2:54:C-D)
Chick-pea: Milesia (2:55:B)
Lentil: Gela (1:30:B)
Lupine: Lacedaemon/Sparta (2:55:E)
Pine nut: General (2:57:B-D)
Walnut: Persia (2:53:D-E)

Oils:
Olive: Samos (2:66:F)
Sesame: General (2:64:E)

Vegetables:
Artichoke: Libya (2:71:C)
Asparagus: Lusitania (8:331:A)
Beet: Sicily (9:37:A)
Cabbage: Megara (7:281:A)
Cactus: Sicily (2:70:E)
Carrot: Dalmatian Coast (9:369:D)
Celery: General (2:69:A)
Colocynth: Magnesia (2:59:B)
Cress: Milesia (1:28:D)
Cucumber: Antioch (2:59:B)
Fern: General (2:71:A)
Iris bulb: General (2:61:C)
Kale: Carthage (1:28:D)
Lettuce: Laconia (2:69:A)
Mallow: General (2:58:E)
Mushroom: Ceos (2:61:D)
Onion: Samothrace (1:28:D)
Palm heart: General (2:71:E)
Radish: Corinth (2:56:F)
Scallion: General (2:68:E)
Sorrel: General (2:61:C)
Squill: Libya (2:64:B)
Turnip: Boeotia (9:369:A)

prepared as thick soups or *etnos*. Vegetables and legumes available included asparagus, beans, chokeweed, clematis, elm-leaf, garlic, lettuce, onion, peas, radish, and
turnip. Combination dishes or special preparations of asparagus, lentils, lupine,
mushrooms, radishes, and peas were sold on the street as "fast foods".[85–86,88]

Common fruits and nuts available would have included almond, apple, blackberry, cherry, chestnut, citron, dates, fig, filbert, grape, mulberry, olive, peach, pear,
pistachio, plum, pomegranate, quince, and walnut.[85,87]

Athenaeus credited Antiphanes of Rhodes, who such identified seasonings and
flavoring agents used to improve combination dishes as chopped acorn, capers,
cashew nut, cheese, cress, cumin, fig leaf, smoked fish, honey, marjoram, boiled
must, olive, raisin, rennet, salt, *silphium,* soda, thyme, vinegar, and various young
greens.[90] Other seasonings and condiments would have included caraway, coriander,
mustard, pepper, and sesame. Honey was the primary sweetener.[11,86]

Water was the most common beverage among both poor and elite, while wine
was associated primarily with the prosperous. Some wines were flavored with cinnamon, mint, or thyme. Regardless of preparation, however, wines were usually
diluted with water before drinking. Water mixed with honey, *hydromel,* was touted
as a refreshing medicinal beverage, while *kykeon* was popular as a beverage among
the poor. It was prepared from barley meal steeped in water, flavored with mint,
pennyroyal, or thyme. Fresh goat's milk was drunk infrequently.[11,85,91]

III. ROMAN FOOD PATTERNS

A. MOST ANCIENT ROMANS

Seeds and plants excavated at Neolithic- through Bronze-Age settlements in the
Italian peninsula permit reconstruction of the food patterns of earliest settlers. Excavations at Monte Còvolo and Monte Leoni have revealed numerous probable foods,
among them acorn, barley, millet, and wheat; fava bean; wild apple, blackberry, wild
cherry, elderberry, wild grape, and sloe.[92]

Virgil of Andes stated that before the harvest deity Ceres brought the gift of
domesticated food to humans and taught them how to plow, the Mediterranean diet
was based on acorns and wild berries.[93] Mythology notwithstanding, archaeological
evidence suggests that early foods present in the Italian peninsula included almond,
apple, fig, grape, olive, pear, plum, and quince.[94]

The pre-Roman Etruscans practiced a sophisticated irrigation agriculture that
focused on wheat as well as millet, oats, and rye. Grapes were cultivated and animal
husbandry included cattle/oxen, horses, lamb, pigs, and sheep. Wild game included
numerous varieties of birds, deer, hare, and wild boar.[95] While little is known about
specific fruits and vegetables grown by the Etruscans, information gleaned from
their tomb art has revealed probable use of artichoke, palm, poppy, and pomegranate.[96] Etruscan cheese, specifically, was lauded and produced in quantities for export.
Martial of Bilbis wrote that a single *caseus* from the Etruscan settlement of Luni
could provide a thousand meals for the slaves of a single family.[97]

B. REPUBLICAN AND EMPIRE PERIODS

1. Dining Patterns

During early centuries, both wealthy and poor Romans lived on simple dietary fare. Cato of Tusculum, surnamed the Elder, reportedly ate little meat and exhibited a food pattern of raw, uncooked items in a frugal attempt to save fuel.[98] The diet of most Romans, rich or poor, was boiled wheat porridge eaten with different vegetable-based flavoring agents and relishes. Contrary to popular 20th to 21st-century views, Romans did not dine regularly on exotic foods such as sparrow's tongues, nor did they engage in nightly food and alcoholic debauches, as suggested by Petronius Arbiter of Rome in his *Satyricon*.[99]

The poet Plautus of Sarsina stressed the simplicity of Roman food and identified his countrymen as a race of porridge-eaters (*pultiphagonidae*). Plautus wrote that most wealthy Romans did not employ slaves or cooks trained in the sophisticated culinary arts, and since most Roman cooks were slaves, their culinary talents, presumably, would have been mediocre. Hence, some scholars have concluded that most Roman meals were limited and dull.[100–101] Nevertheless, Apicius of Rome produced a cookbook that revealed a range of interesting, complicated recipes (Table 2).[8]

Romans commonly ate one meal per day and frequently skipped breakfast or *ientaculum*, which, if eaten, usually was at sunrise. Children and adults ate the same relative fare: wheat biscuits or bread, sometimes served with cheese, dates, eggs, dried fruits such as dates and raisins, honey, olives, and salt. *Ientaculum* generally was *ad hoc*, not family focused, and irregular.[102–106]

Throughout early Roman history, the main meal, or *cena*, was at midday and consisted of heavy fare. In the early years of the Roman Republic, the primary dish served at the cena was wheat porridge or *puls*, eaten with green vegetables or *olera*; meat was rarely served. Among the wealthy, however, the midday cena consisted of three parts. Appetizers, collectively called *gustatio* or *promulsio*, included eggs, mushrooms, oysters, radishes, salads, and sardines, followed by a palate-cleansing drink of *mulsum* or wine sweetened with honey. Main dishes followed in three or more separate courses distinguished by fish, poultry, or meat. Mediterranean fish dominated over freshwater varieties, although wealthy Romans sometimes raised fish in ponds to assure freshness. Common poultry courses included dishes of chicken, crane, dove, duck, fig-pecker, goose, ostrich, partridge, peacock/peahen, pheasant, pigeon, sometimes thrush. Meat courses consisted of game animals, whether wild boar, goat, hare, venison, or domesticated sources such as beef, goat, lamb, and pork. After several courses, came dessert or *secunda mensa*, commonly honey-sweetened cakes and fruits. The cena beverage usually was wine, always drunk diluted or mixed with water.[103,105–106]

During the days of the Roman Empire, the midday meal changed in both name and content. The heavy midday cena meal shifted to evening and was replaced by a light, midday meal, *prandium*, that consisted of leftovers, or light foods such as bread, cheese, fruits, cold meats, nuts, olives, and salads.[102–106]

During early Roman history, the evening meal, or *vesperna*, was a light supper eaten before retiring. During the Empire Period, however, this changed and the heavy

TABLE 2
Roman Foods and Recipes: Selections from *The Art of Cooking* by Apicius[8]

Asparagus (3:3:1[72])	Leeks (3:10:1[93])
Brain with bacon (4:2:21[148])	Lentils and chestnuts (5:2:2[184])
Brain sausage: (2:1:5[45])	Lettuce (4:18:2[110])
Cabbage (3:15:1[103])	Lobster with cumin sauce (9:1:3[399])
Carrots (3:21:1[122])	Milk-fed snails (7:18:1[323])
Chicken (3:4:7[80])	Peaches (4:2:34[160])
Cucumber (3:6:1[82])	Peas (5:3:1[185])
Cuttle-fish croquettes (2:1:2[42])	Pheasant dumplings (2:2:1[48])
Stuffed dormouse (8:9:1[396])	Pumpkin (3:4:1[73])
Duck with turnips (6:2:3[214])	Sardines (4:2:20[147])
Gruel: barley (4:4:1[172])	Scallops (2:1:6[46])
Stuffed hare (8:8:3[384])	Sow's womb and udder (7:1:1[251])
Lamb steak (8:6:4[358])	Veal with leeks (8:5:2[352])

BARLEY GRUEL RECIPE

Crush barley, soaked the day before, well washed, place on the fire to cook . . . when hot add enough oil, a bunch of dill, dry onion, *satury* and *colocasium* to be cooked together because for the better juice, add green coriander and a little salt; bring it to a boiling point. When done take out the bunch [of dill] and transfer the barley into another kettle to avoid sticking to the bottom and burning, make it liquid [by adding broth, milk, and water] strain into a pot, cover the tops of the *colocasia*. Next crush pepper, lovage, a little dry flea-bane, cumin, and sylphium. Stir it well and add vinegar, reduced must and broth; put it back into the pot, the remaining colocasia finish on a gentle fire.

(Apicius, *The Art of Cooking*: 4:4:1[172]).[8]

cena pattern shifted to evening. The evening cena, like its earlier predecessor, consisted of three parts: appetizer or *gustus/gustatio*, alternatively called *antecina* or *promulis*, dinner proper or cena, which consisted of distinct courses called *fercula*, and dessert or *secunda mensa/mensae secundae*. Appetite was stimulated by the gustus/gustatio with finger foods such as sliced egg, fresh marine fish, pickled or salted fish, various herbs, leeks, lettuce, mint, olives, onions, oysters, sea urchins, and snails. The beverage served at the gustus/gustatio continued to be mulsum. The cena proper consisted of several courses characterized by fish, fowl, and meat, served with vegetables. Cena courses were identified as *cena prima/mensa prima, cena secunda/mensa altera, cena tertia/mensa tertia* (and such) numbered up to six or seven. Foods served at various courses included: vegetables in rich sauces, cutlets, goose, ham, hare, young kid, lamprey, pheasant, turbot and in rare instances sow's udders and wild boar. The evening meal finished with secunda mensa/secundae mensae, alternatively called *bellaria*, and typically included fruits such as apples, figs, grapes, and pears, nuts of different varieties, pastries, and sweets. The urban poor and rural peasants continued to eat their "light" vesperna, which usually consisted of cereal-based porridges or breads served with vegetables.[102–107]

Wealthy Roman families ate meals in the *triclinium*, a room with three couches. Traditionally, adult Romans reclined while eating; children sat on stools in front of their parent's couch. Waiters, collectively called *ministratores*, served the food. Dining usually was without utensils, thus, considerable time would have been spent washing hands before, during, and after meals.[102–107]

2. Common Foods

Composition of Roman diet depended on wealth and class. While considerable interest has focused on descriptions of dietary and culinary excesses of the wealthiest Romans, the vast majority of Romans, out of economic necessity, ate simply. Most Roman diets were based on whole-grain wheat products supplemented with legumes, vegetables, and limited quantities of fish and meat. Primary meats included beef, goat, mutton, and pork with wild game such as ass, boar, goat, and hare. Pork was eaten by both wealthy and poor and was the preferred domestic meat. Beef was a mark of luxury, eaten only on festive occasions after the bovines had been sacrificed and their meat dispersed or sold. Three flesh-foods — beef heart, liver, and lungs, collectively called *exta*, were reserved exclusively for sacrificial priests. Dormice, *glis* or *nitedula/nitella*, were considered delicacies and fattened at special farms called *gliraria*. Wild hare and other game animals were maintained on hunting preserves; roast shoulder of hare was thought to enhance the consumer's personal charm. Domesticated fowl such as chickens, ducks, geese, and pigeons were widely eaten. Wild fowl prominent in the Roman diet included crane, white grouse, partridge, peacock/peahen, pheasant, snipe, thrush, and woodcock. Marine and freshwater fish and shellfish also were common — cod, mullet, oyster, pike, and sturgeon. Salted and pickled fish were esteemed and generically categorized by the word *tarichos*. Fish-based condiment sauces, *garum*, *muria*, and *allex*, were prepared from mackerel, sturgeon, or tunny.[108–109]

Numerous invertebrates were used as food and medicine. According to Pliny of Verona, beetle larvae or *cossi* were fattened on wheat flour and eaten as delicacies; cockroaches boiled with oil or rose-oil were eaten by those who suffered from asthma or jaundice; earthworms preserved in honey were eaten as snacks and served with wine; while cooked scorpions were ashed, and the ash eaten to counter bladder stones.[110]

Dairy products included cheese, cream, curd, milk, and whey. Butter — as in ancient Greece — was not eaten by the Romans but was commonly applied externally to soothe wounds. Honey was the primary sweetener.[109,111–112]

Garden crops of both poor and wealthy Romans included herbs and spices, legumes, and vegetables, among them alexander, anise, artichoke, asparagus, basil, bay, bean, beet, cabbage, caper, caraway, carrot, celery, chicory, chive, coriander, cress, cucumber, cumin, dill, fennel, fenugreek, garlic, juniper, lavender, leek, lentil, lettuce, mallow, marjoram, marrow, melon, mint, mustard, onion, parsley, parsnip, pea, pennyroyal, poppy, pumpkin, radish, rosemary, safflower, sage, shallot, silphium, thyme, and turnip. Curiously, beans were considered heavy foods recommended for men engaged in heavy labor, for example, blacksmiths, gladiators, and slaves.[113–115]

Wheat was the staple food grain. Barley was considered poor-man's food, rye was not widely cultivated, and millets and oats served as poverty food or as animal fodder. The Italian peninsula did not have enough land to grow cereals in quantities needed to assure the Roman food supply, therefore, wheat was imported from Roman colonies, especially northwest coastal Egypt.[111,116]

Bread, the mainstay of the Roman diet, was identified by type of grain, fineness of millstone setting, and flour sieve aperture. Best quality, pure wheat flour, *siligo*, produced the bread called *panis siligineus*. Such siligo-based breads were preferred to those made from coarse flour, or breads baked from flour mixed with bran or bran alone. Such second-quality breads had readily identifiable names such as *panis plebeius* or *panis rusticus*.[116–117]

Cooking shops and taverns in Roman urban centers were under political control. Tiberius (14–37 C.E.) restricted cook-shops from selling pastries; Caligula (37–41 C.E.) levied taxes on street foods; Claudius (41–54 C.E.) ordered that no boiled meat or hot water could be sold in Rome; Nero (54–68 C.E.) prohibited sale of all food in taverns except for vegetables and pea soup; and Vespasian (69–79 C.E.) reinforced the tavern food sale bans, and limited food sales to legumes only.[118]

The eruption of Mount Vesuvius in 79 C.E. presented future archaeologists and food historians with a unique opportunity to examine foods preserved in the villas and gardens of the wealthy and in the food shops at Herculaneum and Pompeii. Examination of these foods reveals a numerical simplicity, since very delicate plants and some food preparations would have been incinerated, while others that were more dense were protected, and survived as carbonized remains. Still, the list is enlightening and some of the foods ready for consumption that terrifying day in 79 C.E. included almond, apple or crabapple, barley, broad bean or fava bean, carob, cherry and sour cherry, chestnut, chickpea, date, fig, garlic, grape, filbert, lentil, millet (both broomcorn and foxtail varieties), black mustard, oat, olive, onion, garden pea, pear, pine nut, plum, pomegranate, walnut, and wheat.[3–4,119]

IV. SPECIAL FOOD PATTERNS

A. CONCEPTION AND PREGNANCY

Hippocrates of Cos wrote that, if parents desired a girl baby, the father's diet should include a regimen "inclining to water," defined as foods, beverages, and pursuits of a cold, moist, and gentle nature. But should a male child be desired, the opposite was required.[120]

Soranus of Ephesus prescribed ways to strengthen the mother's appetite during pregnancy and how to enhance dietary assimilation:

[A pregnant woman] ought to partake of foods of neutral character, such as fish which are not greasy, meats which are not very fat, and vegetables which are not pungent ... she should avoid everything pungent, such as garlic, onions, leeks, preserved meat or fish, and very moist foods.[121]

Soranus recommended that pica (geophagia) during pregnancy be countered by a diet based on soft-boiled eggs, porridge, and meat from lean poultry. He also recommended that nausea or vomiting during pregnancy could be reduced by eating wheat groats prepared with cold water or diluted vinegar mixed with pomegranate pips, as well as almonds, baked apples and quinces, olives pickled in brine, and preserves of grapes, medlars (meadowlarks), and pears. Soranus recommended that his nauseated patients also consume a diet pattern of raw and cooked vegetables, specifically wild asparagus, endive, parsnip, plantain, and purslane, as well as meat from lean fowl, specifically blackbird, wild duck, francolin, partridge, pigeon, ring-dove, thrush, and breast-meat of domesticated fowl; meat from wild animals, especially antelope and hare, as well as ears, feet, snout, stomach, and uterus of tender pigs. He also recommended varieties of marine fish and other seafoods including crayfish, red mullet, mussels, oysters, shrimp, trumpet-shell, and fish with a purple hue.[122]

The important medical compilation prepared by Paulus of Aegina, the 7th-century commentator, is commonly overlooked, given ready accessibility to texts of earlier Greco-Roman physicians. Nevertheless, Paulus contributed significantly to Mediterranean medicine and dietetics, as evidenced by his passage on pregnancy:

> Most troublesome [complaints during pregnancy] are continued vomiting, salivation, heartburn, and loathing of food; remedies are exercise on foot, food that is not too sweet, [use of] wines that are yellow, fragrant, and about five years old; these will cure vomiting; for medicines you may give [her] dill at or before a meal; heartburn may be alleviated by drinking warm water … for those who have an aversion to food, whet their appetite with savory foods, and give dry starch, this last is particularly serviceable to those who long to eat earth, which occurs most frequently about the third month after conception … labor and long journeys will contribute to restore a desire for wholesome food; to those who loathe food, they may take acrid substances, particularly mustard.[123]

B. INFANTS

Aristotle of Stageira wrote that newborn children commonly experienced convulsions if overfed with breast milk suckled from obese wet nurses, and that wine given to infants would also cause convulsions.[124]

Galen of Pergamum stated that newborn infants should be provided with food and drink that was moist, and that nature had planned that children's food be mother's milk, which he considered was best for all infants unless the mother was ill.[125]

Soranus of Ephesus wrote that wet nurses typically should be between the ages of 20–40, have already delivered 2–3 infants, be large-framed, in good health with fine complexion, and should regularly abstain from drinking wine.[126] Having identified the characteristics of good wet nurses, he prescribed their diets:

> [They] ought to forgo leek and onions, garlic, preserved meat or fish, radish, pulse, and all preserved food, and most vegetables; and meat of sheep and oxen, and this especially if roasted … [they] should partake of pure bread, carefully prepared and leavened and made from spring wheat, the yolks of eggs, brain, thrushes, the young of pigeons and domestic birds, fishes living among rocks, bass, red mullet and … the meat of suckling pigs.[127]

Soranus emphasized the importance of breast feeding throughout the first 6 months of infancy, identified infant weaning foods, and the timing of weaning:

> When the body has already become firm and ready to receive more solid food, which it will scarcely do successfully before the age of six months, it is proper to feed the child also with cereal food: with crumbs of bread softened with hydromel or milk, sweet wine, or honey wine. Later, one should also give soup made from spelt, a very moist porridge, and an egg that can be sipped ... as soon as the infant takes cereal food readily and ... [after growth of the teeth] ... one must stealthily and gradually take it off the breast and wean it by adding constantly to the amount of other food but diminishing the quantity of milk ... The best season for weaning is the spring.[128]

C. THE ELDERLY

Galen considered health and exercise needs of the elderly, and commented on specific diets appropriate at this life stage. He described the food-intake pattern of an 80-year-old male who exercised, kept himself well, who ate only toasted bread with Attic honey in the morning, dined on laxative foods in moderation at noon (identified as rock-bass and deep-sea varieties of fish), then in the evening ate soft foods such as barley with honey-wine, or game-birds cooked in simple broths.[129] Galen also described another near-centenarian who ate sparingly:

> [The man ate] barley boiled in water mixed with the best raw honey ... who [when dining at lunch] ate vegetables first, and then fish or game ... but in the evening he ate only bread moistened in dilute wine.[130]

Paulus recognized that diets changed with age and recommended specific foods for the elderly:

> Old age is dry and cold [therefore] about the third hour give a small bit of bread with Attic honey; and afterwards about the seventh hour ... [give] fish or fowls; and then for supper, such things as are wholesome, and not apt to spoil in the stomach; we must give [elderly with phlegm] ripe figs in preference to every other kind of food, and if during the winter dried figs, unless they complain of unpleasant symptoms ... it is obvious that all pot-herbs ought to be eaten before all other food, with oil, pickles, or olives and damascenes seasoned with salt.[131]

V. FOOD AND MEDICINE

A. DIETETICS

1. Hippocrates

Hippocrates identified three categories of nutriments required for life: solids, beverages, and air. Health, he explained, was the state of balance of elements and humours, whereas disease represented imbalance. Hippocrates urged dietary moderation and recommended that diet should reflect seasonality:

[During Winter]: Eat as much as possible, drink as little as possible; eat bread; all meat and fish should be roasted; eat as few vegetables as possible;

[During Spring]: Take more to drink [than in winter], increasing quantity a little at a time; take softer cereals, substituting barley cake for bread; boiled meat should replace roasted; eat a few vegetables once Spring has begun, both raw and boiled;

[During Summer]: Live on soft barley-cake, watered wine in large quantities, and all meat should be boiled;

[During Fall]: Cereal [intake] should be increased and made drier, and likewise the meat in the diet. Quantity of drink taken should be decreased and less diluted; take in the smallest quantity of the least diluted drink and the largest quantity of cereals of the driest kind; this will keep the person in good health.[132]

Hippocrates stressed the importance of moderation in diet, that food should be eaten at established meal times, and that illness was caused by incautious diet:

A simple diet of food and drink, if it be preserved in without a break, is on the whole safer for health than a sudden violent change ... Those who are not in the habit of lunching, if they have taken lunch, immediately become feeble, heavy in all the body, weak and sluggish. Should they also dine, they suffer from acid [indigestion]. Diarrhea, too, may occur in some cases because the digestive organs have been loaded ... It is beneficial, then, in these cases [to take] a slow, long walk without stopping. Such a man will suffer yet more if he eat three times a day to surfeit, and still more if he eats more often.[133]

Several Hippocratic dietary recommendations parallel 20th-century approaches to patient care:

Those who eat only once a day become exhausted and weak ... Their mouth becomes salty, or even bitter, and [they] are unable to digest their dinner as they would have if they had had a breakfast. [Such persons] must eat less at dinner than they are used to, [they should] replace bread with quite moist barley-cake and [from] vegetables [select] dock, mallow, peeled barley or beets. With their food, let them drink wine in a reasonable amount and quite dilute ... Let [such people also] eat boiled fish ... pork is the best of all meats; the most nutritious is that which is neither very fat nor very lean, and which has not the age of an old slaughter-animal; eat it without the skin, and slightly cooled.[134]

2. Celsus

The Roman physician Celsus practiced medicine more than 300 years after Hippocrates. Celsus identified foods and drugs used to treat common Mediterranean diseases and wrote that certain categories of food were medically "stronger" than others, an observation that in the 21st century of the Common Era would be correlated with the concept of caloric density:

All pulses and all bread-stuffs made from grain, form the strongest kind of food; to the same class belong: [meat from] all domesticated quadruped animals, all large game such as deer, wild boar, wild ass, all large birds such as crane, goose, and peacock, all sea monsters, among them which is the whale and such, also honey and cheese. Hence, it is [obvious why] pastry made of grain, lard, honey, and cheese is very strong food.[135]

Celsus wrote that bread was more nutritious than any other food, that wheat bread was stronger than millet, and millet bread superior to barley. He wrote that beans and lentils were stronger than peas, that meat from domesticated animals provided different strength options to consumers: beef was strongest, pork weakest. Cuts of meat from larger animals provided "better" nutrition to humans than similar cuts from smaller livestock. He identified middle-strength foods such as pot-herbs, edible bulbs and roots, hare, all varieties of edible birds, and all fish except those that required salting for preservation. Celsus wrote that flightless or "walking birds" were stronger foods than species that flew; large birds more nourishing than small; meat from water fowl weaker than meat from birds unable to swim. Celsus suggested a third category of suitable but weak foods that included stalked vegetables, fruit-like vegetables (i.e., cucumber), orchard fruits including olives, edible land snails, and shellfish.[136]

In his dietary system Celsus claimed that young plants and animals provided less nourishment to humans than older forms of the same species; chickens raised in coops were superior to those allowed to free-range; grain cultivated on hilly slopes was more nutritious than grain harvested from valley flatlands; and rock-swimming fish less nutritious than species swimming over sandy environments. He also wrote that meat from wild animals was lighter and easier to digest than similar cuts from domesticated, tamed animals. Celsus observed that fatty meat provided more nutrition to the human body than lean, and that fresh meats were superior to salted, stewed meats better than roasted.[137]

3. Plutarch

Plutarch — philosopher, traveler, and observer of human nature — was born 9 years after the death of Celsus. Although untrained in medicine, Plutarch wrote extensively on food and dietary topics and proposed several dietary recommendations:

1. We ought especially to guard against excess in eating and drinking, and against all self-indulgence.
2. Let everybody [urge] himself not to make his [food] more ample than lentils, and by all means not to proceed beyond cress and olives to croquettes and fish.
3. Especially to be feared are indigestions arising from meats; for they are depressing at the outset, and a pernicious residue from them remains behind. It is best to accustom the body not to require meat in addition to other food.

4. Milk ought not be used as a beverage but as a food [one that] possesses solid and nourishing power; wine is the most beneficial of beverages. In the course of the daily routine [drink] two or three glasses of water.

5. In regard to food and drink it is expedient to note what kinds are wholesome rather than what are pleasant, and to be better acquainted with those that are good in the stomach rather than in the mouth, and those that do not disturb the digestion rather than those that greatly tickle the palate.[138]

Plutarch suggested that food should be simple. He wrote that moderation kept appetite in check and discouraged eating fancy culinary creations.[139]

4. Galen

Galen, born shortly after the death of Plutarchus, was the most influential Greek physician of the Common Era. He traveled extensively, visited Greece and Egypt, practiced medicine at Pergamum, and retired at Rome. His medical texts provided a rich exposition of Greek and Roman medicine and documented the importance of food and nutrition in the Greco-Roman healing arts.[140]

Galen described the "social disgrace" of contracting gout, kidney stones, or ulcerated bladders. His strongest words, however, were directed toward patients who suffered from arthritis, a disease he believed to be caused by improper diet:

Is it not disgraceful that a person [with arthritis] be unable to use his own hands, and should need somebody else to bring food to his mouth, and to perform his toilet necessities for him? Unless one were an absolute weakling, one would prefer to die a thousand deaths rather than endure such a life.[141]

B. Obesity

Obesity, bane of wealthy Mediterraneans for more than 4,500 years, has an ancient origin that dates to the Central European Mesolithic era, where "earth mother" statuettes such as the famed Venus of Willendorf (ca. 15,000–10,000 B.C.E), accentuated adipose deposition on the upper arms, breasts, stomach, hips, and upper thighs. Male pattern obesity, in turn, can be traced to Ancient Egyptian tomb art dated to ca. 2400 BCE, where a stone-cut tomb relief depicts the super-generous body of the noble Meru-Ka-Ra.[142] Even a cursory inspection of Greek and Roman statuary, vase paintings, and funerary reliefs reveals examples of overweight or obese individuals.

Hippocrates offered a specific treatment for obesity, one that blended exercise with dietary recommendations:

Fat people who want to reduce should take their exercise on an empty stomach and sit down to their food out of breath. They should not wait to recover their breath. They should before eating drink some diluted wine, not too cold, and their meat should be dished up with sesame seeds or seasoning and such-like things. The meat should also be fat as the smallest quantity of this is filling. They should take only one meal a day, go without baths, sleep on hard beds and walk about with as little clothing as may be required.[143]

Galen described a treatment for obesity, but provided few dietary insights except to use "foods of little nourishment":

> I have made any sufficiently stout patient moderately thin in a short time by compelling him to do rapid running ... then massaging him maximally ... [then after an initial washing] ... led him to the second bath and then gave him abundant food of little nourishment, so as to fill him up but distribute little of it to the entire body.[144]

Paulus of Aegina discussed obesity and recommended exercise and a strict food regimen to reduce weight:

> When the body gets to an immoderate degree of obesity, it will be necessary to melt it down and reduce it; active exercises, an attenuant regimen, medicines of the same class, and mental anxiety, bring on the dry temperament and thereby render the body lean; salts from burned vipers attenuate the body; the body may also be reduced and attenuated by having an oil rubbed into it, containing the root of the wild cucumber; one ought not to take food immediately after the bath, but should first sleep for a little time; thin white wines ought to be used; a smaller quantity of food ought to be given in proportion to the exercise taken; it will be best if [patients] eat only once in the day.[145]

C. CARDIOVASCULAR DISEASE

Athenaeus wrote that patients suffering from cardiac disorders should eat cereal food mixed with wine.[146] Celsus, in turn, described a cure for patients suffering from angina and noted that they could be symptom-free for a year if they took a nesting swallow preserved in salt, burned the carcass, stirred the ash into *hydromel*, and drank the product.[147]

A well known ancient dietary treatment for heart disease that used wine intoxication was practiced at Alexandria, Egypt, and attributed to Herophilus of Chalcedon:

> [He] used phlebotomy and applied very harsh clysters; and to warm up the patient's chilled limbs [he] applied warm rags and wool that [had] been steeped in olive-oil and smoked with sulfur. And [he] used acrid and pungent foods: garlic, salted and pickled food, and silphium. And throughout the entire day and night [he] filled the patient with wine to the point of intoxication.[148]

VI. SUMMARY

Ancient Greek and Roman food-related information is widely diversified. While the archaeological record is never complete and literary accounts are biased toward food patterns exhibited by the educated elite, preliminary conclusions can be drawn regarding what constituted Mediterranean dietary patterns through the ages.

In remote antiquity, from Neolithic through Iron ages, most ancient Greek livestock included cattle, goats, pigs, and sheep; mutton and pork, presumably, were the most widely consumed meats. Although ducks, geese, and pigeons appear in Minoan art, they may not have been eaten. While bone evidence or drawings of chickens are not present in Minoan art, an alternative line of evidence suggests their use as food. This assertion is based on tomb art in Egypt, dated to ca. 2000 B.C.E, where a chicken is included as a component of Minoan tribute offerings to the Egyptian king.[149-150] The most ancient Greeks also feasted on seafood, especially, cockles, crab, fish of various types, limpets, lobster, oyster, and both terrestrial and marine snails, while pottery decoration suggests that cephalopods such as octopus and squid were eaten as well.

Despite apparent meat and protein consumption, osteological evidence suggests that the most ancient Greeks were short in stature and the probability remains that their food-intake pattern was based more on grains, fruits, legumes, nuts, and both domesticated and wild vegetables.[151]

During Classical and Hellenistic periods, wealthy urban Greeks followed a vegetable-based food pattern, one based on grains, legumes, olive oil, and wine: barley and wheat were prepared as porridge and bread; fava beans, chickpeas, lentils, lupines, and peas were served as specific dishes or as ingredient flours with breads and porridges; olive oil dominated cooking; while water and wine were beverages of choice.[86-87,152]

Foods of rural and poor urban Greeks, as well as Greeks living in the diaspora in North Africa and elsewhere, were vegetable based and commonly included artichoke, cabbage, celery, cucumbers, garlic, leeks, lettuce, onions, radishes, and turnips (Tables 1 and 3). Domesticated and wild fruits and leaves provided abundant food to the rural poor. Eating patterns of poor Greeks focused on cereals served with edible greens and roots, sometimes lentils and lupines. Still, some scholars have noted that the dietary staples of poor Greeks consisted of barley porridge flavored with salt or honey, barley cakes and loaves, commonly served with beans, cabbage, figs, lentils, olives, onions, and peas. Vegetable foods would have been complemented by cheese, dried and fresh fish, shellfish, also figs and honey. Butter was not used and cooking oil would have been poorer grades of olive oil.[11,153-155]

In ancient Greece — as today — wealth and poverty existed side by side, as noted in this passage on eating behavior recorded by Athenaeus, who credited Alexis of Thurium with the observation:

> When you see an ordinary citizen eating one meal a day, or a poet who has lost his desire for songs and lyrics, then you may be sure the first has lost one half of his life, the other, one half of his art; and both are scarcely alive.[156]

The diet and food patterns of most Romans also was simple fare, usually a monotonous diet based on grains/bread, vegetables, and olive oil. Husked wheat, collectively called *far*, was commonly prepared as porridge or puls. Wheat bread was served with honey or cheese. Among the Roman elite, vegetable consumption was limited, since vegetable consumption was viewed in some circles as a sign of frugality. This view notwithstanding, recipes assembled by Apicius in his *Art of Cooking* (Table 2), reveal the important role of vegetables in Roman diet.[8,102,157-158]

In summary, food patterns of both poor and elite Classical-Hellenistic Greeks and Republican-Empire Romans were based on cereals, legumes, a wide range of fruits, nuts, seeds, and vegetables, with relatively limited meat intake. Simply stated, food was medicine — medicine was food. Expansion of Greeks and Romans into

TABLE 3
Commonly Consumed Foods in Egypt: Greco-Roman Era

Almond (Athenaeus: 15:688:F)[161]
Almond oil/metopium (Pliny: 13:11:8)[110]
Anise (Pliny: 20:73:187)[110]
Barley (Athenaeus: 4:149:F)[161]
Beef: calf/veal (Athenaeus: 9:384:A)[161]
Blackberry (Diodorus Siculus: 1:34:9)[162]
Bulbs (Athenaeus: 2:64:B)[161]
Cabbage (Athenaeus: 9:369:F)[161]
Caper (Pliny: 13:44:127)[110]
Carob (Newberry, 1889)[163]
Celery (Dioscorides: 3:64)[50]
Cheese (Athenaeus: 4:149-F)[161]
Chicken (Gabra et al., 1941; Lefebvre, 1924)[164-165]
Chicken: eggs (Diodorus Siculus: 1:74:4-5)[162]

Cinnamon (Athenaeus: 5:201:A)[161]
Citron (Hunt and Edgar, 1932: 1:18)[166]
Corchorus (Pliny: 21:106:183)[110]
Coriander (Apicius: 3:4:3)[8]
Cucumber/gourd (Apicius: 3:4:3; Lindsey, 1966)[8, 167]
Cumin (Pliny: 19:47:161)[110]
Dates (Plutarchus: *Table Talk*, 8:4:723:C-D)[168]
Dove (Athenaeus: 5:200:C; Columella: 8:8:7-8)[161, 169]
Endive/chicory (Pliny: 20:29:73)[110]
Fig (Pliny: 15:19:70)[110]
Fish (Athenaeus: 3:121:B-C; Martial: 13:85; Strabo: 17:2:4)[97, 161, 170]
Geese (Athenaeus: 9:384:A)[16]
Grapes/raisins (Athenaeus: 1:33:E)[161]

Jubube (Theophrastus: 4:3:3)[49]
Leek (Juvenal: 15)[171]
Lentils (Athenaeus: 4:158:D)[161]
Marjoram (Dioscorides: 3:39)[50]
Mint (Apicius: 3:4:3)[8]
Mustard (Pliny: 12:14:28)[110]
Olive (Pliny: 8:19:63)[110]
Olive: oil (Strabo: 17:1:35)[170]
Parsley (Pliny: 20:47:118)[110]
Peach (Newberry, 1889)[163]
Pear (Newberry, 1889)[163]
Pepper (Theophrastus: 9:20:2)[49]
Persea (Theophrastus: 4:2:5)[49]
Pigeon (Athenaeus: 5:200:C; Columella: 8:8:7-8)[161, 169]
Pomegranate (Pliny: 13:34:113)[110]
Pumpkin (Apicius; 3:4:3)[8]
Radish (Pliny: 19:26:80)[110]
Radish: oil (Pliny: 15:7:30)[110]
Sebsten plum (Theophrastus: 4:2:10)[49]

Sesame oil: (Hunt and Edgar, 1932, 1:98)[166]
Shellfish: mussels (Athenaeus: 3:87:F)[161]
Sycamore fig (Diodorus Siculus: 1:34:8)[162]

Turnip (Hunt and Edgar, 1932: 1:186)[166]
Wheat (Pliny: 18:45:161-162)[110]

adjacent and distant lands produced three important changes in diet. First, soldiers and subsequent colonists were exposed to different foods. Second, following generations of Greek and Roman colonists adopted some of the food practices of their new land and ultimately practiced "blended" diets, for example, combinations of Greek and Libyan or Roman and Egyptian foods. Third, expanded trade networks ultimately reduced food-related differences between the periphery and heartland of the Greek and Roman empires as foods of African, east and south Asian, and northern European origin entered Byzantine and Medieval Mediterranean diets. Mediterranean diets would change even more dramatically following 1492 after food exchanges between Europe and the Americas.[159-160]

Through the centuries, Mediterranean foods have provided more than energy and nutrients. They have served specific cultural functions: use of pork has united or separated peoples; specific recipes and wines have provided social-dining pleasure; certain legumes and meats were identified with political parties, religious sects, social status, or with wealth. Were treatments for obesity identified by Galen, Hippocrates, Paulus and others radically different from those prescribed by 21st-century physicians? While Pliny's treatments for gout seem amusing from a 21st-century observation, ancient Greek and Roman physicians recommended wine as a preventative for cardiovascular disease, a practice that today has proven sound. Indeed, the food classification system of Celsus, divided into strong, medium, and weak categories, has mirrored 20th- and 21st-century concepts of nutrient density. Thus, while ancient and modern views commonly diverge, at other times they converge with an almost uncanny parallel leading one to ponder — is there anything new under the sun?

VI. REFERENCES

1. Bökönyi, S., Faunal remains, in *Excavations at Sitagroi*. Vol. 1. Renfrew, C., Gimbutas, M., Elster, E. S., Eds., University of California Press, Los Angeles, 1986, 63.
2. Vickery, K. F., Food in early Greece, Illinois Studies in the Social Sciences, Vol. 20, Number 3. University of Illinois, Urbana, Illinois, 1936, 15.
3. Meyer, F. G., Carbonized food plants of Pompei, Herculaneum, and the villa at Torre Annunziata, *Econ. Bot.*, 34: 401, 1980.
4. Meyer, F. G. food plants identified from carbonized remains at Pompeii and other Vesuvian sites, in *Studia Pompeiana and Classica in Honor of Wilhelmina F. Jashemski*, Caratzas, A. D., Ed., New Rochelle, New York, 1989, 183.
5. Schmitt-Pantel, P., Sacrificial meal and the symposion, two models of civic institutions in the archaic city?, in *Sympotica*. Murray, O., Ed. Clarendon Press, Oxford, 1990, 14.
6. Richter, G. M. A., *Animals in Greek Sculpture*. Oxford University Press, New York, 1930.
7. Toynbee, J. M. C., *Animals in Roman Life and Art*. Thames and Hudson, London, 1973.
8. Apicius, *The Roman Cookery Book*. Flower, B., and Rosenbaum, E. Translators, George G. Harrap, London, 1958; Apicius, *Apicius. Cookery and dining in Imperial Rome*. Vehling, J. H. D., Translator, Dover Publications, New York, 1977.
9. Brothwell, D., and Brothwell, P., *Food in Antiquity*. The Johns Hopkins University Press, Baltimore, 1998.
10. Norman, B., *Tales of the Table*. Prentice-Hall, Englewood Cliffs, New Jersey, 1972, 12.
11. *Oxford Classical Dictionary*, Hammond, N. G. L., and Scuttard, H. H., Eds., 2nd ed., Clarendon Press, Oxford, 1970, 443.
12. Sandys, J. W., *A Companion to Latin Studies*. Cambridge University Press, Cambridge, 1910, 48.
13. Waterlow, J. C., Diet of the classical period of Greece and Rome, *Eur. J. Clin. Nut.* 43 [Sup. 2], 3, 1989.
14. Whibley, L., *A Companion to Greek Studies*. 4th ed., Revised., Cambridge University Press, Cambridge, 1931, 639.
15. Olck, F., Apfel, in *Paulys Real-Encyklopädie der Classischen Alter-tumswissenschaft*, new ed. Wissowa, G., Ed., Alfred Druckenmüller Verlag, Stuttgart, 1894, 2699.

16. Braun, T., Barley cakes and emmer bread, in *Food in Antiquity*, Wilkins, J., Harvey, D., and Dobson, M., Eds., University of Exeter Press, Exeter, 1995, 25.

17. Pollard, J., *Birds in Greek Life and Myth*, Thames and Hudson, Plymouth, 1977.

18. Cubberley, A., Bread-baking in ancient Italy. In *Food in Antiquity*, Wilkins, J., Harvey, D., and Dobson, M., Eds., University of Exeter Press, Exeter, 1995, 55.

19. Andrews, A. C., The carrot as a food in the classical era. *Class. Phil.*, 44, 182, 1949.

20. Andrews, A. C., Celery and parsley as foods in the Graeco-Roman period, *Class. Phil.*, 44, 91, 1949.

21. Kroll, H., Käse, in *Paulys Real-Encyklopädie der Classischen Alter-tumswissenschaft*, new ed., Wissowa, G., Ed., Alfred Druckenmüller Verlag, Stuttgart, 1932, 1490.

22. West, B., and Zhou, B.-X., Did chickens go north? New evidence for domestication. *J. Arch. Sci.*, 15, 515, 1988.

23. Olck, F., Feige, in *Paulys Real-Encyklopädie der Classischen Alter-tumswissenschaft*, new ed., Wissowa, G., Ed., Alfred Druckenmüller Verlag , Stuttgart, 1909, 2099.

24. Braund, D., Fish from the Black Sea. Classical Byzantium and the Greekness of trade, in *Food in Antiquity*, Wilkins, J., Harvey, D., and Dobson, M., Eds., University of Exeter Press, Exeter, 1995, 162.

25. Purcell, N., Eating fish. The paradoxes of seafood, in *Food in Antiquity*, Wilkins, J., Harvey, D., and Dobson, M., Eds., University of Exeter Press, Exeter, 1995, 132.

26. Richmond, J. A., Chapters on Greek fish-lore, *Zeit. für Klass. Phil.*, Volume 28. F. Steiner, Wiesbaden, 1973.

27. Sparks, B., A pretty kettle of fish, in *Food in Antiquity*, Wilkins, J., Harvey, D., and Dobson, M., Eds., University of Exeter Press, Exeter, 1995, 150.

28. Schuster, M., Mel, in *Paulys Real-Encyklopädie der Classischen Alter-tumswissenschaft*, new ed., Wissowa, G., Ed., Alfred Druckenmüller Verlag, Stuttgart, 1932, 364.

29. Andrews, A. C., Alimentary use of lovage in the Classical period, *Isis*, 33, 514, 1941.

30. Hondelmann, W., The lupine. Ancient and modern crop plant, *Theoret. and App. Gen.*, 68, 1, 1984.

31. Andrews, A. C., Marjoram as a spice in the Classical era, *Class. Phil.*, 56, 73, 1961.

32. Frayn, J., The Roman meat trade, in *Food in Antiquity*, Wilkins, J., Harvey, D., and Dobson, M., Eds., University of Exeter Press, Exeter, 1995, 107.

33. Baird, J., R., and Thieret, J. W., The medlar (*Mespilus germanica*, Rosaceae) from antiquity to obscurity, *Econ. Bot.*, 43, 328, 1989.

34. Andrews, A. C., Melons and watermelons in the Classical period, *Osiris*, 12, 368, 1956.

35. Herzog-Hauser, G., Milch, in *Paulys Real-Encyklopädie der Classischen Alter-tumswissenschaft*, new ed., Wissowa, G., Ed., Alfred Druckenmüller Verlag, Stuttgart, 1932, 1570.

36. Andrews, A. C., The mints of the Greeks and Romans and their condimentary use and thyme as a condiment in the Graeco-Roman era, *Osiris*, 13, 127, 1958.

37. Houghton, W., Notices of fungi in Greek and Latin authors. *Ann. and Mag. Nat. Hist.*, Series 5, Vol. 5, 22, 1885.

38. Andrews, A. C., Alimentary use of hoary mustard in the Classical period, *Isis*, 34, 161, 1942.

39. Runnels, C. N., and Hansen, J., The olive in the prehistoric Aegean. The evidence for domestication in the early Bronze Age. *Oxford. J. Arch.* 5, 299, 1986.

40. Andrews, A. C., Oysters as a food in Greece and Rome, *Class. J.*, 43, 299, 1948.

41. Andrews, A. C., The parsnip as a food in the Classical era, *Class. Phil.*, 53, 145, 1958.

42. Steier, [no initials], Pfeffer, in *Paulys Real-Encyklopädie der Classischen Alter-tumswissenschaft*, new ed., Wissowa, G., Ed., Alfred Druckenmüller Verlag, Stuttgart, 1932, 1421.
43. Andrews, A., C., The opium poppy as a food and spice in the Classical period, *Ag. Hist.*, 27, 152, 1953.
44. Bedigian, D., and Harlan, J. R., Evidence for cultivation of sesame in the ancient world, *Econ. Bot.*, 40, 137, 1986.
45. Andrews, A. C., Orach as the spinach of the Classical period, *Isis*, 39, 169, 1948.
46. Perry, C., What was tracta?, *Petis Propos Culin.*, 12, 37, 1982.
47. Hill, S., and Bryer, A., Byzantine porridge. Tracta, trachanas, and tarhana, in *Food in Antiquity*, Wilkins, J., Harvey, D., and Dobson, M., Eds., University of Exeter Press, Exeter, 1995, 4.
48. Jasny, N., *The Wheats of Classical Antiquity, The Johns Hopkins University Studies in Historical and Political Science*, Series 62, Number 3, The Johns Hopkins Press, Baltimore, 1944.
49. Theophrastus, *Enquiry into Plants*, Hort, A., Translator, 2 Vols., G. P. Putnam's Sons, New York, 1916.
50. Dioscorides, *The Greek Herbal of Dioscorides*, Gunther, R. T. Translator, Hafner, New York, 1959.
51. Douglas, N., *Birds and Beasts of the Greek Anthology*, Jonathan Cape and Harrison Smith, New York, 1929.
52. Thompson, D. W., Fauna, in *A Companion to Greek Studies*, Whibley, L., Ed., 4th ed., University of Cambridge Press, Cambridge, 1931, 34.
53. Thiselton-Dyer, W. T, Flora, in. *A Companion to Greek Studies*, Whibley, L., Ed., 4th ed., University of Cambridge Press, Cambridge, 1931, 52.
54. Keller, H. O., Fauna, in *A Companion to Latin Studies*, Sandys, J. E., Ed., Cambridge University Press, Cambridge, 1910, 48.
55. Thiselton-Dyer, W. T., Flora, in *A Companion to Latin Studies*, Sandys, J. E., Ed., Cambridge University Press, Cambridge, 1910, 66.
56. Thompson, D. W., *A Glossary of Greek Birds*, George Olms, Hildersheim, 1966.
57. Thompson, D. W., On Egyptian fish names used by Greek writers, *J. of Egypt. Arch.*, 14, 22, 1928.
58. Anderson, J. K., *Hunting in the Ancient World*. University of California Press, Berkeley, California, 1985.
59. Fox, R. L., Ancient hunting: from Homer to Polybios. In *Human Landscapes in Classical Antiquity*. Shipley, G., and Salmon, J., Eds., Routledge, London, 1996, 119.
60. Hearn, L., *Insects and Greek Poetry*, W. E. Rudge, New York, 1926.
61. Beavis, I. C., *Insects and Other Invertebrates in Classical Antiquity*, University of Exeter Press, Exeter, 1988.
62. Renfrew, J. M., *Palaeoethnobotany*, Columbia University Press, New York, 1973, 203.
63. Renfrew, J. M., The first farmers in southeast Europe. In *Festschrift Maria Hopf*. Körber-Grohne, Ed., Rheinland-Verlag GMBH, Köln, 1979, 243.
64. Renfrew, J. M., 1973, pp. 40–103, 107–119, 125–160, 164–189, *(See* reference 62).
65. Vickery, K. F., 1936, pp. 29–39, *(See* reference 2).
66. Hansen, J. M., Agriculture in the prehistoric Aegean. Data versus speculation, *Am. J. Arch.*, 92, 39, 1988.
67. Jarman, M., R., and Jarman, H. N., The fauna and economy of early Neolithic Knossos, in *Ann. Brit. Sch. Athens*, Vol. 63, 1968, 241.

68. Bisel, S. C., and Angel, J. L., Health and nutrition in Mycenaean Greece. A study in human skeletal remains, in *Contributions to Aegean Archaeology. Studies in Honor of William A. McDonald.* Wilkie, N. C., and Coulson, W. D. E., Eds. Center for Ancient Studies, University of Minnesota Publications in Ancient Studies, Minneapolis, 1985, 197.

69. Angle, J. L., Skeletal change in Ancient Greece, *Am. J. Phys. Anthro.* New Series. 4, 69, 1946.

70. Homer, *The Iliad.* Murray, A. T., Translator, 2 Vols., G. P. Putnam's Sons, New York, 1924-1925.

71. Homer, *The Odyssey,* Dimock, G. E. Translator, Harvard University Press, Cambridge, Massachusetts, 1995.

72. Minchin, E., Food fiction and food fact in Homer's *Iliad, Petis Propos Culin.,* 25, 42, 1987.

73. Athenaeus, *The Deipnosophists,* Gulick, C. B., Translator, 7 Vols., G. P. Putnam's Sons, New York, 1927-1941, 1:12:D-E.

74. Athenaeus, 1927–1941, 1:11:B–D, *(See* reference 73).

75. Athenaeus, 1927–1941, 1:11:C–E, *(See* reference 73).

76. Felton, C. C., *Greece, Ancient and Modern. Lectures Delivered Before the Lowell Institute.* 2 Vols., James R. Osgood and Company, Boston, 1877, 362.

77. Tucker, T. T., *Life in Ancient Athens,* The Macmillan Company, New York, 1918, 108.

78. Athenaeus, 1927–1941, 2:47:E, *(See* reference 73).

79. Whibley, L., 1931, pp. 641–642, *(See* reference 14).

80. Flacelière. R. *Daily Life in Greece at the Time of Pericles,* Green, P., Translator, The Macmillan Company, New York, 1965, 167.

81. Dalby, A., *Siren feasts. A History of Food and Gastronomy in Greece.* Routledge, London, 1996, pp. 12, 22–23.

82. Athenaeus, 1927–1941, 1:16:B–C; 2:54:F; 2:58:B; 2:60:A–B; 2:64:F; 2:66:C, *(See* reference 73).

83. Athenaeus, 1927–1941, 1:127:F, 1:18:A, *(See* reference 73).

84. Athenaeus, 1927–1941, 2:63:D–E, *(See* reference 73).

85. Felton, C. C., 1877, pp. 359–361, *(See* reference 76).

86. Blümner, H., *The Home Life of the Ancient Greeks.* Zimmern, A. S., Translator, Russell and Company, London, 1895, 202.

87. Whibley, L., 1931, pp. 638–639, *(See* reference 14).

88. Flacelière. R. 1965, pp. 169–170, *(See* reference 80).

89. Pollard, J., 1977, pp. 87–95, 104–109, *(See* reference 17).

90. Athenaeus, 1927–1941, 2:68:A, *(See* reference 73).

91. Flacelière. R., 1965, p. 172, *(See* reference 80).

92. Pals, J.-P., and Voorrips, A., Seeds., fruits and charcoals from two prehistoric sites in northern Italy, in *Festschrift Maria Hopf.* Körber-Grohne, Ed., Rheinland-Verlag GMBH, Köln, 1979, 217.

93. Virgil, *Georgics,* in *Virgil's works. The Aeneid, Eclogues, Georgics,* Mackail, J. W., Translator, The Modern Library, New York, 1950, 1: 6-8.

94. Johnston, H. W., *The Private Life of the Romans,* Scott, Foresman and Company, Chicago, 1932, 204.

95. Keller, W., *The Etruscans,* Henderson, A., and Henderson, E., Translators, Alfred A. Knopf, New York, 1974, 52.

96. Heurgon, J., *Daily Life of the Etruscans,* Kirkup, J., Translator, The Macmillan Company, New York, 1964, 113.

97. Marital, *Epigrams*, Ker, W. C. A., Translator, 2 Vols., G. P. Putnam's Sons, New York, 1919-1920, 13:30.
98. Cowell, F. R. , *Everyday Life in Ancient Rome*, G. P. Putnam's Sons, New York, 1961, 76.
99. Petronius Arbiter, *Satyricon*. Arrowsmith, W. Translator, University of Michigan Press, Ann Arbor, Michigan, 1959.
100. Cowell, F. R., 1961, p. 77, *(See* reference 98).
101. Johnston, H. W., *The Private Life of the Romans*, Scott, Foresman and Company, Chicago, 1932, 222.
102. Adkins, L., and Adkins, R. A., *Handbook to Life in Ancient Rome*. Facts on File, New York, 1994, 343.
103. Balsdon, J. P. V. D., *Life and Leisure in Ancient Rome*. McGraw-Hill Book Company, New York, 1969, 41.
104. Carcopino, J., *Daily Life in Ancient Rome. The People and The City at the Height of the Empire*. Lorimer, E. O., Translator, Yale University Press, New Haven, 1940, 264.
105. Cowell, F. R., 1961, pp. 77-80, *(See* reference 98).
106. Johnston, H. W., 1932, pp. 230-231, *(See* reference 101).
107. Marshall, F. H., Daily Life, in *A Companion to Latin Studies*, Sandys, J. E., Ed., Cambridge University Press, Cambridge, 1910, 205.
108. Cowell, F. R., 1961, p. 80, *(See* reference 98).
109. Preston, H. W., and Dodge, L., *The Private Life of the Romans*. Benjamin H. Sanborn and Company, Chicago, 1927, 82.
110. Pliny, *Natural History*, Rackham, H., and Jones, W. H. S., Translators, 8 Vols., Harvard University Press, Cambridge, 1938-1956, 17:37:220; 29:39:142; 30:21:66; 30:30:100.
111. Johnston, H. W., 1932, pp. 206–210, *(See* reference 101).
112. Keller, H. O., 1910, p. 51, *(See* reference 54).
113. Adkins, L., and Adkins, R. A., 1994, p. 342, *(See* reference 102).
114. Johnston, H. W., 1932, pp. 205–206, *(See* reference 101).
115. Preston, H. W., and Dodge, L., 1927, p. 81, *(See* reference 109).
116. Preston, H. W., and Dodge, L., 1927, pp. 78–79, *(See* reference 109).
117. Johnston, H. W., 1932, pp. 213–214, *(See* reference 101).
118. Toner, J. P., *Leisure and Ancient Rome*, Oxford University Press, Oxford, 1995, 79.
119. Jashemski, W. F., The discovery of a market-garden orchard at Pompeii, *Am. J. Arch.*, 78, 391, 1974.
120. Hippocrates, Regimen, in *Hippocrates*, Vol. 4. Jones, W. H. S. Translator, G. P. Putnam's Sons, New York, 1931, 1:27.
121. Soranus, *Gynecology*, Temkin, O., Translator, the Johns Hopkins Press, Baltimore, 1956, 1:14:46.
122. Soranus, 1956, 1:14:50-51, *(See* reference 121).
123. Paulus Aegineta, *[Epitome] The Seven Books of Paulus Aegineta*. 3 Vols., Adams, F., Translator, Sydenham Society, London, 1844, 1:1.
124. Aristotle. *Historia Animalium*. Peck, A. L., Translator, 3 vols., William Heinemann, London, 1970, 7:11.
125. Galen, *De Sanitate Tuenda*, Green, R. M., Translator, Charles C. Thomas, Springfield, Illinois, 1951, 1:7.
126. Soranus, 1956, 2:12:19, *(See* reference 121).
127. Soranus, 1956, 1:14:25–26, *(See* reference 121).
128. Soranus, 1956, 2:21:46–48, *(See* reference 121).
129. Galen, 1951, 5:3, *(See* reference 125).

130. Galen, 1951, 5:4, *(See* reference 125).
131. Paulus Aegineta, 1844, 1:23, *(See* reference 123).
132. Hippocrates, Regimen in Health, in *Hippocrates*, Vol. 4, Jones, W. H. S. Translator, G. P. Putnam's Sons, New York, 1959, 1.
133. Hippocrates, Regimen in acute disease, in *Hippocrates*, Vol. 2, Jones, W. H. S. Translator, William Heinemann, London, 1923, 30-33.
134. Hippocrates, 1923, 44–47, 49–50, *(See* reference 133).
135. Celsus, *On Medicine*. Spencer, W. S. Translator, 3 Vols. Harvard University Press, Cambridge, 1935–1938, 2:18:2.
136. Celsus, 1935–1938, 2:18:3–7, *(See* reference 135).
137. Celsus, 1935–1938, 2:18:8–10, *(See* reference 135).
138. Plutarch, Advice about keeping well, in *Plutarch's Moralia*, Vol. 2, Babbitt, F. C. Translator, Harvard University Press, Cambridge, Massachusetts, 1956, 123:E–137:A.
139. Plutarch, 1956, 125:F–126A, *(See* reference 138).
140. Grivetti, L. E., Nutrition past — Nutrition today. Prescientific origins of nutrition and dietetics. Part 2. Legacy of the Mediterranean. *Nut. Today.* 26(4), 18, 1991.
141. Galen, On the preservation of health, in *Greek Medicine. Being Extracts Illustrative of Medical Writers from Hippocrates to Galen*, Brock, A. J., Translator, J. M. Dent, London, 1929,:5:1.
142. Darby, W. J., Ghalioungui, P., and Grivetti, L. E., *Food: The Gift of Osiris*. 2 Vols. Academic Press, London, 1977, Vol. 1., 60.
143. Hippocrates, On the nature of man, in *Hippocrates*, Vol. 4, Jones, W. H. S. Translator, William Heinemann, London, 1959, pp. 2-41, 4.
144. Galen, 1951, 6:8, *(See* reference 125).
145. Paulus Aegineta, 1844, 1:57, *(See* reference 123).
146. Athenaeus, 1927–1941, 1:10:D, *(See* reference 73).
147. Celsus, 1935–1938, 4:7:5, *(See* reference 135).
148. Herophilus of Chalcedon, *Herophilus. The Art of Medicine in Early Alexandria*, von Staden, H., Translator and Ed., University Press, Cambridge, 1989. 312.
149. Müller, W. M., *Asien und Europa nach altägyptischen Denkmälern*, Engleman, Leipzig, 1893, 348.
150. Darby, W. J., Ghalioungui, P., and Grivetti, L. E., 1977, Vol. 1, 301, 306, *(See* reference 142).
151. Vickery, K. F., 1936, pp. 74-84, 88–89, *(See* reference 2).
152. *Oxford Classical Dictionary*, 1970, p. 603, *(See* reference 11).
153. Tucker, T. T., 1918, pp. 149–150, *(See* reference 77).
154. Whibley, L., 1931, p. 640, *(See* reference 14).
155. Dalby, A., 1996, pp. 24–25, *(See* reference 81).
156. Athenaeus, 1927–1941, 2:47:C, *(See* reference 73).
157. Preston, H. W., and Dodge, L., 1927, p. 77, *(See* reference 109).
158. Toner, J. P., 1995, pp. 81–82, *(See* reference 118).
159. Grivetti, L. E., Clash of cuisines. Notes on Christoforo Colombo 1492-1503, *Nut. Today*, 26(2), 13, 1992.
160. Matalas, A. -L., and Grivetti, L. E., The diet of nineteenth-century Greek sailors. An analysis of the log of the Konstantinos, *Food and Foodways*. 5, 353, 1994.
161. Athenaeus, 1927-1941, *(See* reference 73).
162. Diodorus Siculus, *Library of History*, Oldfather, C. H., Sherman, C., Welles, C. B., Geer, R. M., and Walton, F. R., Translators, 12 Vols., G. P. Putnam's Sons, New York, 1933–1967.

163. Newberry, P., On the vegetable remains discovered in the cemetery of Hawara, in *Hawara, Biahmu, and Arsinoe*, Petrie, W. M. F., Ed., Trubner and Company, London, 1889, 46.

164. Gabra, S., Drioton, E. T., Perdrizet, P., and Waddell, W. G., *Rapport sur les fouilles d'Hermoupolis Ouest (Touna el Gebel)*, l'Institut Français d'Archéologie Orientale, Cairo, 1941.

165. Lefebvre, G., *Le Tombeau de Petosiris*, Service des Antiquités de l'Egypte, Institut Français d'Archéologie Orientale, Cairo, 1924, Vol. 3, Plate 35.

166. Hunt, A. S., and Edgar, C. C., *Select Papyri*, 2 Vols., G. P. Putnam's Sons, New York, 1932–1934.

167. Lindsey, J., *Leisure and Pleasure in Roman Egypt*, Barnes and Noble, New York, 1966.

168. Plutarchus, *Table talk*, in *Moralia*, Minar, E. L., Sandbach, F. H., and Helmbold, W. C. Translators. Vol. 9, Harvard University Press, Cambridge, Massachusetts, 1959, 142.

169. Columella, *On Agriculture*. Forster, E. S., Heffner, H. H., and Ash, H. B. Translators, 3 Vols., Harvard Uaniversity Press, Cambridge, Massachusetts, 1948.

170. Strabo, *Geography*, Jones, H. L., Translator, 8 Vols., G. P. Putnam's Sons, New York, 1917–1932.

171. Juvenal, The satires of Juvenal, in *Juvenal and Persius*, Ramsay, G. G., Translator, Heinemann, London, 1957.

2 The Mediterranean Diet: Historical Background and Dietary Patterns in Pre-World War II Greece

Antonia-Leda Matalas

CONTENTS

0-8493-0110-6/01/$0.00+$.50
© 2001 by CRC Press LLC

I. INTRODUCTION AND SOURCES

A. Rationale for Studying the Historical Background of the Greek Diet

The diets followed by people living in southern European regions in the 1960s have formed the basis for a healthy-eating model called the Mediterranean diet. The rationale for the promotion of Mediterranean dietary patterns and foodways among non-Mediterranean peoples lies in the ability of these dietary patterns to reduce chronic disease risk.[1] The major source of information regarding traditional Mediterranean diets has been the Seven Countries Study,[2,3] conducted in the 1960s and 1970s. It has been argued, however, that the historical, social, and cultural features underpinning the Mediterranean Diet have been largely ignored, and thus, the proposed food models constitute artifacts that cannot be of benefit to non-Mediterranean populations.[4] Regarding the Greek version of the Mediterranean Diet specifically, available information describes the diets followed on Greek islands since the 1940s,[5-7] but no information is available in the medical literature on Greek dietary patterns prior to World War II.

Revealing the characteristics of the Greek diet before World War II is important for appreciating the historical and social perspectives of the traditional Mediterranean diet and, therefore, understanding how it has evolved. It has been argued that insight on how the Mediterranean Diet has developed over time is required in order to formulate effective food guides for Mediterranean populations.[8] A historical insight into the Greek diet will also facilitate any attempt to define the unifying characteristics among traditional diets followed in different regions of the Mediterranean. The scope of this chapter is to examine the dietary patterns prevailing in Greece prior to World War II. Specific questions addressed are: what were the dietary patterns of the Greeks during the 19th and early 20th centuries? How did Greek dietary patterns differ among social classes? How did they differ from the diets followed in other European regions? Were the dietary patterns followed by Greeks before World War II similar to those recorded in the 1960s?

B. Sources

Any attempt to reveal dietary patterns of past centuries is complicated by a number of factors, among which the scarcity of reliable data on food availability and consumption is of primary importance. The geographical and economic diversity of the region under consideration further complicates the task of reconstructing dietary patterns of past times. To estimate food availability and examine foodways of the Greeks during late modern times, historical sources were called upon. Data presented in this chapter have been extracted from sources that fall into four categories:

   (a) Surveys on family budgets conducted by Greek state agencies with the aim of estimating the cost of living among rural and urban Greek citizens
   (b) Archival documents, i.e., detailed logs accounting food expenses executed by prosperous households

(c) Monographs by physicians and other expert scientists written before World War II that aimed at evaluating the dietary habits of the Greeks

(d) Published studies on agricultural production, import-export activities, and prices of foods, as well as essays on agricultural and folklore issues and descriptions written by tourists

The dietary patterns followed by Greek peasants in past centuries are derived from two historical sources: first, the results of a survey that provides estimates on food availability in the typical Greek rural household in the mid19th century, conducted by official Greek agents among households in southern Greece in 1853.[9] These estimates provided food availability figures for the average rural household that practiced small scale agriculture and consisted of two adults and five children. The second source is a monograph on the economic structure and subsistence conditions of an extended family of herders in the northern region of Greek Macedonia that accounted food produced and purchased by the family during 1930.[10] The family consisted of eight adults and ten children.

Data on the diet followed in Greek cities and towns in the early 20th century are derived from two family-budget surveys conducted by Greek State officials with the aim of identifying consumption patterns and cost of living in urban centers. The first survey was conducted among 55 working-class and middle-class families of Athens and the neighboring town of Piraeus that were selected from a mailing list during the period 1926–1927.[11] The second survey was conducted in 1930 among 473 low-income households in 28 Greek cities and towns, with the laboring class representing 69% of the sample.[12]

Archival household logs were used to analyze the dietary patterns followed by urban upper-class families in the 19th century. The logs used come from the period 1834–1891 and provide accounts of expenses disbursed by urban families residing either in Athens or in Hermoupolis, the capital of the island of Syros in the Aegean Sea.[13-16] The accounts typically provide the amount of money spent for food, with the common exception of vegetable items.

All of the above historical sources have been previously analyzed for the information they provide on prices of goods, economic indices, and consumption trends. None, however, has been previously studied for elucidating the diets followed in the region during past times.

II. GREEK FOOD PATTERNS IN MODERN TIMES

A. OVERVIEW OF FOOD AVAILABILITY AND FOOD SHORTAGE

Greece has been a predominantly agricultural society through the 1970s. In the mid 1800s, the Greek State was limited to the southern part of its current lands and had a population of approximately one million.[17] About 90% of the active Greek population was composed of peasants, including small-scale farmers, ranchers, and peasant laborers.[9,18,19] Greek farmers grew crops primarily for sustaining themselves and their families, and secondly for earning some income.[20,21] Crops and products that the farmers were selling were mainly grapes, wine, honey, and beeswax, and, to a smaller degree, cereal crops.

The core diet of the Greek peasants in the mid 19th century consisted of cereals, dry legumes, vegetables, wine, and fruits and was supplemented with quantities of meat, cheese, olive oil, and olives, salted fish and seafood — known under the generic term *almyra,* meaning salty. Subsistence agriculture provided a great portion of the food consumed — in particular, legumes, vegetables, cereals, wine, and, often, some honey. Meat, dairy, and eggs came from animals raised by the household.[9] According to official sources,[9] a typical rural household kept for subsistence purposes ten goats and maybe one or two cows that served plowing purposes. In most cases, olive oil, preserved fish, cheese, and dry onions were purchased. According to official statistics,[9] the members of an average rural household consisting of five to seven people consumed, year round, 25 kg of grain. During harvest time, however, the farmers relied on purchased meat, dairy products, and, sometimes, cereals, to cover their food needs.

By the 1930s, the Greek population had increased to approximately 6.4 million and 61% of the active population were peasants.[22] Besides the natural population growth, the expansion of sovereign territory that occurred in the early 20th century, and the influx of one million migrants from Asia Minor, contributed to the population growth noted.[17] The dietary patterns of the Greeks in the early 20th century did not differ greatly from those that prevailed a century ago. The diet was based on cereals, vegetables, legumes, wine, and fruits.[23-25] In rural areas, grains, beans, wine, and vegetables were produced by the household.[23] Small quantities of cheese, salted fish and meat supplemented the regimen of the poorer classes.[26-27] Olive oil and olives were consumed mainly in the olive-oil-producing regions. Availability of milk and dairy products among the higher social classes appears to have increased in the early years of the 20th century as compared with the 19th century.

A large portion of the Greek population, especially in the mountainous areas, specialized in sheep- and goat herding. Data on the food resources of an 18-member family of herders in northern Greece reveal that, besides sheep and goats, the family also kept 23 pigs (out of which two were fed in a special manner in order to be fattened), two cows, and several hens for subsistence purposes.[10] Cereal crops, potatoes (by the early 20th century, the potato had gained an important position as a crop in the mountainous areas of Greece)[25] and other vegetables were also produced by the family to support its food needs and that needed for its animals.

Food availability among Greek peasants was at its highest during the periods that followed the harvest of cereal crops, i.e., during summer and autumn months. Available food, however, decreased markedly in winter and spring months. Areas particularly vulnerable to famine were the islands and the mountainous regions. During the period between 1670 and 1800, ten cases of famine were traced in various Greek regions.[28] Specifically, archival sources mention hunger periods accompanied by several deaths on the islands of Cephalonia, Chios, Crete, and Hydra, as well as in some northern regions of the country (such as the region of Pelion and the town of Kozani).[28,29] During periods of food scarcity, there were outbreaks of infectious diseases, as reflected by the documented malaria cases.[28] To obtain some nutrition during hunger periods, islanders were even resorting to sea pebbles; the peasants in

Corfu collected pieces of stone that had attached various little shells and seaweed, boiled them, and used the broth as the basis of their meal.[30] By the 19th century, however, according to modern Greek historians, the phenomenon of hunger was the exception, at least in the grain-producing areas.[28]

In the 1930s, several Greek public health experts maintained that the majority of the Greek population was chronically undernourished, basically "due to a regimen that was deficient in high-quality protein".[26,27] Life expectancy in 1928 was 49 years, a figure that was significantly lower than that reported for the United States and northern European countries. However, life expectancy increased by 13 years during the period 1837 to 1928. In the 1930s, infant mortality was still high: 38.0% and 26.5% of the children in rural and urban regions, respectively, died before the age of five.[31] Infant mortality accounted at that time for 34% of total deaths in Greece, and Greece ranked seventh among 24 European regions in total unadjusted death rate. Among death causes, tuberculosis ranked first, accounting for 9% of all deaths. Diarrhea and other gastrointestinal complications ranked second, while malaria came third as a death cause.[26]

B. Staple Foods

1. Cereals and Cereal Products

a. The old cereals: wheat, barley, rye, millet

Wheat was the cereal preferred by the Greeks since ancient times, however, it represents only one of the cereals consumed in Greece. The French tourist de Pouponne, who visited the island of Chios in the 1600s, was impressed by the scarcity of wheat and wrote that "on the island abandons everything but the wheat".[32] Wheat production in the mid 19th and early 20th centuries was not sufficient to meet the consumption needs of the Greek State (limited in the southern part of Greece) and most of the wheat consumed was imported.[17] In the northern region of Macedonia, which was occupied by the Turks until 1922, however, cereal production exceeded needs and a substantial proportion was exported.[33] In the late 1920s, cereal crops occupied about 60% of all cultivated land in Greece.[19,34] Wheat occupied 25%, and barley 12% of the total cultivated land, while another 10% was occupied by corn.[19] Barley was cultivated extensively in dry areas, whereas rye was the grain with higher yield rates in cold, mountainous regions.[28] Millet was another cereal that was grown and consumed in some Greek regions, especially during periods of food shortage. On the island of Crete, during medieval times, peasants prepared their bread from a mixture of barley, wheat, and millet flour.[35] Extensive use of millet by the Cretans has been documented during the 1591 famine, at a time when the island was under Venetian occupation.[29]

b. The new cereals: corn and rice

Wheat and barley are winter crops, and reliance on these plants created a pattern that was associated with significant risk of food shortage. Greek farmers cultivated corn, as this was a cereal that could support them during the springtime, thus reducing food-shortage risk.[28] Corn, a New World food, was cultivated in western and northern regions such as the Ionian islands, Epirus, and Etolia.[9,36] On the other hand, on the islands of the eastern Aegean, corn remained unknown until the 20th century.[37,38]

Bread made from corn was used extensively by peasants and herders in western and northern Greece and was less expensive than wheat bread.[36] Corn was used by itself or mixed with wheat to prepare small unleavened breads and soups. The bread that was made of mixed wheat and corn flour was known as *mixed-bread (anaka-totos)*.[39] Corn meal, often referred to as *boukouvala,* was a common food in western Greece.[39] Corn, however, was viewed by the Greeks as a second-choice grain. Corn flour was known in Corfu as *barbaralevro,* a colloquial term for "barbarians' flour".[40] Corn bread was also referred to as *alitourgito,* for not having been blessed in church, thus being distinguished from wheat bread, which was the bread used during the procession of the Holy Communion (*litourgia*).[40] In the southeastern parts of the country, corn was hardly consumed, and its sole use in human nutrition was in the form of a street-food item; in the late 19th century, boiled corn-on-the-cob was sold by street vendors in Constantinople and the towns of Asia Minor.[41]

Rice became part of the Greek diet in recent times. Though some rice was grown in a few Greek regions such as the island of Crete, since the 17th century,[29] almost all rice consumed in Greece until the 1940s was imported. In the 19th and early 20th centuries, rice was an expensive commodity and only prosperous families could afford it.[15,16] Unlike dry legumes and other cereal grains, which were typically purchased in large quantities, rice was procured by urban families on a day-to-day basis. From evidence that household logs provide, we can conclude that rice was invariably eaten as part of meat dishes.[13]

c. Breads consumed

Bread has been the main dietary staple for the Greeks since ancient times.[42,43] Periods of famine were marked by the shortage of this commodity.[44]

Preparation of fresh bread was done by villagers on a weekly basis.[29] Various types of dry-flour products were used when out of fresh bread, mainly toasted bread (*paximadi*) and a type of dry bread, the *kouloura.* In medieval Crete, a particular type of dry bread, the *frisopo,* was also used.[35] According to Kostis,[28] poor Greek farmers subsisted on a coarse bread that contained more barley, corn, or millet than wheat. Use of bread made of barley as well as other cereals, besides wheat, has been also documented in accounts written by early tourists who traveled in Greece in the 17th century.[45] The same pattern regarding the composition of bread has been reported for many other European areas during the Middle Ages.[46]

In 19th- and early 20th-century Greek cities, two types of bread were available, premium bread and second-quality bread.[14,22] Premium bread, known as *hasiko* or *kathario* (a colloquial term for pure), was an all-wheat white bread and was the bread of choice of prosperous Greeks.[39] All-wheat bread was also highly esteemed by poor Greek peasants, who considered it a luxury food. The second-quality bread was a whole-flour bread, usually made from mixed wheat and barley flour.

Available evidence indicates that the dietary importance of bread and cereal products was inversely related to affluence and urban environment. The amount of money typically spent toward bread and wheat products by prosperous 19th-century Greeks fell behind that spent for meat. According to historical sources, expenses made by wealthy households toward meat purchases were as much as 2.5-fold higher than expenses toward procuring bread and other wheat products.[15,16]

2. Dry Legumes and Vegetables

Dry legumes constituted an important dietary item for the Greeks during past centuries. The lentil, the broad bean, the garbanzo bean, and the dry pea were the legumes most commonly eaten. In certain areas such as the island of Crete, the horse bean (*lathouri*) was also consumed by peasants.[35] French beans were introduced in the Greek diet long before the other New World vegetable items, such as the tomato and the potato. Medieval sources provide evidence that French beans were imported in Crete from Venice as early as the 1700s[35,47] On the islands of the eastern Aegean Sea however, French beans became available only during the 1900s.[37] "French beans" (*fragofasoula*) was the term adopted initially for this new type of beans in most Greek regions;[14] later on however, French beans were simply named "beans" (*fasolia*), a fact that illustrates the popularity this legume gained among Greeks.

Legumes were very popular among rural people, but were deemed of low value by urban Greeks. During the early 20th century, legume consumption by Athenians inversely mirrored their income.[11] Dry legumes' value as a source of protein and amino acids was not fully appreciated by Greek scientists before the 1940s.[26,48] It is noteworthy that a prominent Greek physician in her treatise on Foods and Nutrition,[49] maintained that consumption of legumes should be avoided, and even more so by the poor people, as it results in an increased protein requirement!

Vegetables hold an important role in the traditional Greek diet. Of great dietary significance were wild greens. Collection of wild greens constituted a major food resource for rural Greek families. The German geographer Josef Partsch, in his accounts of rural life on the Ionian island of Corfu, wrote in late 1800s that villagers "depend for their nutrition on wild vegetables and other strange greens to which they add some olive oil and sometimes, lemon juice."[50] Twenty seven species of wild greens are reported to have been collected and consumed routinely on the eastern Aegean island of Samos in the beginning of the 20th century.[37] Wild greens were available in urban markets throughout the Greek mainland and the Aegean islands in the 19th century,[38] but were generally considered a lesser food item by urban Greeks.[29] Wild greens were usually consumed plain-boiled as salad, but occasionally were also eaten fried, braised, or as the main ingredient in pies and dishes. Greens and herbs were collected by the villagers, not only for food, but also for their medicinal and cosmetic properties.[29]

Among cultivated vegetable species, of most widespread use during the 19th and early 20th centuries were onions, leeks, cabbage, carrots, endive, chard, okra, artichoke, purslane, and parsley.[14,27,35,38] Several other vegetables were available in the markets of Athens and other urban centers in 19th century, but they were expensive.

Zucchinis were available in the Greek markets as early as 1800s, but were expensive and sold by the piece.[14] Also highly priced were the tomato, the pepper, and the potato, all items that were originally introduced from the Americas. While most of the vegetables are mentioned in household logs collectively under a generic term for salad items (such as *salatika* or *kipeftika),* zucchini, potato, and the tomato were typically mentioned by name. Cultivation of tomatoes spread in the islands of the Aegean Sea during the mid 19th century.[29] The potato was unknown in the Greek mainland until the 1800s. Use of potatoes was first adopted by the poor peasants in mountainous areas and soon acquired a significant dietary role.[51] Potatoes were sold in the Athenian market as early as 1834,[14,52] but were introduced to Crete and the islands of the eastern Aegean Sea after the 1860s.[29,38]

3. Olive Oil

The Greek diet is, above all, characterized by the type of added fat it involves — olive oil. Olive oil has been highly esteemed and considered a very nutritious food by the Greeks since medieval times.[53] Besides being an important food commodity, olive oil found several non-nutritional uses in past centuries, mainly as a fuel and cosmetic.[47] Olive oil was, though, an expensive commodity because its production offered a low yield and was produced through a laborious process.[47,54] Olive oil's liberal consumption was considered a privilege that only rich people could have. The widespread belief that spilling olive oil brings bad luck[55] illustrates the scarcity of the product. Olive oil is the only vegetable food that, according to Christian Orthodox doctrines, devoted Christians should remove from their regimen during the days of Lent. However, consumption of olives is not restricted during Lent. This tradition must have aimed at reducing the demand for olive oil.

Historical sources reveal that olive oil's production and consumption in medieval Crete were far less than current levels.[54,56] Prices of olive oil in Crete during the 1300s were extremely high; the cost of one kilo of olive oil matched a laborer's monthly wage.[56] During this period, it was forbidden by law for Cretans to sell retail quantities of olive oil that exceeded one kilo per person.

Archival sources provide evidence that, in the mid 18th century, in the monastery of St. George Ragousi, located on the island of Chios, the quantity of olive oil secured for the operational needs of the church (i.e., as fuel for oil candles) surpassed the quantity that was used for the nourishment of the ten monks (61.5 kg/year vs. 46.0 kg/year).[57] Prices of olive oil in the 1840s are also indicative. Olive oil was sold in the Greek cities at prices two to four times higher than the price of meat, one and a half times higher than the price of cheese, and five to twelve times higher than the price of wine.[15] The price of olive oil, however, was half the price of butter, in contrast to other areas of Europe, such as France, where olive oil was sold at prices comparable to those of prime quality butter.[58]

Following the establishment of the New Greek State in the 1820s, production of olive oil in Greece exhibited a continuous increase throughout the 19th century. [60] First, because of an increase in the number of cultivated olive trees, and second, because of advancements in olive-oil-extraction techniques. The new techniques allowed for the yield rate to increase by up to 10–12%.[59,60] These changes made olive oil a less expensive food item and, in the 1920s, its price in Athens was comparable to the prices of meat and salted cod, and only three times higher than the price of wine.[11] In the 1930s, Greece exported about 9% of its total olive oil production.[61]

4. Wine

Wine has been a staple food for the Greeks since ancient times. Grapes were the main export item for the Greek State throughout the 19th century. In 1860, vineyards occupied 21.4% of all arable land in Greece. Most of these vineyards (76%) represented wine-producing varieties, while the rest were table grapes.[17] Grape production was high in southern Greece but relatively limited in northern Greece. In the early 20th century, two thirds of the grape production came from the regions of the Peloponnese (southern Greece), Sterea Hellas (southern central Greece) and the island of Crete.[17] In the northern regions, however, the main alcoholic beverage consumed was not wine, but *raki* or *tsipouro*, alcoholic beverages made from distilled grapes or pomace, similar to the French *eau de vie.*[33]

5. Meat

Most of the meat produced and consumed in 19th-century Greece was lamb and goat.[35] Beef was a commodity hardly used in most rural Greek areas before the 1920s.[37] In the early 20th century, production of beef was increased to represent 35% of total meat production, while goat and lamb represented 38%, pork 15%, and poultry 13% of the total meat produced in the country.[25] Among the labor classes in Athens, beef was the major type of meat eaten in the early 20th century. Laborers in Athens preferred beef over lamb and goat, as it was less expensive.[22] The meat of choice among prosperous urban Athenians during spring and summer months was lamb, while beef was preferred during winter months,[14] a period when the price of meat was generally higher.

Pork provided valuable nutrients to peasants who often raised one pig at home.[29] Most of the pork was consumed in preserved form rather than fresh. Several traditional dried and cured pork products, such as smoked cuts, sausages, and blood sausages (*hematites*) were prepared in most of rural Greek regions.[47,49] Greeks used extensively the various lesser cuts of meats and offal.[37] In urban centers, pork consumption was limited and was substantially lower than that of beef,[14] a consumption pattern that persisted throughout the 20th century.

In sharp contrast with the situation in western European urban centers,[62,63] most of the meat consumed in 19th-century Greek cities and towns was fresh. Dried and cured forms of meat in the Greek markets were exceptionally expensive. In the mid 1800s, pork sausage was the only available type of preserved meat sold in the markets of Athens, at prices that were more than double the price of fresh beef.[14]

Rural Greeks resorted regularly to game birds to supplement their diet. In urban centers, only prosperous people could afford to buy game meat. Rabbit and partridge were especially esteemed. Rabbit meat was often preserved in salt, much the same as fish.[29]

5. Fish and Seafood

Greeks who did not reside in areas neighboring the sea consumed salted and dried fish and seafood. Salted sardines and octopus were sold widely in the Greek markets in the 1800s.[18] Octopus and other kinds of molluscs, such as squid and snails, were consumed extensively during Lent, when all other animal food was restricted.

IV. DIETARY PATTERNS AMONG RURAL AND URBAN PRE-WORLD WAR II GREEKS

A. MACRONUTRIENT AND ENERGY AVAILABILITY

To better understand the characteristics of the diets followed by Greeks in the past, the macronutrient composition of the diets should be examined. Although the data used here are derived from populations that cannot be regarded as statistical samples, some generalizations can be drawn about the diet of pre-World War II Greece. Total per capita energy availability and the composition of available energy in terms of macronutrients in two rural and three urban groups are shown in Table 1. Values presented reflect average per capita nutrient availability in populations composed of adults and children, with the adult to children ratio ranging for the rural working-class and middle-class urban populations from 0.40 to 1.0, while it was up to 5.5 for upper-class families. Energy and macronutrient values were estimated on the basis of previously published data derived from family-budget surveys for the rural groups and the first two urban groups, and from household logs for the upper class group.

The amount of daily per capita available energy differed according to economic environment. For the 19th-century peasants in southern Greece, available energy was estimated at 1926 kcal/day, while for the 20th-century herders, it amounted to 2310 kcal/day. For members of the urban working class, the per capita energy availability was 2336 kcal/day, for the middle-class city inhabitants, 2903 kcal/day, and for the members of the 19th-century upper class, 3335 kcal/day. These differences can be explained to some extent by the differences in mean age (or the adult to children ratio), however, it is apparent that total energy availability increased with affluence.

The composition of diets followed by rural Greeks, whether specializing in agriculture or in animal husbandry, exhibit common characteristics. Protein represented almost 18% of the total available energy for rural Greeks in previous decades. The largest part of the available protein (70% and 84%, for peasants and herders, respectively) was derived from vegetable sources and mainly from cereals. Availability of lipids, on the other hand, was low and represented 22.0% and 27.2% of the total available energy for the southern peasants and the herders, respectively. Though quantities of lipid calories differed significantly between southern peasants and northern Greeks specializing in animal husbandry (47 g vs. 70 g), the contribution of the three types of fatty acids to caloric availability reveals unifying characteristics. Saturated fatty acids accounted for less than 10% of total calories in both groups (6.1% and 9.6% in southern peasants and northern herders, respectively). Monounsaturated fatty acids contributed 8.2% and 9.0% of the energy, while contribution of polyunsaturated fatty acids was limited to 4.3–4.4%. The diets of the urban populations were characterized by higher proportions of lipid calories and lower proportions of protein and carbohydrate than the diets of rural Greeks. Protein

TABLE 1
Daily Nutrient Availability and Regimen Composition In Rural and Urban Greeks During the Nineteenth and Early Twentieth Century[a]

	Type of Economic Environment; Date				
	Rural, Peasants; 1855	Rural, Herders; 1930	Urban, Working Class; 1926-27	Urban, Middle Class; 1926-30	Urban, Upper Class; 1830-91
Adult to children ratio in the population[b]	0.40	0.80	0.65	1.0	5.5
Energy[c], kcal/capita	1,926	2,310	2,336	2,903	3,335
Protein, % energy	17.8	17.9	13.9	13.2	13.3
(g/capita)	(86)	(104)	(81)	(96)	(111)
Animal pr., % energy	2.9	5.3	3.5	4.4	6.6
(g/capita)	(14)	(31)	(20)	(32)	(55)
Vegetable pr., % energy	14.9	12.6	10.4	8.8	6.7
(g/capita)	(72)	(73)	(61)	(64)	(56)
Carbohydrate, % energy	57.0	54.9	53.8	48.3	39.6
(g/capita)	(293)	(338)	(335)	(374)	(352)
Lipid, % energy	22.0	27.2	30.9	35.5	43.1
(g/capita)	(47)	(70)	(80)	(116)	(160)
SFA, % energy	6.1	9.6	11.2	9.9	15.1
(g/capita)	(13)	(25)	(29)	(32)	(56)
MUFA, % energy	8.2	9.0	15.1	18.1	21.0
(g/capita)	(18)	(23)	(39)	(59)	(78)
PUFA, % energy	4.3	4.4	4.1	4.3	4.2
(g/capita)	(9)	(11)	(11)	(14)	(15)
P:S ratio	0.70	0.46	0.37	0.44	0.30
Alcohol, % energy	3.2	—	1.6	3.0	4.0
(g/capita)	(9)	—	(5)	(12)	(18)
Cholesterol, mg/cap.	59	139	119	175	340

SFA = saturated fatty acids
MUFA = monounsaturated fatty acids
PUFA = polyunsaturated fatty acids

[a] For a presentation of the original sources used, see section 1B.

[b] Energy and macronutrient availability figures are derived from values that refer to the average household and not to the average individuals and therefore the relationship between adult and young members differs from one study to the other.

[c] Energy and nutrient content of foods procured were calculated on the basis of the values provided in *McCance and Widdowson's The Composition of Foods*, (5th ed.), The Royal Society of Chemistry, Cambridge, 1991 (ref. 74). Energy values for macronutrients were taken as follows: protein, 4 kcal/g; carbohydrate, 3.75 kcal/g; fat, 9 kcal/g; alcohol, 7 kcal/g. The caloric contribution of vegetables, other than the potato and fruits, is not included as it cannot be estimated with accuracy.

represented 13–14% of the energy available to urban representatives. Among urban Greeks, the higher the degree of affluence, the lower the contribution of vegetable protein to energy availability. Carbohydrate accounted for 53.8, 48.3, and 39.7% of total energy for working-middle and upper-class urban Greeks, respectively.

An overview of all five groups reveals that the higher the degree of affluence, the higher the percentage of calories derived from lipids as a whole, as well as from monounsaturated fatty acids. For the representatives of the working class, total lipids and monounsaturated fatty acids accounted for 30.9% and 15.1% of available energy, respectively. Middle-class Greeks derived higher proportions of their energy from lipids, as well as monounsaturated fats (35.3% and 18.1%, respectively). Prosperous 19th-century Greeks showed an even greater reliance on fats, deriving an impressive 43.2% of their total calories from fat, and a 21.0% from monounsaturates. For all three urban groups, half of the total available fat came in the form of monounsaturated fatty acids. In contrast, monounsaturated fats represented about a third of total fat grams for the two rural populations. Availability of polyunsaturated fatty acids among the three urban groups remained at the same low levels found in the rural Greeks, representing approximately 4% of the total calories. Cholesterol availability was low among rural Greeks and representatives of the working and middle class, with the southern rural group exhibiting the lowest (59 mg) and the urban middle-class group the highest value (175 mg). In contrast, the estimated cholesterol available to the prosperous 19th-century urbanites reached 340 mg/day.

It is worth mentioning that the daily per capita saturated fat and cholesterol availability observed among northern herders was only 25 g and 139 mg, respectively, a fact due to a limited use of animal products, despite their involvement in animal husbandry.

B. Food Availability

Some points regarding the availability of foods among rural and urban Greeks deserve mention. Based on the examination of the sources presented above,[9-16] cereals were the foods that provided more energy than any other food group to the populations examined. Energy from cereals represented about two thirds of the total available energy for the rural groups. The dietary importance of cereals however, diminished with increasing affluence and urban environment. Urban representatives of the working, middle, and upper class derived 60%, 48% and 43% of their total food energy, respectively, from cereals. Cereals consumed by peasants in southern Greece were wheat, barley, and corn. Peasants in northern Greece based their diet on corn, rye, and wheat, deriving somewhat more food energy from corn than either rye or wheat, and approximately equal energy amounts from rye and wheat. Urban Greeks, on the other hand, consumed wheat and barley as well as substantial amounts of rice. Rice consumption appears to have paralleled economic affluence.

Southern peasants relied heavily on legumes to meet their food needs and derived 16% of their calories from broad beans and other dry legumes. For the urban Greeks, however, legumes contributed much less to energy intake, and represented 3–5% of the total available energy, with members of the prosperous class exhibiting the most limited use of these food commodities.

Olive oil was available to urban Greeks at much higher quantities than to their rural counterparts. Among the former, olive oil contributed 14% to 18% to total available energy, while it accounted for only 5% and 2% of the available energy in southern 19th-century peasants and 20th-century herders, respectively. A limited availability of olive oil among 19th-century Greek peasants has also been previously reported; availability estimates for peasants on the island of Evea ranged between 6.5 and 10.2 g/capita/day.[60] The increased olive oil consumption among middle- and upper-class urban representatives was responsible for the higher availability of monounsaturated fatty acids, as well as for a good portion of the saturated fatty acids' availability. Middle-class and prosperous urban Greeks used butter on a regular basis, while this item was not used by southern peasants.

Contribution of animal products to the regimens varied according to economic environment and degree of affluence. A remarkable difference emerges regarding consumption of meat. The per capita meat availability among southern 19th-century peasants was, on the average, 30 g/day whereas among working- and middle-class urban Greeks, it was 55 g/day and 77 g/day, respectively. Meat and eggs provided 4%, 6% and 8% of the total available energy to peasants, working-class, and middle-class city inhabitants, respectively. For northern herders, meat and eggs provided 11% of the total calories. Use of milk was greater among 20th-century Greeks than in their 19th-century counterparts. Cheese, however, was consumed in higher quantities by rural Greeks than by urban Greeks; and accounted for 4% and 5% of the total available energy for southern peasants and northern herders, respectively.

Wine contributed significantly to energy intake in all populations except the northern herders, accounting for 2–5% of the total available energy. These figures do not reflect consumption levels among adults, especially males, for whom actual availability must have been considerably higher. Sugar and honey were used by all groups. Consumption of these sweeteners was limited among 19th-century Greeks (10 g/capita/day among rural; 21 g/capita/day among prosperous urban). Sugar availability however, was greatly increased among the 20th-century urban Greeks and reached 48 g/capita/day among representatives of the middle class.

Evidence for an extensive use of vegetables is provided by all household logs and survey results used in our analysis. For northern herders, for instance, it is mentioned that onions, peppers, and various green vegetables were produced by the household, while herb tea was collected by the children of the family.[10] For representatives of the working and middle class, daily vegetable (other than the potato) and fruit availability ranged between 160 g and 170 g per capita. The sources, however, provide incomplete accounts on production and purchases of vegetable and fruit items and, furthermore, do not allow for identification of the particular species used. For this reason, vegetables, other than the potato, were excluded from the analyses on energy and macronutrient availability.

V. PRE-WORLD WAR II GREEK DIETARY PATTERNS IN PERSPECTIVE

A. COMPARISON WITH CONTEMPORARY EUROPEAN PATTERNS

Although further work is required before these data can be accepted as definitive, there are substantial grounds for taking them as a basis for discussion. In that context, Greek dietary patterns can be compared against published information on the diets followed by contemporary rural and urban populations in other European countries. Such a comparison allows a better appreciation of the characteristics of the traditional Mediterranean diet.

Descriptions of the diets followed by low-income rural and urban French and English in the 19th and early 20th centuries were examined.[62-64] Contribution of macronutrients and the major staple food item, bread, to the diets followed by low-income French and English as well as Greek representatives are shown in Table 2. Data shown for the French and English populations are derived from the same types of sources as those used for the elucidation of the Greek patterns, i.e., either family-budget surveys or archival household logs.

Rural Greeks and French exhibited patterns characterized by higher availability of protein (86–119 g/capita/day) than their English counterparts (56 and 70 g/capita/day). Data presented in Table 2 also show that rural groups, with the exception of Greek herders and French fishermen, derived lower proportions of their calories from fat than their low-income urban counterparts.

Compared with the English and the French, low-income urban Greeks derived a higher percentage of their energy from fat and a lower one from carbohydrate. This observation is in agreement with the increase in availability and consumption of olive oil that occurred in the late 19th century in Greece. It has been well documented that diets in England throughout the 19th century were based on cereals and tubers.[63,65] Furthermore, consumption of bread and animal foods by English laborers dropped throughout the 19th century, compared with 18th-century consumption.[63] For members of the working class in England, the typical response to salary increase in the 1800s was an increased consumption of alcohol and beer, but not of meat or dairy.[63] Potato consumption, however, showed a dramatic rise during the 19th century and, for working classes, ranged from 270 g to 400 g daily. It has been maintained, therefore, that during the first half of the 19th century, a deterioration in the diet of working classes in England occurred, despite an increase in overall food supplies.[63,64] Bread consumption was high among low-income French; available evidence indicates that poor laborers in mid 19th-century France were eating one to two kilograms of bread daily.[66,67]

This pattern of reliance on cereals and potato was reversed in England as well as other western European regions at the end of the 19th century with the dawning of economic growth and the improvement of transportation and food-storage techniques. The transition was marked by a decline in cereal and potato consumption and a concomitant increase in consumption of animal foods,[64,68] resulting in a higher fat intake. Economic growth in Greece occurred at a later time than in western

TABLE 2
Daily Nutrient Availability and Regimen Composition Among Low Income Greeks Compared to Published Diets of Other Europeans During Nineteenth and Early Twentieth Century

Nationality; Date	Protein	% Energy from[a] (Quantity/Capita) Carbohydrate	Lipid	% Energy from Bread	Energy kcal/Capita
Rural Environment					
Greek peasants; 1855[b]	18	57	22	62	1,926
	(86 g)	(293 g)	(47 g)		
Greek herders; 1930[b]	18	55	27	65	2,310
	(104 g)	(338 g)	(70 g)		
French fishermen; 1879[c]	19	56	25	59	2,300
	(110 g)	(353 g)	(67 g)		
French peasants; 1856[c]	11	73	10	86	4,161
	(119 g)	(811 g)	(48 g)		
English; 1863[d]	10	63	18	39	2,760
	(70 g)	(460 g)	(54 g)		
English; 1902-13[d]	10	64	22	41	2,172
	(56 g)	(370 g)	(53 g)		
Urban-Working Class					
Greek; 1926-1930[b]	14	54	30	56	2,336
	(81 g)	(335 g)	(80 g)		
French (carpenters); 1856[c]	14	58	20	59	2,627
	(89 g)	(404 g)	(58 g)		
French; 1860[c]	13	67	14	63	1,638
	(52 g)	(293 g)	(26 g)		
French (porcelain workers); 1891[c]	12	62	21	50	2,500
	(75 g)	(416 g)	(58 g)		
French; 1901[c]	12	46	35	33	2,064
	(60 g)	(252 g)	(81 g)		
English; 1863[d]	10	63	22	39	2,190
	(55 g)	(370 g)	(53 g)		
English; 1902-1913[d]	11	59	27	43	2,431
	(67 g)	(380 g)	(73 g)		

[a] Energy contribution of macronutrients was calculated on the basis of the following values: protein, 4 kcal/g; carbohydrate, 3.75 kcal/g; fat, 9 kcal/g.

[b] Data are derived from family-budget surveys. For a presentation of the original sources, see section 1B.

[c] Adapted from Dauphin C. and Pezerat, P., Annalles E.S.C., 30, 537, 1975 (ref. 62); reported data are derived from logs.

[d] Adapted from Oddy, D.J., Proc. Nutr. Soc., 29, 150, 1970 (ref. 63); reported data are derived from family-budget surveys.

European countries, and the availability of animal products among rural and low-income Greeks increased only after the 1960s.[69,70]

Further differences between the European and Greek 19th-century diets that are not obvious from the data in Table 2 should be noted. Specifically, the Greek diet was enriched with generous quantities of vegetables and fruits, including several wild species. In contrast, in 19th-century England, consumption of vegetables and fruits items is known to have been limited, due to a sheer scarcity as well as an ingrained distrust and prejudice held toward these items by the working classes.[63,71,72]

B. COMPARISON OF THE DIETARY PATTERNS OF RURAL GREEK MEN IN THE 1960s

Features of the diets followed by rural Greek men in the 1960s (as assessed by the Seven Countries Study[6,7,73]) as well as by 19th- and early 20th-century rural Greeks, are presented in Table 3. Though these data are derived by two very different methods (detailed dietary assessment techniques on one hand, and family budget surveys on the other) it is informative to examine the similarities and differences between the two populations.

The diets followed by rural Greeks prior to World War II were characterized by levels of fat intake substantially lower than those observed among Greek peasants in the 1960s (Table 3). Among the former, percent of available energy from fat ranged between 22% and 27%; among the latter, fat represented 33–36% of the total energy intake. In terms of the relative contribution of the various types of fatty acids to available energy in the four populations, there are no significant differences regarding the contribution of saturated fatty acids, but a great difference is seen regarding the contribution of monounsaturated fatty acids. The above differences are primarily due to the much higher consumption of olive oil exhibited by peasants in the 1960s than by their counterparts who lived before World War II. Mean daily consumption of olive oil by Cretan and Corfu men was 95 g/capita and 75 g/capita, respectively,[7] accounting for 31.4% and 23.9% of the total energy. In contrast, for the 19th-century peasant families, available olive oil amounted to 10 g/capita on the average, accounting for 2.3–4.7% of total energy. An inverse relationship is observed for cereals and bread: Greek islanders in the 1960s consumed less cereals than their 19th-century counterparts, as revealed by the observed differences in percent energy derived from bread (27–40% vs. 62–65%). Differences in protein can be attributed to the differences in cereal consumption; groups that had a higher consumption of bread and cereals also exhibited higher percentages of food energy from protein.

VI. CONCLUSIONS

The diets followed at large in Greece prior to World War II were characterized by the limited use of animal products and a concomitant high intake of grains and other vegetable food sources. For this reason, they represent dietary patterns that are in line with the Cretan diet of the 1960s, which has formed the basis for the Greek version of the Mediterranean Diet.

TABLE 3
Regimen Composition in Rural Greeks In Nineteenth and Early Twentieth Century Compared to Diets of Rural Greek Men in the 1960s[a]

	Region; Date			
	South Greece 1853	North Greece 1930	Crete 1960-65[b]	Corfu 1960-63[b]
Adult to children ratio in the population[c]	0.40	0.80	—[d]	—[d]
Protein, % energy	17.8	17.9	10.5	11.5
Animal pr. % energy	2.9	5.3	3.1	3.3
Lipid, % energy	22.0	27.2	36.1	35.5
SFA, % energy	6.1	9.6	7.7	6.4
MUFA, % energy	8.2	9.0	25.8	18.3
PUFA, % energy	4.3	4.4	2.5	3.5
P:S ratio	0.70	0.46	0.32	0.55
Alcohol, % energy	3	—	4	8
% Energy from bread	62.1	65.4	26.5	39.5
% Energy from olive oil	4.7	2.3	31.4	23.9

SFA = saturated fatty acids

MUFA = monounsaturated fatty acids

PUFA = polyunaturated fatty acids

[a] For a presentation of the original sources used, see section 1B.

[b] Adapted from Keys, A., Aravanis, C. and Sdrin, H., Voeding, 11, 575, 1966 (ref. 6) and Keys, A., Djordjevic, B.S., Dontas, A.S.,m Fidanza, F., Keys, M., Kromhout, D., Nredjkovic, S., Pusnar, S., Seccareccia, F., and Toshima, H., Am. J . Epidem., 124, 903, 1986 (ref. 73).

[c] Energy and macronutrient availability figures are derived from values that refer to the average household and not to the average individuals and therefore, the relationship between adult and young members differs from one study to the other.

[d] Values refer to middle-aged men.

The data presented above, however, suggest that important differences can also be traced between the diets that persisted in Greece during late modern times and the Cretan diet of the 1960s; the major difference being the lower intake of olive oil and, consequently, of monounsaturated fatty acids, by Greeks during the 19th and early 20th century. The dietary use of olive oil by the Greeks before World War II was widespread although levels of consumption were moderate, when compared with those observed among Cretans in the 1960s. Socio-economic factors are related to the dietary transition from a low olive oil intake to a high one. During the decades after World War II, Greek rural society completed its transition from a subsistence economy to a market economy. The economic and social shift was accompanied by drastic changes in food availability and, consequently, in dietary patterns. Changes initially involved an increased production and consumption of olive oil. Consumption of olive oil increased in all regions and social classes, with more marked changes observed among the lower socio-economic groups and the inhabitants of the non-olive-producing areas, resulting in an increased fat intake. A parallel phenomenon of an increase in fat consumption among low-income people also occurred in western European countries in the late 19th century as a result of economic changes. In contrast with the Greek case however, fat intake in western Europe increased because of an increased availability of animal foods, rather than a vegetable fat source.

REFERENCES

1. Wilson, C.S., Mediterranean diets: once and future?, *Nutrition Today,* 33, 246, 1998.
2. Keys, A., Aravanis, C., Blackburn, H., Buzina, R., Djordjevic, B.S., Dontas, A.S., Fidanza, F., Karvonen, M.J., Kimura, N., Menotti, A., Mohacek, I., Nedeljkovic, S., Puddu,V., Punsar, S., Taylor, H.L., and van Buchem,.F.S.P., *Seven Countries. A Multivariate Analysis of Death and Coronary Heart Disease,* Harvard University Press, Cambridge MA, 1980.
3. Keys, A., Aravanis, C., van Buchem, F. S. P., Blackburn, H., Buzina, R., Djordjevic, B. S., Fidanza, F., Karvonen, M.J., Kimura, N., Menotti, A., Nedeljkovic, S., Puddu, V., Punsar, S., and Taylor, H.L., The diet and all-causes death rate in the Seven Countries Study. *Lancet,* II, 58, 1981.
4. Crotty P., The Mediterranean Diet as a food guide, *Nutrition Today,* 33, 227, 1998.
5. Allbaugh, L. G., *Crete. A Case Study of an Undeveloped Area,* Princeton University Press, Princeton, NJ, 1953, 124.
6. Keys, A., Aravanis, C., and Sdrin, H., The diets of middle-aged men in two rural areas of Greece, *Voeding,* 11, 575, 1966.
7. Kromhout, D., Keys, A., Aravanis, C., Buzina, R., Fidanza, F., Giampaoli, S., Jansen, A., Menotti, A., Nedeljkovic, S., Pekkarinen, M., Simic, B. S., and Toshima Taylor, H., Food consumption patterns in the 1960s in the seven countries, *Am. J. Cl. Nutr.,* 49, 889, 1989.
8. Simopoulos, A., The Mediterranean food guide, *Nutrition Today,* 30, 54, 1995.
9. Psichoyios, D.K., *Dowries, Taxes, Raisin and Bread,* EKKE eds, Athens, 1987, 113 (in Greek).
10. Karavidas, K. D., *Agrotika: A Comparative Study,* Athens,1931 (reprint of the Agricultural Bank of Greece, Athens, 1978), 385 (in Greek).
11. Pratsikas, N., *Studies on the Cost of Living and Price Fluctuation in Athens During the Years 1923-27,* Athens, 1927 (in Greek),.
12. Aiphantopoulos, T., Les conditions d'existence des classes ouvrieres en Grece. *Bulletin Economique et Financier de la Banque d'Athenes,* June 1932, 2042.
13. Kremmidas, V., Urban dietary patterns: a paradigm from the Greek island of Syros in 1837, *Historica,* 14, 352, 1988 (in Greek),
14. Papayeorgiou, S. and Pepelasi-Minoglou, I., *Prices and Commodities in Athens (1834),* National Bank Educational Institute, in the series: Sources of Economic History, Athens, 1988 (in Greek).
15. Liata, E., *Prices and Commodities in Athens (1839-1846),* National Bank Educational Institute, in the series: Sources of Economic History, Athens, 1984 (in Greek).
16. Loukos, C., and Samiou, D., *Economic Behavior, Psychology and Living Standard of a Banker From Syros: Stefanos Rigas,* E.M.N.E.- Mnimon, Athens, 1991 (in Greek).

17. General Greek Statistical Office, *Statistics Bulletin of Greece*, Greek Government Printing Office, Athens, 1938 (in Greek).
18. Skaltsa, M.C., Social Life and Public Sites of Social Gathering in 19th Century Athens, Thesis Dissertation, Thessaloniki University, 1983, 66 (in Greek).
19. Raftakis, G.G., How to increase the national income, *Georgiki Epitheorisi*, 1,74, 1932 (in Greek).
20. Chalkiopoulos, P.I., *On the Improvement of the Greek Agriculture*, Athens, 1880, 89 (in Greek).
21. Raftakis, G.G., The management of agricultural production, *Georgiki Epitheorisi*, 1,102, 1932 (in Greek).
22. Riyinos, M., *Structures of Production and Labor Wages in Greece, 1909–1936*, Research and Education Institute of the Commercial Bank of Greece, in the series: Studies on Modern Greek History, Athens,1987, 255 (in Greek).
23. Bournova, E., Rapsani Dans la Première Motié du XXème Siècle: Essaie d' Economie Sociale d' un Village Grec, Thesis Dissertation, Lyon II University, 1986.
24. Exarhos, I., *A Contribution to the Investigation of the Nutrition of the World and of Greece*, Thessaloniki University eds., Thessaloniki, 1973, 218 (in Greek).
25. Zannos A., *Two Studies for a Healthier Diet and the Food Sufficiency of the Greeks*, Athens, 1932, 11 (in Greek).
26. Dontas, A.S., Nutrition and mortality statistics for the Greek population, *Proc. Acad. Athens*, 12, 448, 1937 (in Greek).
27. Ioakimoglou, G. and Yianousis, S., On the cost of securing adequate food for the poor classes, *Proc. Acad. Athens,* 8, 223, 1933 (in Greek).
28. Kostis, K., *Infertility, Costliness and Hunger,* Alexandria, Athens, 1993 (in Greek).
29. Psilakis, N., Foods of the poor and the prosperous in Venetian-occupied Crete, in the *Proceedings of the International Conference On the Prosperous and the Poor in the Eastern Greek-Latin Society*, Venetia, Athens, 1998, 319 (in Greek).
30. Koder, J., *The Kipouros and the Everyday Cuisine in Byzantium*, Goulandri-Horn, Athens, 1992 (in Greek).
31. Valaoras, V., A reconstruction of the demographic history of Modern Greece, *Milbank Mem. Fund Quart.*, April 1960, 115.
32. de Pouponne, N., *Voyageur d' Europe*, Paris, 1676.
33. Vakalopoulos, K., *Financial Function of the Macedonian and Thracean Region in the Middle Nineteenth Century Within the International Commerce*, Society of Macedonian Studies eds, Thessaloniki, 1980, Chap. 3 (in Greek).
34. Kypriadis, E.M., *Management of Cereal Crops*, State Printing Office, Greek Ministry of Agriculture, Athens, 1931 (in Greek).
35. Papadakis. M.M., The foods of the Cretans in the 15th and 16th century, *Kretologia*, 7, 52, 1978 (in Greek).
36. Andreadis, A., *The Eptanesian State Economy During the Years 1797–1814*, Meza, B., Ed., Corfu, Greece, 1936 (in Greek).
37. Dimitriou, N., *Folklore Issues of the Island of Samos*, Samos, Greece, 1982 (in Greek).
38. Matalas, A-L. and Grivetti, L.E., Dietary assessment of 19th-century Greek sailors. Analysis of the log of the Konstantinos, *Food and Foodways*, 5, 353, 1994.
39. Loukopoulos, D., *Home Appliances and Foods of the Etolea*, Athens, 1925, (reprint by Dodoni, 1984), chap. 3 (in Greek).
40. Laskari, N., *Kerkyra During the Period 1204–1864*, Sideris, Athens, 1998 (in Greek).
41. Matalas, A-L., and Yannakoulia, M., Greek street food vending: an old habit turned new, *World Rev. Nutr. Diet.*, 86,1, 2000.

42. Foxhall, L., and Forbes, H.A., Sitometria: the role of grain as a staple food in classical antiquity, *Chiron,* 12, 41, 1982.
43. Lawrence Angel, J. Paleoecology, paleodemography and health, *Population, Ecology and Social Evolution,* Polgar, S., Mouton Publishers, the Hague-Paris, 1975, 167.
44. Kostis, K., *In the Era of Plague,* University of Crete eds., Heraklion, Greece, 1995, chap. 16 (in Greek).
45. de Thevenot, J., *Relation d' un Voyage Fait au Levant,* Paris, 1665, 203.
46. Ashtor, E., Essai sur l'alimentation des diverse classes sociales dans l' Orient medieval, *Annalles E.S.C.,* 23, 1017, 1968.
47. Koukoules, F. *Byzantine Everyday Life and Culture,* Athens, 1952 (in Greek).
48. Eleftheriadis, D. *Controversial Issues on Nutrition,* Athens, 1939 (in Greek).
49. Katsigra, A., *Greek Food Products and the Greek Way of Nutrition,* N.D. Frantzeskakis, Athens, 1940 (in Greek).
50. Partsch, J., *The Island of Corfu,* Nohamouli editions, Corfu-Greece, 1892 (Greek translation).
51. Zographos, D., *The History of the Greek Agriculture,* Agricultural Bank editions, Athens, 1976 (in Greek).
52. Luth, C., *Athens in 1847–1848,* Ermis, Athens, 1991 (Greek translation from Danish).
53. Landos, A., *Geoponikon* [1st ed. Venice,1643], Tenos, Volos, Greece,1991, 190 (in Greek).
54. Gasparis, C., Olive tree and olive oil: production and commerce in medieval Crete, *Olive Tree and Oil,* The Cultural and Technological Foundation of ETBA, Athens, 1996 (in Greek).
55. Argenti, P., Manuscripts of Chian Folklore, Vol. II, Chios Archives, ca. 1890.
56. Gasparis, C., *Land and Farmers in Medieval Crete,* EIE eds., Athens,1997, 87 (in Greek).
57. Code of the monastery St. Georgios Ragousis for the years 1711–1866, Historical Archives of Chios, manuscript no. 215.
58. Flandrin, J. L., Le goût et la necessité: sur l'usage des graisses, *Annalles E.S.C.,* 33, 369, 1983.
59. Rionde, A., *On the Olive Tree* , Printing Off. of A. Koromila, Athens, 1882, 273 (in Greek).
60. Mathas-Demathas, Z. and Sapounaki-Drakaki, L., Olive oil in 19th-century Greece: consumption and prices, *Olive Tree and Oil,* Cultural and Technological Foundation of ETBA editions, Athens, 1996 (in Greek).
61. Mikeli, N. *The Greek Industry In the Year 1938,* B. Xinos eds., Athens, 1939, 15 (in Greek).
62. Dauphin, C. and Pezerat, P., Les consommations populaires dans la second moitié du 19ème siècle a travers les monographies de l'école de le Play, *Annalles E.S.C.,* 30, 537, 1975.
63. Oddy, D.J., Food in nineteenth century England: nutrition in the first urban society, *Proc Nutr. Soc.* 29, 150, 1970.
64. Razzell, P., An interpretation of the modern rise of population in Europe—A critique, *Pop. Studies,* 28, 5, 1974.
65. Knapp, V. J., Major dietary changes in nineteenth-century Europe, *Perspect. Biol. Med.,* 31, 188, 1988.
66. Montanari, M., *Famine and Affluence. The History of Nutrition in Europe* , Ellinika Grammata, Athens, 1997, 187 (Greek translation from Italian).
67. Toutain, J-C., La consommation alimentaire en France de 1789 a 1964, *Economies et Sociétés,* 5, 1909, 1971.

68. Aymard, M., Pour l' histoire de l'alimentation: quelques remarques de methode, *Annalles E.S.C.*, 30, 431, 1975.
69. Kafatos, A., Kouroumalis I., Vlachonicolis I., Theodorou, Labadarios D. Coronary-heart-disease risk-factors status of the Cretan urban population in the 1980s, *Am. J. Clin. Nutr.*, 54, 591, 1991.
70. Matalas, A-L., Franti C.E., and Grivetti, L.E., Comparative study of diet and disease prevalence in Greek Chians: Part I, rural and urban residents of Chios, *Ecol. Fd and Nutr.*, 38, 351, 1999.
71. Knapp, V. J., The coming of vegetables, fruit and key nutrients to the European diet, *Nutr. Health*, 10, 313, 1996.
72. Knapp, V. J., Life expectancy, infant mortality and malnutrition in preindustrial Europe: a contemporary explanation, *Nutr. Health*, 12, 89, 1998.
73. Keys, A., Djordjevic B. S., Dontas, A.S., Fidanza, F., Keys, M., Kromhout, D., Nredeljkovic, S., Punsar, S., Seccareccia, F., and Toshima, H., The diet and 15-year death rate in the Seven Countries Study, *Am. J. Epidem.*, 124, 903, 1986.
74. McCance, and Widdowson, *The Composition of Foods* (5th ed.), Ministry of Agriculture, Fisheries and Food, The Royal Society of Chemistry, Cambridge, 1991.

3 The Mediterranean Diet: Definition, Epidemiological Aspects, and Current Patterns

Antonia Trichopoulou and Pagona Lagiou

CONTENTS

I. THE MEDITERRANEAN DIET

The dietary patterns that prevail in the Mediterranean have many common characteristics, most of which stem from the fact that olive oil occupies a central position
in all of them. Thus, although different regions in the Mediterranean basin have their

own diets, it is legitimate to consider these as variants of a single entity, the Mediterranean Diet. The Mediterranean Diet can be defined as the dietary pattern found in the olive-growing areas of the Mediterranean region in the late 1950s and early 1960s, when the consequences of World War II were overcome, but the fast-food culture had not yet invaded the area. It can be thought of as having eight components:

(a) High monounsaturated–to–saturated lipid ratio
(b) Moderate ethanol consumption
(c) High consumption of legumes
(d) High consumption of cereals (including bread)
(e) High consumption of fruits
(f) High consumption of vegetables
(g) Low consumption of meat and meat products
(h) Moderate consumption of milk and dairy products[1]

Olive oil is important both because of its several beneficial properties and because it allows the consumption of large quantities of vegetables in the form of salads and equally large quantities of vegetables and legumes in the form of cooked foods. Other essential components of the Mediterranean Diet are wheat, olives, and grapes and their various derivative products. Total lipid intake may be high, around, or in excess of, 40% of total energy intake, as in Greece, or moderate, around 30% of total energy intake, as in Italy. In all instances, however, the ratio of monounsaturated to saturated lipids is much higher than in other parts of the world, including northern Europe and North America.

The Italian variant of the Mediterranean Diet is characterized by higher consumption of pasta, whereas in Spain, fish consumption is particularly high. In the traditional Greek diet, foods include large quantities of whole grain bread, and cooked foods and salads (in which legumes and vegetables are consumed in large amounts) rich in olive oil. Intake of milk is moderate, but consumption of cheese and, to a lesser extent, yogurt is high; feta cheese is regularly added to most salads and accompanies vegetable stews. Meat used to be expensive and rarely consumed, whereas fish consumption was a function of proximity to the sea. The high dietary content of vegetables, fresh fruits, and cereals and the liberal use of olive oil guarantee a high intake of ß-carotene, vitamin C, tocopherols, various important minerals, and several possibly beneficial non-nutrient substances like polyphenols. Wine has been consumed in moderation and almost always during meals.[2-6]

In the context of the International Conference on the Diets of the Mediterranean, which was organized in Boston in January, 1993, international experts on nutrition and health reviewed the evidence on the composition and health implications of the Mediterranean Diets consumed in the first half of the 20th century. The Mediterranean Diet of the early 1960s was generally described as providing an abundance of plant foods (fruits, vegetables, bread, cereal products, legumes, nuts, and seeds), favoring the consumption of locally grown, seasonally fresh, and minimally processed foods, and being consumed by physically active people. It was pointed out that the Mediterranean Diet is not a vegetarian diet. It includes modest amounts of foods from animal sources and this assures the necessary intake of vitamin B_{12} and

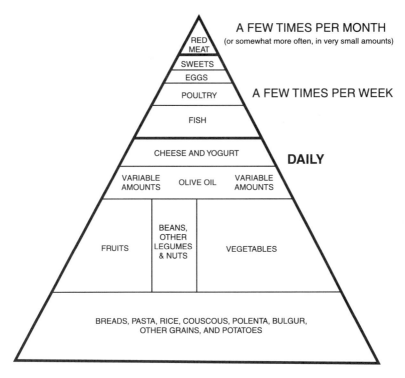

A FEW TIMES PER MONTH
(or somewhat more often, in very small amounts)

A FEW TIMES PER WEEK

DAILY

RED MEAT
SWEETS
EGGS
POULTRY
FISH
CHEESE AND YOGURT
VARIABLE AMOUNTS
OLIVE OIL
VARIABLE AMOUNTS
FRUITS
BEANS, OTHER LEGUMES & NUTS
VEGETABLES
BREADS, PASTA, RICE, COUSCOUS, POLENTA, BULGUR, OTHER GRAINS, AND POTATOES

FIGURE 1 The Traditional Healthy Mediterranean Diet Pyramid, developed in the International Conference on the Diets of the Mediterranean, held in Boston in January, 1993.

iron, while keeping saturated lipid low. Furthermore, it was stressed that people in the Mediterranean basin in the early '60s were physically active. In this conference, a Mediterranean Diet pyramid was developed jointly by the World Health Organization, the Harvard School of Public Health, and the Oldways Preservation and Exchange Trust, with substantial input from Greek scientists (Figure 1). Similar to the pyramid of the Department of Agriculture of the United States,[7] the Mediterranean Diet pyramid was designed as a dietary guide for the general adult population. It was meant to provide an overall sense of the relative proportions and frequency of consumption of the respective food groups and give a broad impression of healthy food choices.[8]

II. DIET AND HEALTH OF THE MEDITERRANEANS

A. THE EARLY EVIDENCE

Mortality statistics provided the earliest evidence that something unusual was favorably affecting the health of the Mediterranean populations. Even though health care for many of these populations has been inferior to that available to people in northern Europe and North America, and the prevalence of smoking has been unusually high among the Mediterraneans,[9] the death rates from various diseases in the Mediterra-

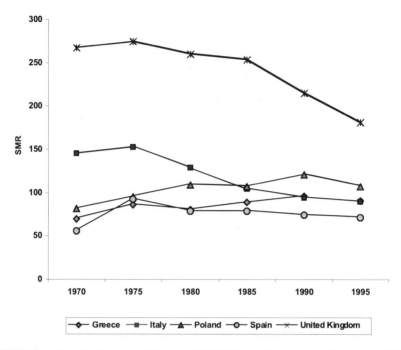

FIGURE 2   Standardized mortality rates (SMR) from ischemic heart disease per 100,000 people from 1970 to 1995 in five European countries. (Based on data from reference 9)

nean region have been, and still are, generally lower than those prevailing in the economically more developed countries of northern Europe and North America, particularly among men.[10] Figures 2, 3, and 4 present standardized mortality rates from ischemic heart disease, all cancers, and all causes from 1970 to 1995 in three Mediterranean, one western, and one eastern European country for both genders. The advantage of the Mediterranean countries is obvious.[11] Cause-specific mortality statistics indicate that the health advantage of the Mediterranean populations is mainly accounted for by lower mortality rates from coronary heart disease (CHD), as well as from cancers of the large bowel, breast, endometrium, ovary, and prostate. Ecological interpretations are, of course, beset by difficulties, but it is clear that widespread factors should be held responsible, and such candidate factors, after discounting population genetic influences as unlikely, could be linked to diet, physical activity, or climate. The relationship of the Mediterranean Diet to CHD, cancer, and diabetes mellitus are discussed extensively elsewhere in this volume.

B. THE ANCEL KEYS STUDY

The classic international study launched by Keys[12] in the 1950s involved 12,763 men aged 40 to 59 years. The men were enrolled in 16 sub-cohorts: two in Greece, three in Italy, five in the former Yugoslavia, two in Japan, two in Finland, one in The Netherlands, and one in the U.S. For logistical reasons, the dietary data in the Seven Countries Study were analyzed only as sub-cohort averages and not for each

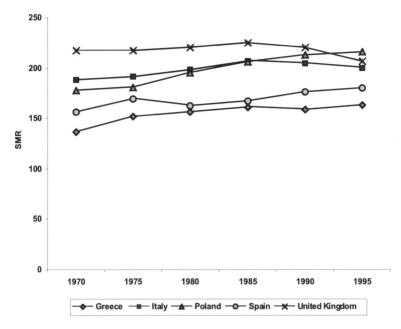

FIGURE 3   Standardized mortality rates (SMR) from all cancers per 100,000 people from 1970 to 1995 in five European countries. (Based on data from reference 9)

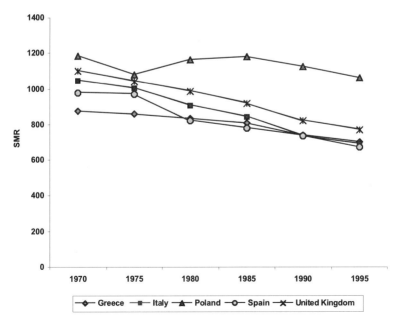

FIGURE 4   Standardized mortality rates (SMR) from all causes per 100,000 people from 1970 to 1995 in five European countries. (Based on data from reference 9)

individual subject in the study. Although this is not an optimal analysis, there can be no doubt that many of the differences in disease occurrence between Mediterranean groups on the one hand and northern European and North American groups on the other were due to differences in dietary patterns. For age-adjusted data, only major differences in other important disease-causing factors or conditions could explain the observed large differences in disease incidence. Such factors are genes, widespread epidemics, tobacco smoking, and low socio-economic class. None of these factors, however, is likely to have played a major role. Migrant studies eliminated a gene-based explanation, no major infectious epidemic had selectively affected northern Europe and North America, and poverty and tobacco smoking were, if anything, more common in the Mediterranean countries.

Over a period of 30 years, Keys and various collaborators[12-17] reported follow-up findings that were mostly focused on the role of diet in the occurrence of CHD. The results of the Keys study were interpreted as indicating that saturated lipids could largely account for the variation of total cholesterol and, inferentially, the incidence of coronary heart disease — lipoprotein fractions were not, during that period, considered as critical intermediate variables with different impact on CHD risk. Although it was clear that Mediterranean populations had lower incidence, not only of CHD, but also of other important causes of morbidity and mortality, the lasting conclusion was that Mediterraneans were privileged by having low rates of coronary heart disease simply because they consumed diets with low saturated lipid content. The argument of several scientists from Mediterranean countries that the diet of their region is more than a low saturated lipid diet and has implications for diseases other than CHD, was not appreciated by the wider scientific community.[1]

C. Recent Epidemiological Studies and Mechanistic Considerations

In the last two decades, scientific research in the fields of clinical medicine, epidemiology, and biochemistry has provided converging evidence on the health benefits of the Mediterranean Diet and has set a solid biologic foundation for the understanding of the mechanisms underlying these benefits.

1. Evidence on the Health Properties of the Main Constituents of the Mediterranean Diet

a. Vegetables and fruits

Consumption of vegetables and fruits has been systematically found to reduce the risk of most forms of cancer, although the responsible compounds or processes have not yet been established.[18] High consumption of vegetables and fruits is typical among Mediterraneans and helps explain the relatively low incidence of several forms of cancer in the region. Some of the earliest studies demonstrating this inverse association have been reported from Mediterranean countries, particularly from Greece, where the consumption of vegetables has been and remains exceptionally high. Thus, in 1983, it was reported that high consumption of vegetables and, independently, low consumption of red meat substantially reduce the risk for cancer of the large bowel.[19] Two years later, the results of another study[20] indicated that individuals consuming high quantities of raw vegetables and citrus fruits, as well as whole-grain bread, were less likely to be affected by cancer of the stomach. Another study from Greece[21] was the first to point out that consumption of vegetables was inversely associated with breast cancer risk, an association that was later confirmed by several researchers. The connection was also noticed in a larger investigation in Greece.[22] A protective effect of vegetables and fruits against cancer of various sites has been documented in a number of epidemiological studies in the Greek population. An effect of fruits was more evident with respect to lung cancer,[23] whereas crude fiber, mostly from vegetables, was the discriminatory protective agent in studies of ovarian[24] and pancreatic cancers.[25] Fruits and vegetables were also the only food groups inversely associated with cancer of the endometrium[26] and adenocarcinoma of the esophagus,[27] although these associations were not always significant.[26] It should be pointed out that, in most of the previously mentioned studies, the associations with particular micronutrients, including ß-carotene and vitamin C, were generally not as strong as those with vegetables and fruits as a whole. The protective effect of vegetables and fruits against malignancies of various sites has also been documented in a series of case-control studies conducted in Italy. The results of these studies are summarized in a review by La Vecchia and Tavani,[28] who point out that the association is generally most marked for epithelial cancers, apparently stronger for those of the digestive and respiratory tracts, and somewhat weaker for hormone-related cancers. Studies conducted in other parts of the world have also supported a protective role of fruits and vegetables against different forms of cancer. In fact, such associations represent the main thrust of nutritional epidemiology of cancer.[18]

With respect to cardiovascular diseases, studies in Greece have also provided evidence that high intake of total carbohydrates and crude fiber, reflecting a high intake of vegetables and fruits, is beneficial against atherosclerosis, as manifested in peripheral arterial occlusive disease[29] and CHD.[30] These findings have been supported by the results of other large and sophisticated investigations[31, 32] and are compatible with a generalized beneficial effect of a diet rich in antioxidant substances.[33] They could, however, also be explained in terms of the homocysteine hypothesis. Recently, accumulated evidence on the deleterious role of plasma homocysteine levels on CHD risk[34,35] provides solid biologic foundation for the inverse association between consumption of vegetables on the one hand, and CHD and peripheral arterial disease on the other, as homocysteine levels are reduced by folic acid, which is found mainly in vegetables.

b. Olive oil

By definition, olive oil is a central component of the diet in the Mediterranean basin. The Greek version of the Mediterranean Diet and, to a lesser extent, the other versions of this diet, are dominated by the consumption of olive oil. Olive oil is the only vegetable oil obtained from whole fruit rather than from seeds. As compared with other vegetable oils, olive oil has a peculiar fatty acid composition (percentage (mol/mol) of methyl esters): oleic acid (56.0–83.0), palmitic acid (7.5–20.0), linoleic acid (3.5–20.0), stearic acid (0.5–3.5), palmitoleic acid (0.3–3.5), linolenic acid

(0.0–1.5), myristic acid (0.0–0.05), and other fatty acids in minute amounts. Olive oil also contains, in total concentration of about 2% of the oil, several other minor compounds, among which tocopherols, carotenoids, and phenolic compounds have powerful antioxidant properties.[36] Extra virgin olive oil is particularly rich in phenols.[37] The exact mechanism of action of flavonoids and other polyphenols has not been established, but they are believed to act as free radical scavengers that may play a role in forfeiting some early steps in the carcinogenic process.[38]

There is converging evidence that olive oil conveys some form of protection against breast cancer,[22,39-41] as well as data suggesting that olive oil may reduce the risk of endometrial[26] and ovarian cancers.[24] A recent report indicates that monounsaturated lipids, mostly from olive oil, is associated with a statistically significant decrease in the risk of sporadic colorectal cancer with wild-type ki-ras genotype.[42]

With respect to cardiovascular diseases, it has been established that monounsaturated lipids, the main type of lipid in olive oil, affect HDL cholesterol more favorably than do polyunsaturated lipids,[43] and substantially more favorably than do carbohydrates,[44,45] making olive oil an optimal energy-generating nutrient.[45,46] Furthermore, vitamin E, which exists in olive oil, has been reported to reduce the risk of CHD.[47] The antioxidant activity of olive oil has been clearly demonstrated *in vitro* and it is likely that the responsible compounds also block oxidation of low density lipoprotein (LDL) cholesterol, the preeminent risk factor for atherosclerosis.[48]

Finally, with respect to other chronic conditions, a study from Greece suggests that consumption of olive oil-derived monounsaturated lipids may increase bone mineral density and reduce the risk of osteoporosis.[49]

c. Fish

Though fish consumption varied widely both between and within Mediterranean countries, fish was by far preferred over meat in the traditional Mediterranean Diet.[50] Fish consumption is associated with reduced coronary heart[51,52] and cerebrovascular[53] mortality, though a recent review of cohort studies suggests that the effect is more evident among high-risk groups only.[54] A possible mechanism is the beneficial role of n-3 fatty acids on blood clotting and triglyceride levels.[55]

d. Cereals and legumes

Cereals form the basis of the Mediterranean Diet pyramid and legumes are listed among the important compounds of diet in the Mediterranean region. Overall, there is substantial epidemiologic evidence that whole grains are associated with decreased risk of coronary artery disease and some cancers.[56-58] The role of legumes in these diseases appears promising, but is as yet inconclusive, although it appears that frequent consumption of legumes and derivatives is associated with reduced levels of LDL cholesterol in the blood.[59] Complex carbohydrates derived from whole wheat bread, other cereal products, and legumes, which are plentiful in the Mediterranean Diet, are only weakly conducive to postprandial hyperglycemia, which could be important in the pathogenesis of metabolic and other diseases.

e. Alcohol

Moderate wine drinking in the context of meals has been a long-standing tradition in the Mediterranean basin.[2] It has been established that moderate drinking of alcoholic beverages reduces the risk of coronary heart disease,[60] probably by increasing levels of serum high density lipoprotein (HDL) cholesterol, which is probably as important for the prevention of CHD as low levels of serum low density lipoprotein (LDL) and total cholesterol.[61] It is also possible, although not yet established, that some of the beneficial effect of moderate wine consumption may be due to antioxidant substances, particularly catexin, which is found in higher concentrations in red, rather than white, wine.[62,63]

2. Evidence on the Role of the Mediterranean Diet as a Whole in Longevity

In a study undertaken in Greece,[6] an overall nutritional score describing the traditional Mediterranean Diet and particularly the Greek version of it, and based on the eight characteristics of this diet, was *a priori* defined. The investigators reported that adherence to the traditional diet, as reflected by the nutritional score, favorably affected life expectancy among elderly people. Furthermore, when the individual components of this score were examined, they had weak and generally nonsignificant associations with survival, in contrast to the overall score, which had a substantial and significant effect. The favorable effect of the Mediterranean Diet on the survival of the elderly, assessed again through a score based on the eight characteristics of this diet, was also shown in a study conducted in Spain.[64]

Results of studies of the Mediterranean Diet in Mediterranean populations, however, may be confounded by the likely association of adult diet with early life nutritional patterns and culture-specific psychosocial variables such as social support. A study performed in Denmark, however, provided similar results,[65] and so did a study examining the diets of Greek-Australians and Anglo-Celt Australians.[66]

III. CURRENT PATTERNS

The evolution of dietary patterns in the Mediterranean and the adherence to the traditional diet is an issue of utmost importance, as it means serious implications in the disease patterns of the populations.[18,67] Data from the Food and Agricultural Organization (FAO) food balance sheets, the DAFNE databank,[68] and surveys at the individual level, including the large European Prospective Investigation into Cancer and nutrition (EPIC),[69-74] provide information on the evolution of dietary patterns.

We have examined trends for Greece, Italy, and Spain, three Mediterranean European countries. What is striking is an increase in the availability of red meat,[3] which has approximately doubled, according to FAO data, followed by a smaller increase in the availability of dairy products.[10] Olive oil remains the main type of added lipid,[68] though availability of seed oils has increased in the last 30 years.[10] A slight reduction is observed with respect to cereal products and legumes,[2] while availability of fruits and vegetables has, if anything, increased.[10] Figures 5–12 are

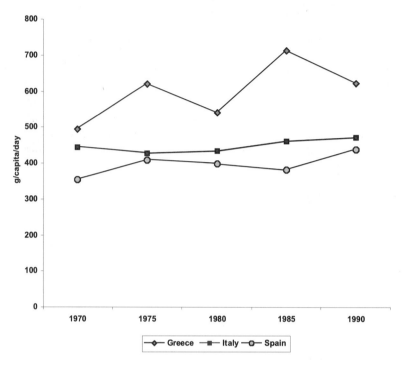

FIGURE 5   Trends in vegetable availability in three Mediterranean countries from 1970 to 1990. (Based on data from reference 10)

based on data from the FAO food balance sheets and present trends in the availability of selected food groups and their products in Greece, Italy, and Spain.[10]

Differences in current nutrition patterns are observed even within countries. Figures 13 and 14 are based on data from the DAFNE databank and present examples of differences in adherence to the traditional Mediterranean Diet by degree of urbanization and education level in Greece and Spain. Based on DAFNE data, we have detected a tendency of the Greeks and Spaniards residing in rural areas to better adhere to their traditional diet than those living in the urban areas.[68]

IV. CURRENT DIETARY GUIDELINES BASED ON THE TRADITIONAL MEDITERRANEAN DIET — THE EXAMPLE OF DIETARY GUIDELINES FOR ADULTS IN GREECE

The first attempt to develop dietary guidelines based on the principles of the traditional Mediterranean Diet was that of the Harvard-led group, with substantial input from Greek scientists.[8] Another example of contemporary dietary guidelines based on the same principles can be found in the Dietary Guidelines for Adults in Greece recently developed by the Supreme Scientific Health Council of the Hellenic Ministry of Health and Welfare.[75] A list of reasons is given in the official document justifying the need for the development of dietary guidelines for a population with

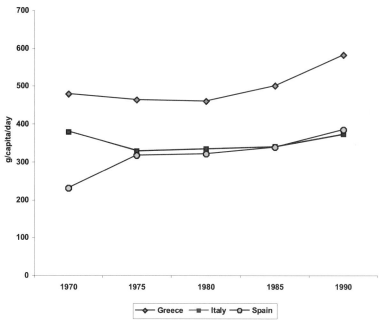

FIGURE 6 Trends in fruit availability in three Mediterranean countries from 1970 to 1990. (Based on data from reference 10)

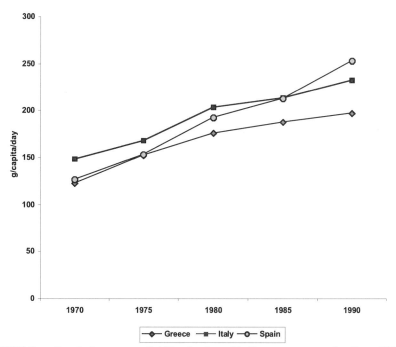

FIGURE 7 Trends in meat availability in three Mediterranean countries from 1970 to 1990. (Based on data from reference 10)

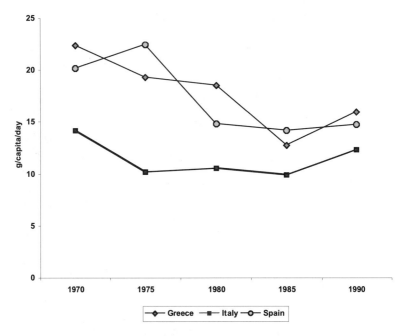

FIGURE 8   Trends in legume availability in three Mediterranean countries from 1970 to 1990. (Based on data from reference 10)

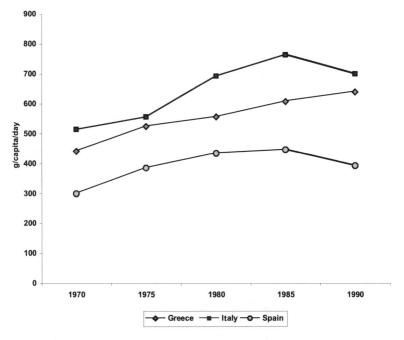

FIGURE 9   Trends in milk availability in three Mediterranean countries from 1970 to 1990. (Based on data from reference 10)

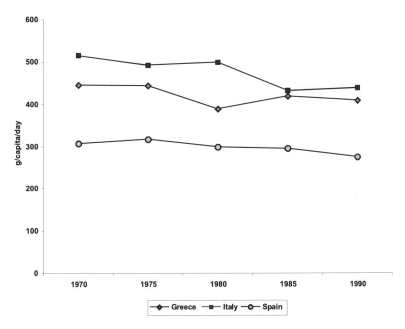

FIGURE 10   Trends in cereal availability in three Mediterranean countries from 1970 to 1990. (Based on data from reference 10)

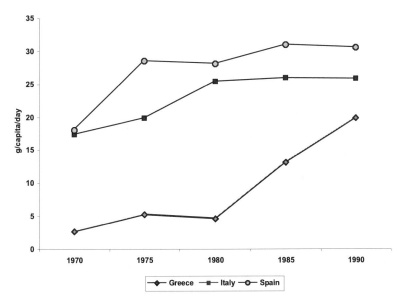

FIGURE 11   Trends in polyunsaturated oil availability in three Mediterranean countries from 1970 to 1990. (Based on data from reference 10)

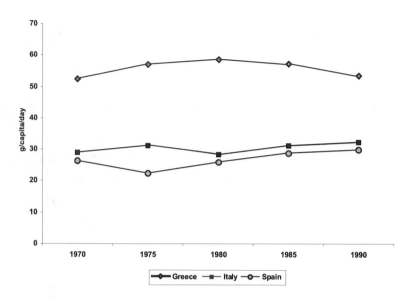

FIGURE 12   Trends in olive oil availability in three Mediterranean countries from 1970 to 1990. (Based on data from reference 10)

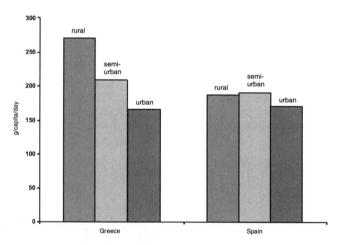

FIGURE 13   Bread availability by degree of urbanization in Greece and Spain, circa 1990. (Based on data from reference 68)

traditionally good health indices, the most important of which is the increasing mortality from diseases such as cardiovascular and cancer over the last three decades, which has followed the westernization of the dietary patterns of a large segment of the Greek population and could be considered as evidence that the model diet for the Greek population closely approximates the traditional Greek diet in the late 1950s and early 1960s.

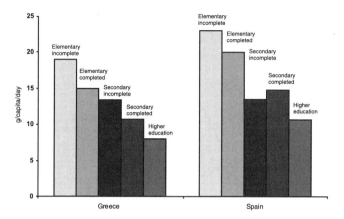

FIGURE 14   Legumes availability by education level of the household head in Greece and Spain, circa 1990. (Based on data from reference 68)

The dietary advice included in the guidelines for Greek adults strongly reflects the principles of the traditional Mediterranean Diet, with emphasis on foods of plant origin, but without excluding foods of animal origin, which should nevertheless be consumed more rarely. Some slight adjustments in the Mediterranean Diet pyramid as developed by Willett et al.[8] have been introduced, however, based on the most recent scientific evidence. In this context, the use of whole grain cereal products is stressed because of their high content of dietary fiber and micronutrients, and their lower glycemic index.[76,77] Potatoes have been removed from the base of the pyramid and the suggestion is that they should be consumed on a weekly rather than a daily basis, as they contribute to the glycemic load of a diet.[78] Special reference is made to wild greens (horta), which are abundant in Greece, so that people do not forget that they are an important part of the vegetable group and they realize that they are an excellent source of antioxidants.[79,80] As in the initial pyramid, people are advised to use olive oil for the preparation of raw and cooked dishes and they are reminded of the benefits of moderate wine drinking during meals and the necessity of being physically active. A note is made of the importance of water in the diet and Greeks are advised to replace salt with the herbs widely available in the flora of their country.

When the Greek version of the Mediterranean Diet pyramid was first developed by the Hellenic National Center for Nutrition and printed by the Hellenic Ministry of Health in 1996, the feedback from the public indicated that they wished for a better sense of relative quantities in the guidelines. To accommodate this, the concept of "serving" was introduced in the recent dietary guidelines for adults in Greece and an indicative list of portion sizes equal to one serving was given. According to this list, one serving is equal to: one slice of bread (25g); 100 g potatoes; half a cup (i.e. 50–60 g) of cooked rice or pasta; a cup of raw leafy vegetables or half a cup of other vegetables, cooked or chopped (i.e. ~ 100 g of most vegetables); one apple (80 g), one banana (60 g), one orange (100 g), 200 g of melon or watermelon, 30 g of grapes;

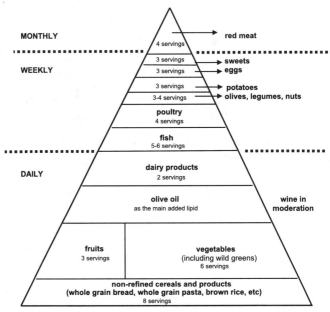

MEDITERRANEAN DIET

FIGURE 15   The Mediterranean Diet Pyramid as it appears in the official Dietary Guidelines for Adults in Greece. (Source: Supreme Scientific Health Council, Hellenic Ministry of Health)

one cup of milk or yogurt; 30 g of cheese; 1 egg; ~ 60 g of cooked lean meat or fish; one cup (i.e. 100 g) of cooked dry beans. Figure 15 presents the Mediterranean Diet pyramid as it appears in the dietary guidelines for Greek adults.

V. CONCLUSIONS

The Mediterranean Diet and life-style of the early 1960s were shaped by climatic conditions, poverty, and hardship, rather than by intellectual insight or wisdom. Nevertheless, results from methodologically superior nutritional investigations have provided strong support to the dramatic ecological evidence represented by the Mediterranean natural experiment. Today, more than ever before, we are well under way to understand and explain what nature has been trying to tell us through the otherwise unexplained good health of the Mediterranean people. The current momentum toward the Mediterranean Diet has solid biological foundation and does not represent a transient fashion. What is even more important is that the Mediterranean Diet, in its several variations, can be considered a realistic model of a prudent diet that fits the current understanding of healthy nutrition and can be adopted by modern populations accustomed to higher intakes of lipids, like the European and North American populations. In any case, even if other populations do not choose to adopt the Mediterranean dietary pattern, the Mediterraneans themselves should be strongly encouraged to adhere to their nutritional traditions.[1,81]

REFERENCES

1. Trichopoulou, A. and Lagiou, P. Healthy traditional Mediterranean Diet: An expression of culture, history and lifestyle. *Nutr. Rev.*, 55, 383, 1997.
2. Helsing, E. and Trichopoulou, A., Eds. The Mediterranean Diet and food culture: a symposium. *Eur. J. Clin. Nutr.*, 43 (suppl 2), 1, 1989.
3. Trichopoulou, A., Katsouyanni, K., and Gnardellis, Ch. The traditional Greek diet. *Eur. J. Clin. Nutr.*, 47 (suppl), 76, 1993.
4. Trichopoulou, A., Toupadaki, N., Tzonou, A., Katsouanni, K., Manousos, O., Kada, E., and Trichopoulos, D. The macronutrient composition of the Greek diet: estimates derived from six case-control studies. *Eur. J. Clin. Nutr.*, 47, 549, 1993.
5. Trichopoulou, A., Lagiou, P., and Trichopoulos, D. Traditional Greek diet and coronary heart disease. *J. Cardiovascular Risk*, 1, 9, 1994.
6. Trichopoulou, A., Kouris-Blazos, A., Vassilakou, T., Gnardellis, Ch., Polychronopoulos, E., Venizelos, M., Lagiou, P., Wahlqvist, M. L., and Trichopoulos, D. The diet and survival of elderly Greeks; a link to the past. *Am. J. Clin. Nut.*, 61, 1346S, 1995.
7. U.S. Department of Agriculture — U.S. Department of Health and Human Services. *Nutrition and Your Health: Dietary Guidelines for Americans* — 4th ed., Washington, DC, 1995.
8. Willett, W. C., Sacks, F., Trichopoulou, A., Drescher, G., Ferro-Luzzi, A., Helsing, E., and Trichopoulos, D. Mediterranean Diet pyramid: a cultural model for healthy eating. *Am. J. Clin. Nutr.*, 61(6 Suppl), 1402S, 1995.
9. World Health Organization. Health for all — Statistical database. WHO, Regional Office for Europe, 1997.
10. World Health Organization. Health for all — Statistical database. WHO, Regional Office for Europe, 1993.
11. World Health Organization. Tobacco or health: a global status report. Geneva, WHO, 1997.
12. Keys, A. *Seven Countries: A Multivariate Analysis of Death and Coronary Heart Disease*, Harvard University Press, Cambridge, 1980.
13. Keys, A., Menotti, A., Aravanis, C., Blackburn, H., Djordevic, B.S., Buzina, R. Dontas, A.S., Fidanza, F., Karvonen, M.J., Kimura, N., et al. The Seven Countries Study: 2289 deaths in 15 years. *Prev. Med.*, 13, 141, 1984.
14. Keys, A., Menotti, A., Karvonen, M. J., Aravanis, C., Blackburn, H., Buzina, R., Djordjevic, B. S., Dontas, A. S., Fidanza, F., Keys, M.H., et al. The diet and 15-year death rate in the Seven Countries Study. *Am. J. Epidemiol.*, 124, 903, 1986.
15. Aravanis, C., Mensink, R. P., Corcondilas, A., Ioanidis, P., Feskens, E. J., and Katan, M. B. Risk factors for coronary heart disease in middle-aged men in Crete in 1982. *Int. J. Epidemiol.*, 17, 779, 1988.
16. Menotti, A., Keys, A., Aravanis, C., Blackburn, H., Dontas, A., Fidanza, F., Karvonen, M. J., Kromhout, D., Nedeljkovic, S., Nissinen, A., et al. Seven Countries Study: First 20-year mortality data in 12 cohorts of six countries. *Ann. Med.*, 21, 175, 1989.
17. Dontas, A.S., Menotti, A., Aravanis, C., Corcondilas, A., Lekos, D., and Seccareccia, F. Long-term prediction of coronary heart disease mortality in two rural Greek populations. *Eur. Heart J.*, 14, 1153, 1993.

18. Willett, W. C. and Trichopoulos, D. Nutrition and cancer: A summary of the evidence. *Cancer Causes Control*, 7, 178, 1996.
19. Manousos, O., Day, N. E., Trichopoulos, D., Gerovassilis, F., and Tzonou, A. Diet and colorectal cancer: a case-control study in Greece. *Int. J. Cancer*, 32, 1, 1983.
20. Trichopoulos, D., Ouranos, G., Day, N. E., Tzonou, A., Manousos, O., Papadimitriou, Ch., and Trichopoulou, A. Diet and cancer of the stomach: a case-control study in Greece. *Int. J. Cancer*, 36, 291, 1985.
21. Katsouyanni, K., Trichopoulos, D., Boyle, P., Xirouchaki, E., Trichopoulou, A., Lisseos, B., Vasilaros, S., and MacMahon, B. Diet and breast cancer: a case-control study in Greece. *Int. J. Cancer*, 38, 815, 1986.
22. Trichopoulou, A., Katsouyanni, K., Stuver, S., Tzala, L., Gnardellis, Ch., Rimm, E., and Trichopoulos, D. Consumption of olive oil and specific food groups in relation to breast cancer risk in Greece. *J. Natl. Cancer Inst.*, 87, 110, 1995.
23. Kalandidi, A., Katsouyanni, K., Voropoulou, N., Bastas, G., Saracci, R., and Trichopoulos, D. Passive smoking and diet in the etiology of lung cancer among nonsmokers. *Cancer Causes Control*, 1, 15, 1990.
24. Tzonou, A., Hsieh, C-C., Polychronopoulou, A., Kaprinis, G., Toupadaki, N., Trichopoulou, A., Karakatsani, A., and Trichopoulos, D. Diet and ovarian cancer: a case-control study in Greece. *Int. J. Cancer*, 55, 411, 1993.
25. Kalapothaki, V., Tzonou, A., Hsieh, C-C., Karakatsani, A., Trichopoulou, A., Toupadaki, N., and Trichopoulos, D. Nutrient intake and cancer of the pancreas: a case-control study in Athens, Greece. *Cancer Causes Control*, 4, 383, 1989.
26. Tzonou, A., Lipworth, L., Kalandidi, A., Trichopoulou, A., Gamatsi, I., Hsieh, C-C., Notara, V., and Trichopoulos, D. Dietary factors and the risk of endometrial cancer: a case-control study in Greece. *Brit. J. Cancer*, 73, 1284, 1996.
27. Tzonou, A., Lipworth, L., Garidou, A., Signorello, L., Lagiou, P., Hsieh, C-C., and Trichopoulos, D. Diet and risk of esophageal cancer by histologic type in a low-risk population. *Int. J. Cancer*, 68, 300, 1996.
28. La Vecchia, C. and Tavani, A. Fruit and vegetables and human cancer. *Eur. J. Cancer Prev.*, 7, 3, 1998.
29. Katsouyanni, K., Skalidis, Y., Petridou, E., Polychronopoulou-Trichopoulou, A., Willett, W., and Trichopoulos, D. Diet and peripheral arterial occlusive disease: the role of poly-, mono- and saturated fatty acids. *Am. J. Epidemiol.*, 133, 24, 1991.
30. Tzonou, A., Kalandidi, A., Trichopoulou, A., Hsieh, C-C., Toupadaki, N., Willett, W., and Trichopoulos, D. Diet and coronary heart disease: a case-control study in Athens, Greece. *Epidemiology*, 4, 511, 1993.
31. Gramenzi, A., Gentile, A., Fasoli, M., Negri, E., Parazzini, F., and La Vecchia, C. Association between certain foods and risk of acute myocardial infarction in women. *Brit. Med. J.*, 300, 771, 1990.
32. Rimm, E.B., Ascherio, A., Giovannucci, E., Spiegelman, D., Stampfer, M.J., and Willett, W.C. Vegetable, fruit, and cereal fiber intake and risk of coronary heart disease among men. *J. Am. Med. Assoc.*, 275, 447, 1996.
33. Pappas, A.M., Ed. *Antioxidant Status, Diet, Nutrition, and Health.* CRC Press LLC, Boca Raton, Florida, 1998.
34. Stampfer, M.J., Malinow, M.R., Willett, W.C., Newcomer, L. M., Upson, B., Ullmann, D., Tishler, P.V., and Hennekens, C.H. A prospective study of plasma homocyst(e)ine and risk of myocardial infarction in U.S. physicians. *J. Am. Med. Assoc.*, 268, 877, 1992.

35. Nygard, O., Nordrehhaug, J.E., Refsum, H., Ueland, P.M., Farstad, M., and Vollset, S.E. Plasma homocysteine levels and mortality in patients with coronary artery disease. *New Engl. J. Med.*, 337, 230, 1997.
36. Trichopoulou, A., Lagiou, P., and Papas, A. Mediterranean Diet: are antioxidants central to its benefits? in Pappas A.M., Ed. *Antioxidant Status, Diet, Nutrition and Health.* pp 107–118. CRC Press, Boca Raton, Florida, 1998.
37. Visioli, F. and Galli, C. Natural antioxidants and prevention of coronary heart disease: the potential role of olive oil and its minor constituents. *Nutr. Metab. Cardiovasc. Dis.*, 5, 306, 1995.
38. Afanasev, I.B., Dorozhko, A.I., Brodskii, A.V., Kostyuk, V.A., and Potapovitch, A.I. Chelating and free radical scavenging mechanisms of inhibitory action of rutin and quercetin in lipid peroxidation. *Biochem. Pharmacol.*, 38, 1763, 1989.
39. Martin-Moreno, J.M., Willett, W.C., Gorgojo, L., Banegas, J.R., Rodriguez-Artalejo, F., Fernandez-Rodriguez, J.C., Maisonneuve, P., and Boyle, P. Dietary fat, olive oil intake and breast cancer risk. *Int. J. Cancer,* 58, 774, 1994.
40. La Vecchia, C., Negri, E., Franceschi, S., Decarli, A., Giacosa, A., and Lipworth, L. Olive oil, other dietary fats, and the risk of breast cancer (Italy). *Cancer Causes Control,* 6, 545, 1995.
41. Lipworth, L., Martinez, M.E., Angeli, J., Hsieh, C-C., and Trichopoulos, D. Olive oil and human cancer: an assessment of the evidence. *Prev. Med.*, 26, 181, 1997.
42. Bautista, D., Obrador, A., Moreno, V., Cabeza, E., Canet, R., Benito, E., Bosch, X., and Costa, J. Ki-ras mutation modifies the protective effect of dietary monounsaturated fat and calcium on sporadic colorectal cancer. *Cancer Epidemiol., Biomarkers, and Prevention,* 6, 57, 1997.
43. Mattson, F.H. and Grundy, S.M. Comparison of effects of dietary saturated, monounsaturated, and polyunsaturated fatty acids on plasma lipids and lipoproteins in man. *J. Lipid Res.*, 26, 194, 1985.
44. Mensink, R.P. and Katan, M.B. Effect of monounsaturated fatty acids versus complex carbohydrates on high-density lipoproteins in healthy men and women. *Lancet*, I, 122, 1987.
45. Sacks, F.M. and Willett, W. Chewing the fat: how much and what kind. *New Engl. J. Med.*, 324, 121, 1991.
46. Willett, W.C. Diet and health: what should we eat? *Science*, 264, 532, 1994.
47. Stampfer, M.J., Hennekens, C.H., Manson, J.E., Colditz, G.A., Rosner, B., and Willett, W.C. Vitamin E consumption and the risk of coronary disease in women. *New Engl. J. Med.*, 328, 1444, 1993.
48. Visioli, F., Bellomo, G., Montedoro, G.F., and Galli, C. Low density lipoprotein oxidation is inhibited *in vitro* by olive oil constituents. *Atherosclerosis*, 117, 25, 1995.
49. Trichopoulou, A., Georgiou, E., Bassiakos, Y., Lipworth, L., Lagiou, P., Proukakis, Ch., and Trichopoulos, D. Energy intake and monounsaturated fat in relation to bone mineral density among women and men in Greece. *Prev. Med.*, 26, 395, 1997.
50. Kromhout, D., Keys, A., Aravanis, C., Buzina, R., Fidanza, F., Giampaoli, S., Jansen, A., Menotti, A., Nedeljkovic, S., and Pekkarinen, M., et al. Food consumption patterns in the 1960s in seven countries. *Am. J. Clin. Nutr.,* 49, 889, 1989.
51. Mizushima, S., Moriguchi, E.H., Ishikawa, P., Hekman, P., Nara, Y., Mimura, G., Moriguchi, Y., and Yamori, Y. Fish intake and cardiovascular risk among middle-aged Japanese in Japan and Brazil. *J. Cardiovasc. Risk*, 4, 191, 1997.

52. Albert, C.M., Hennekens, C.H., O'Donnell, C.J., Ajani, U.A., Carey, V.J., Willett, W.C., Ruskin, J.N., and Manson, J.E. Fish consumption and risk of sudden cardiac death. *J. Am. Med. Assoc.,* 279, 23, 1998.
53. Rodriguez Artalejo, F., Guallar-Castillon, P., Banegas Banegas, J. R., Manzano, B.A., and del Rey Calero, J. Consumption of fruit and wine and the decline in cerebrovascular disease mortality in Spain (1975-1993). *Stroke,* 29, 1556, 1998.
54. Marckmann, P. and Gronbaek, M. Fish consumption and coronary heart disease mortality. A systematic review of prospective cohort studies. *Eur. J. Clin. Nutr.,* 53, 585, 1999.
55. Ulbricht, T.L. and Southgate, D.A. Coronary heart disease: seven dietary factors. *Lancet,* 338, 985, 1991.
56. Kushi, L.H., Meyer, K.A., and Jacobs, D.R. Jr. Cereals, legumes, and chronic disease risk reduction: evidence from epidemiologic studies. *Am. J. Clin. Nutr.,* 70(Suppl 3), 451S, 1999.
57. Liu, S., Stampfer, M.J., Hu, F.B., Giovannucci, E., Rimm, E., Manson, J. E., Hennekens, C.H., and Willett, W.C. Whole-grain consumption and risk of coronary heart disease: results from the Nurses' Health Study. *Am. J. Clin. Nutr.,* 70, 412, 1999.
58. Slavin, J.L., Martini, M.C., Jacobs, D.R. Jr., and Marquart, L. Plausible mechanisms for the protectiveness of whole grains. *Am. J. Clin. Nutr.,* 70 (Suppl. 3), 459S, 1999.
59. Kingman, S.M. The influence of legume seeds on human plasma lipid concentrations. *Nutr. Res. Rev.,* 4, 97, 1991.
60. Rimm, E.B., Giovannucci, E. L., Willett, W. C., Colditz, G. A., Ascherio, A., Rosner, B., and Stampfer, M. J. Prospective study of alcohol consumption and risk of coronary disease in men. *Lancet,* 331, 464, 1991.
61. Gordon, D.J. and Rifkind, B.M. High-density lipoprotein: the clinical implications of recent studies. *New Engl. J. Med.,* 321, 1311, 1989.
62. Fuhrman, B., Lavy, A., and Aviram, M. Consumption of red wine with meals reduces the susceptibility of human plasma and low-density lipoprotein to lipid peroxidation. *Am. J. Clin. Nutr.,* 61, 549-54, 1995.
63. Carbonneau, M.A., Leger, C.L., Monnier, L., Bonnet, C., Michel, F., Fouret, G., Dedieu, F., and Descomps, B. Supplementation with wine phenolic compounds increases the antioxidant capacity of plasma and vitamin E of low-density lipoprotein without changing the lipoprotein Cu^{2+}-oxidizability: Possible explanation by phenolic location. *Eur. J. Clin. Nutr.,* 51, 682, 1997.
64. Lasheras, C., Fernandez, S., and Patterson, A.M. Mediterranean Diet and age with respect to overall survival in institutionalized, nonsmoking elderly people. *Am. J. Clin. Nutr.,* 71, 987, 2000.
65. Osler, M., and Schroll, M. Diet and mortality in a cohort of elderly people in a north European community. *Int. J. Epidemiol.,* 26, 155, 1997.
66. Kouris-Blazos, A., Gnardellis, C., Wahlqvist, M. L., Trichopoulos, D., Lukito, W., and Trichopoulou, A. Are the advantages of the Mediterranean Diet transferable to other populations? A cohort study in Melbourne, Australia. *Brit. J. Nutr.,* 82, 57, 1999.
67. Serra-Majem, L., La Vecchia, C., Ribas-Barba, L., Prieto-Ramos, F., Lucchini, F., Ramon, J.M., and Salleras, L. Changes in diet and mortality from selected cancers in southern Mediterranean countries, 1960–1989. *Eur. J. Clin. Nutr.,* 47 (Suppl 1), S25, 1993.
68. Trichopoulou, A., and Lagiou, P., Eds. *Methodology for the Exploitation of HBS Food Data and Results on Food Availability in 6 European Countries.* European Commission, Luxembourg, EUR 18357, pp 1–162, 1998.

69. Trichopoulos, D., Tzonou, A., Katsouyanni, K., and Trichopoulou, A. Diet and cancer: the role of case-control studies. *Ann. Nutr. Metab.*, 35(Suppl 1), 89, 1991.

70. Riboli, E. Nutrition and cancer: Background and rationale of the European Prospective Investigation into Cancer and Nutrition (EPIC). *Ann. Oncology*, 3, 783, 1992.

71. Trichopoulou, A., Kouris-Blazos, A., Walhqvist, M.L., Gnardellis, Ch., Lagiou, P., Polychronopoulos, E., Vassilakou, T., Lipworth, L., and Trichopoulos, D. Diet and overall survival in elderly people. *Brit. Med. J.*, 311, 1457, 1995.

72. D'Avanzo, B., La Vecchia, C., Braga, C., Franceschi, S., Negri, E., and Parpinel, M. Nutrient intake according to education, smoking, and alcohol in Italian women. *Nutr. Cancer*, 28, 46, 1997.

73. Gnardellis, C., Boulou, C., and Trichopoulou, A. Magnitude, determinants and impact of under-reporting of energy intake in a cohort study in Greece. *Publ. Hlth. Nutr.*, 1, 131, 1998.

74. Agudo, A. and Pera, G. Vegetable and fruit consumption associated with anthropometric, dietary and lifestyle factors in Spain. EPIC Group of Spain. European Prospective Investigation into Cancer. *Publ. Hlth. Nutr.*, 2, 263, 1999.

75. Supreme Scientific Health Council, Hellenic Ministry of Health. Dietary Guidelines for Adults in Greece. *Arch. Hellenic Med.*, 16, 516, 1999.

76. Jacobs, D.R. Jr., Meyer, K.A., Kushi, L.H., and Folsom, A.R. Whole-grain intake may reduce the risk of ischemic heart disease death in postmenopausal women: the Iowa Women's Health Study. *Am. J. Clin. Nutr.*, 68, 248, 1998.

77. Nantel, G. Carbohydrates in human nutrition. *FAO-Food, Nutr Agric*, 24, 6, 1999.

78. Willett, W.C. The dietary pyramid: does the foundation need repair? *Am. J. Clin. Nutr.*, 68, 218, 1998.

79. Trichopoulou, A., Vasilopoulou, E., and Lagiou, A. Mediterranean Diet and coronary heart disease: are antioxidants critical? *Nutr. Rev.*, 57, 253, 1999.

80. Trichopoulou, A, et al. Nutritional composition and flavonoid content of edible wild greens and green pies: a potential rich source of antioxidant nutrients in the Mediterranean Diet. *Fd. Chem.*, 70, 319, 2000.

81. Trichopoulou, A., and Lagiou, P. Options for dietary development based on science and reason, in *Nutrition in Europe: Nutrition Policy and Public Health in the European Union and Models for European Eating Habits on the Threshold of the 21st Century*. Scientific and Technological Options Assessment (STOA) Report to the European Parliament, PE Number 166.481. European Union. Luxembourg, Directorate General for Research, pp. 39–51, 1997.

Part II

Dietary Constituents

4 Fats and Oils

Apostolos K. Kiritsakis, Konstantinos A. Kyritsakis and Maria-Nectaria Mavroudi

CONTENTS

I. INTRODUCTION

Fats and oils, which can originate either from animal or vegetable sources, are essential nutritive elements for the human diet. Fats mainly exist as solids at normal room temperature, while oils remain liquid. Both can be used as salad and cooking oils, as well as raw materials for margarine and shortenings.[1-4]

Fatty acids and other constituents existing in fats, and mainly in oils, such as phenols, tocopherols, chlorophylls, sterols, squalene, aroma, and flavor play a significant role in human nutrition and health.

This chapter refers to the production, usage, composition, quality, and nutritional value of fats and oils, with emphasis given to olive oil, because of its important role as a basic component of the Mediterranean Diet.

II. PRODUCTION OF FATS AND OILS

A. SOURCES

Animal fats are derived almost entirely from three kinds of domestic animals — cattle, sheep, and pigs. The bulk of the world's production of butter fat is obtained from the milk of cows.[2]

The largest source of vegetable oils is the seeds of annual plants such as soybean, cottonseed, peanut, sunflower, corn, and rape. Other sources of vegetable oils are the fruit and nuts of some trees — olive oil, coconut oil, palm oil, and palm kernel oil.[1]

B. HISTORY OF THE PRODUCTION OF FATS AND OILS

Mutton, tallow, lard, butter, and fish oils were known from prehistoric times. When fire was discovered, men used it to melt animal fat. Vegetable oils from olives and sesame seed and possibly flax were also known from ancient days. Olive oil is known as the oldest vegetable oil. Excavations in Tunis show that fat technology was known in Northern Africa many years ago. When the European seafaring nations conquered the world, unfamiliar types of fat and oils were brought back to Europe.[3]

During the industrial revolution, which resulted in a great increase in population of the industrialized countries, there were new requirements for fat production and for new fatty products such as margarine and shortenings.

C. PRODUCTION OF FATS AND OILS IN OUR CENTURY

In recent years, the production of fats and oils has grown at a faster rate than the population (Figure 1). Mielke[4] estimated a 14-fold increase in oil production from 1958 to 2000. Since 1935, there has been a shift from the consumption of animal fat to vegetable oils (Figure 2). This occurred partly because the animal fats, and especially butter, are more expensive.[3] and also because animal fats, being saturated, were not considered, and still are not considered, good for health.

Table 1 shows an increase in the total world production of olive oil in recent years. This is due to the expansion of olive cultivation, favorable climatic conditions, and progress in the technology of olive cultivation and production.

Of the total olive oil production, almost 84% derives from the European Union (EU), especially from Spain, Italy, and Greece. During the years 1985 to 1994 the average production of olive oil in Greece was around 358,000 MT. However, the average production of oilseeds and margarine during the same period was lower (Table 2).

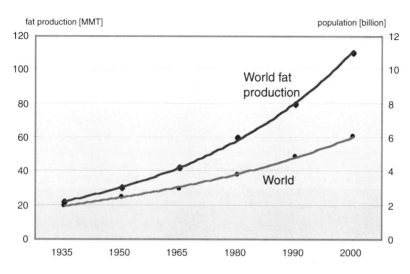

FIGURE 1   World population growth in relation to oil and fat production. (From Bockish, M., *Fats and Oils Handbook*, AOCS Press, Champaign, IL, 1998. With permission.)

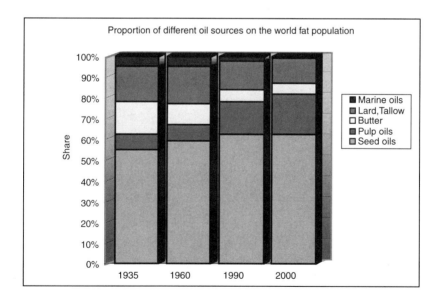

FIGURE 2   Proportion of world oil and fat production from different sources. (From Bockish, M., *Fats and Oils Handbook*, AOCS Press, Champaign, IL, 1998. With permission.)

The U.S. produces less than 3% of the olive oil consumed by Americans.[8] The rest is imported mainly from Italy, Spain, and Greece. During the 1990s, EU exports of olive oil showed an overall increase of 19%.

Most of the American olive crop is used for canning. Recently, there has been increasing interest in California to produce more olive oil. Along with its small olive

TABLE 1
World Production of Olive Oil[5,6]

Years	Production of Olive Oil (Thousand MT)
1980s	1,655 (average)
1990/91	1,453
1991/92	2,205
1992/93	1,705
1993/94	1,943
1994/95	1,800
1995/96	1,637
1996/97	2,635
1997/98	2,500

TABLE 2
Production of Olive Oil, Oilseeds and Margarine in Greece for the Years 1985 to 1994[6,7]

Oil or Fat	Production (Thousand MT)				
	1985-90	1991	1992	1993	1994
Olive	262	430	314	323	464
Soybean		49	51	48	46
Cottonseed		24	33	26	32
Sunflower		25	15	17	20
Corn		3,5	3,5	3,5	3,5
Other seed oils		1,5	1,6	2	2,5
Margarine	30	32	34	34	35

oil production, the U.S. produces an enormous amount of soybean oil. The U.S., Brazil, Argentina, and Asia are the dominant supplying countries for soybean and other seed oils.[4] Almost all European countries import oilseeds because they are not all self-sufficient. Greece mainly imports corn oil, sunflower, and soybean oil.[7] Although the exports of olive oil have increased in recent years, there is now a world olive oil surplus and, as a result, prices have dropped.

III. TRENDS IN AVAILABILITY OF OLIVE OIL AND OTHER FATTY SUBSTANCES

The world availability data for fats and oils differ depending on the source. According to Sharpe,[9] the annual world consumption, per capita, of the 11 major vegetable and marine oils for the year 1989 was 10 kg. In India, the world's largest importing country of vegetable oils, the per capita consumption is estimated around 6 kg. In China,

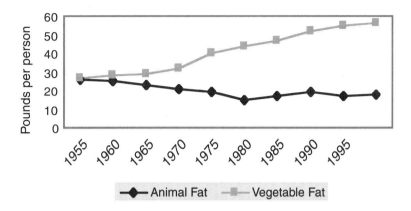

FIGURE 3   U.S. consumption of fats and oils per capita.

however, the consumption is estimated at less than 5 kg. In the higher-income countries of Europe, in Japan, and in the U.S., the consumption of fats and oils is high,[9] especially in The Netherlands, where the consumption is about 47 kg/person. In the U.S., edible vegetable oil consumption per capita has increased during the last four decades from 9.98 to 24.5 kg. During the same period, however, the consumption of animal fats declined (Figure 3).[10]

It is interesting to note that the consumption of olive oil in the U.S. increased from 112,000 MT (251,000,000 pounds) in 1995 to 130,000 MT in 1996, representing 6% of the world olive oil consumption.

The European Union accounts for 69% of the world's olive oil consumption. The European countries with the highest consumption of olive oil are Greece, Italy, and Spain.[5,6] Greeks, at 20 kg per capita per year, have the highest consumption of olive oil in the world.[6] Lately, the consumption of seed oils and margarine in Greece has increased. During the period 1991–1995 the consumption of seed oils increased from 150,000 MT to 165,000 MT (Table 3). During the same period, margarine

TABLE 3
Consumption of Seed Oils in Greece During the Years 1991 to 1995[7]

Oil	Annual Consumption (Thousand MT)				
	1991	1992	1993	1994	1995
Soybean	44	43	29	50	55
Sunflower	43	41	37	39	38
Corn	23	28	18	29	28
Cottonseed	22	33	23	24	25
Rest	18	20	23	18	19
Total	150	165	130	160	165

consumption increased from 37,000 MT to 43,000 MT. This great consumption of seed oils in Greece began in 1986, when Greek restrictions for the protection of domestic olive oil were lifted, followed by advertisement of seed oils

Seed oils represent a high percentage of the total edible fats consumption, but the percentage covered by olive oil remains small in spite of recent increases. However, this situation must be changed by making known its beneficial health effects.

IV. GLYCEROL AND NON-GLYCEROL SYNTHESIS OF FATS AND OILS

A. GLYCEROL SYNTHESIS

Edible fats and oils are mainly composed of mixed triglycerides (triacylglycerols), which are saponifiable. Triglycerides are esters of fatty acids with glycerol. The carbon length, number, and position of the double bonds of the individual fatty acid and the position of the fatty acids in the glycerol molecule determine to a large extent the different properties of fats and oils. Generally, the degree of saturation affects the form — solid or liquid. When there is a high degree of saturation, the fats are solid. A high degree of unsaturated fatty acids results in liquid oils at normal room temperatures. Table 4 gives the fatty acid composition of some common edible fats and oils.

Climate, soil, plant maturity, genetic variation of the plant, and fruit or seed maturity are some of the factors that affect the fatty acid composition of vegetable oils. [8,11-13] For example, olive oil from northern cool Mediterranean countries contains more liquid glycerides (glycerides of unsaturated fatty acids) than southern dry, warm Mediterranean countries' olive oil, which is richer in solid glycerides (mainly glycerides of the saturated fatty acids, palmitic and stearic).[6] Also, the animal fat composition varies according to the animal species, the diet, the location of fat on the carcass, and other factors.[12]

B. NON-GLYCEROL SYNTHESIS

Fats and oils also contain small quantities of several non-glycerol constituents that are unsaponifiable. They include hydrocarbons, sterols, pigments, flavor compounds, phenols, vitamins, non-glycerol esters of fatty acids, triterpenes, alcohols, and acids. These are considered minor constituents, and most are of important nutritive value. Table 5 gives the unsaponifiable composition of some vegetable oils.

Some of the minor constituents such as phenols give olive oil a qualitative superiority over seed oils. They contribute to its flavor quality and increase its oxidative stability and its nutritive value.[8,15] Phenols cover a significant part of the unsaponifiable fraction of olive oil.[6]

1. Hydrocarbons

Hydrocarbons are present in fats and oils in the form of aliphatics, terpenoids, and polycyclics. The latter may originate from the environment.[3] The hydrocarbon

TABLE 4
Fatty Acid Composition of Some Edible Fats and Oils (%)[3,11]

Fatty Acids	Olive Oil	Peanut Oil	Coconut Oil	Corn Oil	Cottonseed Oil	Sunflower Oil	Palm Kernel Oil	Milk Fat
C4:0								3–5
C6:0			<1					<3
C8:0			3–4				<3	<2
C10:0			6–9					3–4
C12:0			45–50				45–50	
C14:0	<1		15–17	<1	<1	<1	15–17	
C14:1								<1
C16:0	7–20	6	7–10	9–17	17–25	6–8	7–10	20–30
C16:1	<3.5			<1	<1.5	<1		<5
C17:0	<1							
C17:1	<1							
C18:0	0.5–5	5	<3.5	<3	<3	3-6.5		16–24
C18:1	55–85	45–65	4–8	20–40	14.5–22	14–38		
C18:2	3.5–21	22	<2	39.5–65	46.5–58	48–74		
C18:3	<1			0.6-1.4	<1	<1		
C20:0	<1.5	5–7		<1	<1	<1	2–4	
C20:1	<1							
C20:2								
C20:3								
C22:0	<1	5–7				<1.5		
C22:1		5–7						
C24:0	<1	<3	<1	<1		<1		

TABLE 5
Unsaponifiable Composition of Some Well Known Vegetable Oils[8,14]

Oils	Hydrocarbons	Squalene	Aliphatc Alcohols	Terpenic Alcohols	Sterols
Olive	2.8–3.5	32–50	0.5	20–26	20–30
Linseed	3.7–14.0	1.0–3.9	2.5–5.9	29–30	34.5–52
Teaseed	3.4	2.6	–	–	22.7
Soybean	3.8	2.5	4.9	23.2	58.4
Rapeseed	8.7	4.3	7.2	9.2	62.6
Corn	1.4	2.2	5.0	6.7	81.3

squalene, which facilitates metabolism and may also work as antioxidant, is a representative terpenoid form.[3] Squalene is present in substantial amounts (20–88mg/100g) in shark liver oil.[3] Olive oil contains the largest amount of squalene among vegetable oils and other edible fats (Table 6).

TABLE 6
Squalene Content of Olive Oil and Other Vegetable Oils[8,16]

Oil	Squalene (mg/100g)
Olive	136–708
Corn	19–36
Cottonseed	4–12
Peanut	13–49
Soybean	7–17
Sunflower	8–19
Teaseed	8–16
Sesame	3
Rapeseed	28
Mustard	7

2. Sterols

Sterols are polycyclic alcohol having sterane as a basic structure. Phytosterols, present in vegetable oils, have recently gained attention as food additives in margarine.[3] The main sterols found in olive oil, are: ß-sitosterol, Δ-5-avenasterol, and campesterol. Stigmasterol, cholesterol, Δ-7-campesterol, and other types of sterols also exist in olive oil but in smaller quantities.[17,18] The total sterol content of olive oil is in the range of 180–265 mg/100g. Figure 4 shows the structure of three sterols present in some oils.

3. Pigments

The color of fats and vegetable oils depends on the presence of the pigments carotenoids, chlorophylls, and pheophytins. These pigments, which are sensitive to oxygen and light, are natural colorants for food. Between carotenoids, α-, ß-, and γ-carotenes are distinguished.[3] Figure 5 shows the structures of some important carotenoids present in oils.

Palm oil and olive oil both contain ß-carotene in high levels.[3] The concentration of ß-carotene in olive oil is 0.33.6 (mg/kg).[8] Chlorophyll mainly exists in those oils that are produced from rape, olive, and avocado.[3] Olive oil contains chlorophyll–a and chlorophyll–b, which impart the green color to the oil. These pigments are easily degraded to pheophytins–a and –b. Fresh olive oil contains chlorophylls–a and –b at a concentration of 1 to 10 ppm, and pheophytins–a and –b at 0.2 to 24 ppm.[8] Both chlorophylls and pheophytins have a pro-oxidant effect on lipids in the presence

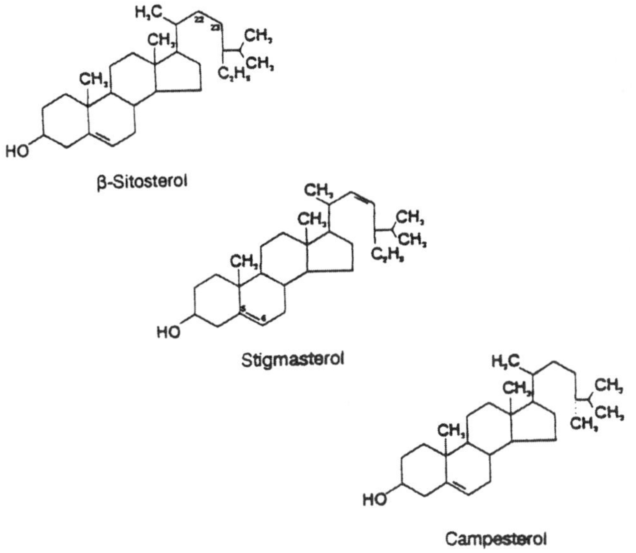

FIGURE 4   Chemical structure of sterols present in olive oil and other oils.

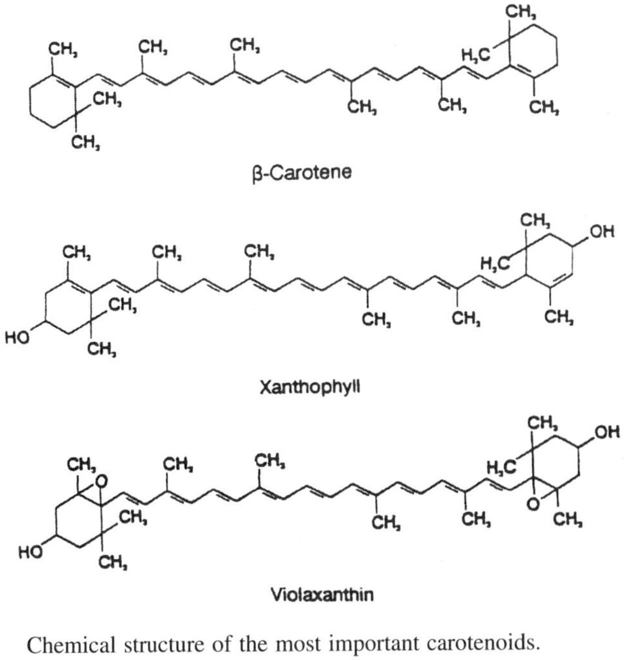

FIGURE 5   Chemical structure of the most important carotenoids.

of light, but they act as antioxidants in darkness.[8,19] Chlorophyll, as well as squalene, can be used in local application against skin diseases.[20]

4. Flavor compounds

Aroma and flavor are distinctive features of olive oil.[11] Hexanal, trans-2-hexanal, 1-hexanol, and 3-methylbutan-1-ol are the major flavor compounds of olive oil.[6,21] Kiritsakis and Min[22] reported that the flavor compounds in olive oil are influenced by many factors such as climatic and soil conditions, cultivation practices, maturity of fruits, and storage and processing conditions.

5. Phenols

Tyrosol, hydroxytyrosol, and several phenolic acids like benzoic and cinamic acids have been identified as the main phenolic compounds in olive oil.[23,24] Tyrosol and hydroxytyrosol are derived from the hydrolysis of oleuropein, while benzoic and cinamic acids are derived from the hydrolysis of flavonoids (anthocyanins, flavones), which are found in considerable amounts in fruits.[25,26] Phenolic compounds increase the oxidative stability of olive oil and improve its flavor considerably.[6,13]

6. Tocopherols

There are different types of tocopherols. These are α–, β–, γ–, δ–, ε–, and ζ-tocopherols. Tocopherols are found in most vegetable oils (Table 7) and in animal fats. Olive oil contains α-tocopherol in higher amounts than other tocopherols. The oxidative stability of fats and oils is related to the presence of tocopherols.[6] Tocopherol-α, known as vitamin E, represents one of the essential radical scavengers in lipid membranes.[6] It was applied in clinical trials to confront illnesses caused by oxidation. Other experiments suggest that vitamin E may have anticarcinogenic effects.

TABLE 7
Tocopherol Content of Certain Vegetable Oils[6,27]

Oil	Tocopherols (mg/g)			
	α	β–γ	δ	Total
Olive	0,24	Traces	Traces	0,24
Cottonseed	0,56	0,38	Traces	0,94
Corn	0,26	0,92	Traces	1,18
Soybean	0,07	0,78	0,24	1,09
Peanut	0,23	0,31	Traces	0,54

7. Vitamins

Vitamin A, which can be derived from carotenoids, is usually found in large quantities in oils extracted from marine liver.[3] Vitamin A is necessary for regular growth. Moreover, it has an important role in the stability of the cell membranes. Vitamin D belongs to the family of sterols. Butter contains 0.0003–0.0015% vitamin D, but vegetable oils, fats, and animal fats do not contain vitamin D in considerable amounts. Therefore, vitamin D is added to many fat products such as margarine.[3]

8. Phosphatides

Seed oils contain phosphatides (phospholipids), one of which is lecithin, which works as an emulsifier in margarines, baked products, ice cream etc.[3] There are three main classes of phosphatide compounds: phosphatidylcholine (PC), phosphatidyle-thanolamine (PE, and phosphatidylinositol (PI).

There are additional constituents present in fats and oils that are not described here.

V. CALORIC ENERGY AND NUTRITIONAL VALUE OF FATS AND OILS

A. Caloric Energy

Fats and oils are sources of energy for humans and both provide the 9.3 cal/gr. When they are not used, they are stored in the lipid tissue until there is an energy need. The caloric energy of fats and oils is produced during the ß-oxidation of the unsaturated fatty acids which takes place in muscles, heart, and liver.[28]

B. Nutritional Value

Fats and oils are also essential nutritive elements for the human diet as they provide essential fatty acids and vital substances. Essential fatty acids, which are unsaturated, are very important for the human body. Unsaturated fatty acids consist of three groups characterized by the position of the first double bond of the fatty acid chain, counted from the methyl group. Representative unsaturated fatty acids are the **polyunsaturated** acids (C18:3, n-3 or ω–3 known as linolenic acid and C18:2, n-6 or ω-6, known as linoleic acid) and the **monounsaturated** acids (C18:1, n-9 or ω-9, known as oleic acid).

The essential fatty acids, which are necessary for growth, contribute substantially to the building of cell walls and form a structurally essential component of phospholipids. They can be found in the brain and nerves and participate in many metabolic processes including those of the mitochondria. Furthermore, fatty acids participate in the structure of cellular membranes. Consequently, they affect membrane penetration and control the metabolism and the hormonal system of cells.[28] An insufficient supply of essential fatty acids leads to disorders.[3] The ω-3 polyunsaturated fatty acids (e.g, linolenic) are vital in our diet, and they compete for the same enzymes with ω-6 polyunsaturated acids (e.g, linoleic), for the formation of eicosanoids.

Cholesterol, a known sterol, can positively or negatively influence heart disease, depending on the type of the lipoprotein[29] by which it is transported in the body. Low density lipoproteins (LDL) are responsible for transporting cholesterol to the peripheral tissues and are directly related to heart disease. High density lipoproteins (HDL), on the other hand, are responsible for transporting cholesterol from the periphery to the liver. The LDL contains the greatest portion of the total cholesterol, as shown in Table 8.

TABLE 8
Composition of LDL and HDL Lipoproteins[30]

Lipoproteins	Composition (%)			
	Triglycerides	Cholesterol	Phospholipids	Proteins
LDL	10	50	15	25
HDL	5	20	25	50

The fatty acids have different effects on the composition, secretion, catabolism, and transport of lipoproteins that carry cholesterol. Thus, the saturated fatty acids, except stearic acid, increase the levels of LDL. On the other hand, polyunsaturated and monounsaturated fatty acids reduce the levels of LDL in blood plasma.[3,15,28] When the supply of saturated fatty acids is reduced from 16% to 9%, the amount of cholesterol in the blood serum drops by 1.9 mg/ml. The fundamental factor is not the amount per se, but the ratio between polyunsaturated (P), monounsaturated (M) and saturated (S) fatty acids.

Oils rich in oleic acid (e.g., olive oil) can be as suitable for the diet as the high-polyunsaturated-content,[3,15] vegetable oils, which have the advantage of reducing cholesterol levels. Animal products, especially animal fats, contain substantial amounts of cholesterol.[31] Vegetable oils are almost cholesterol free, as they contain < 50 ppm.[32] Trans fatty acids, like the saturated ones, increase LDL cholesterol and reduce HDL cholesterol.[33] When olive oil (rich in monounsaturated fatty acids) is heated, a considerably lower amount of trans acid is formed than in other vegetable oils (rich in polyunsaturated fatty acids) (Table 9).[34]

TABLE 9
Effect of Heating on the Formation of Trans Fatty Acids[34]

Oil	% Trans Acids	
	Heating at 200°C	Heating at 200°C
	time = 0 hrs	time = 7 hrs
Olive	0.5	5.5
Sunflower	0.5	12.0
Corn oil	0.6	12.5
Safflower oil	0.6	13.5
Partial hydrogenated vegetable oil	5.5	12.0

Fatty acids present in the body are protected by the body's antioxidants.[15,35] The deficiency of antioxidants and the high quantity of polyunsaturated fatty acids in food could lead to oxidation. Based on the ratio of polyunsaturated fatty acids to vitamin E, olive oil offers to the human organism the needed resistance against oxidation.[6] Furthermore, olive oil is more resistant to oxidation than other oils, due to its high monounsaturation and to the presence of other antioxidants such as phenols and sterols. Even squalene may work as an antioxidant.

C. CONTRIBUTION OF FATS AND OILS IN THE IMPROVEMENT OF FOOD QUALITY AND ABSORPTION BY THE HUMAN BODY

Fats and oils improve the taste and flavor of many dishes, and give a pleasant sense of satisfaction after their consumption. This is particularly true of olive oil, which, as a natural juice obtained by physical or mechanical means, preserves all the taste and flavor characteristics of the olive fruit.

Fats and oils also increase food digestion and absorption by the body.[3,13] In olive oil, the flavor and aroma compounds, as well as the pigments chlorophyll and pheophytin, facilitate food's absorption into the human body. The latter differentiate the gastric fluid composition of the stomach and increase digestive activity. The great assimilation of olive oil by the body facilitates the absorption of vitamins and phenols as well.[8,15]

VI. CONTRIBUTION OF NON-GLYCEROL CONSTITUENTS TO DIET AND HEALTH

A. VITAMIN E, CAROTENOIDS, AND PHENOLS
AS ANTIOXIDENT AGENTS

Oxidation is the result of the reaction of oxygen with unsaturated fatty acids or even, when the temperature is too high, with saturated fatty acids.[36-38] Fatty acids exist in foods and in human lipid tissues. Oxidation, an autocatalytic mechanism, includes three stages.[37] The whole mechanism is related to the formation of free radicals ($R\cdot$, $ROO\cdot$), hydroperoxides (ROOH), and other undesirable compounds.

The accumulation of free radicals ($R\cdot$, $ROO\cdot$) in the body, as a result of oxidation, causes serious problems in human health. In particular, free radicals destroy polyunsaturated fatty acids of the membranes and harm DNA[38] (Figure 6), proteins, and lipids. Thus, the products of oxidation are responsible for many diseases such as cancer, heart disease, cataracts, neuropathies, and enzymatic diseases.[31] Furthermore, free radicals may facilitate the aging process.[15]

Our bodies are protected from free radicals by scavengers such as vitamin E and phenols, which are natural antioxidants.[15] Thus, the natural antioxidants retard the oxidation of fatty foods and act protectively for the human organism as they restrain the oxidation of lipid tissues.[31] They retard oxidation by supplying hydrogen atoms or electrons to the free radicals. In this way, products that do not have the character of free radicals are formed.[8]

$$AH + ROO\cdot \longrightarrow ROOH + A\cdot$$

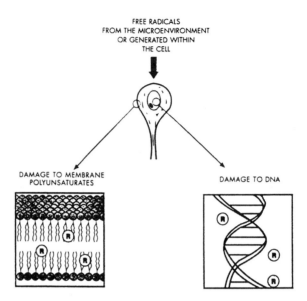

FIGURE 6   Effect of free radicals in the polyunsaturated fatty acids of membranes and in the DNA.[38]

where AH: antioxidant, ROO·: hydroperoxide free radicals, ROOH: hydroperoxides, A·: antioxidant free radical

The antioxidant free radicals react in two ways.

$$A\cdot + A\cdot \longrightarrow AA$$

$$A\cdot + ROO\cdot \longrightarrow ROOA$$

That is, the antioxidant radicals either annihilate each other or react with a peroxide free radical.

Natural antioxidants such as the phenols present in olive oil prevent LDL–cholesterol oxidation, which promotes the atherosclerotic plaque formation.[39-40] Greeks, who have the highest consumption of virgin olive oil in the world and the lowest number of deaths from coronary diseases,[41] take in almost 25 gr of phenols per day, which is a significant amount toward preventing LDL-cholesterol oxidation.[15]

One of the main lipid antioxidants is vitamin E (tocopherol). It reacts with hydroperoxide radicals to produce hydroperoxide and one tocopherol radical that is less active than the hydroperoxide one. Therefore, tocopherols protect the human organism from the negative impacts of lipid oxidation.

Carotenoids are also antioxidants present in fats and oils. There is a variety of carotenoids,[31] with β-carotene the main representative. Carotenoids react with oxygen and with hydroperoxide radicals.[31] Carotenoids, as lipophylic antioxidants, are found in HDL and LDL lipoproteins. They are consumed only during the oxidation of LDL.

Phenols are very important natural antioxidants. They bind free radicals (hydro-peroxide, hydroxide, oxygen) and form phenol radicals, [31] protecting lipid tissues from oxidation. Phenols mainly exist in olive oil, with their concentration depending on several factors such as cultivar, maturity stage of olive fruit, storage period of fruit before processing, and conditions applied during processing. [6,8]

VII. QUALITY CATEGORIES OF OLIVE OIL

The quality of olive oil is decided by a group of characteristics. The acidity, the degree of oxidation, as well as the taste, color, and aroma are the basic criteria for grading olive oil. [6] The International Olive Oil Council (IOOC)[42] proposed the following categories for olive oil and olive pomace oil:

1. **Virgin olive oil**: oil obtained from the fruit of the olive tree by mechanical or other physical means under thermal conditions that do not lead to alterations. This oil has not undergone treatment other than washing, decantation, centrifugation, and filtration. Virgin olive includes the following:
   a. *Extra virgin olive oil*: virgin olive oil with perfect flavor and aroma (sensory score > 6.5) having a maximum acidity, in terms of oleic acid of 1g/100g.
   b. *Virgin olive oil — Fine*: virgin olive oil with perfect flavor and aroma (sensory score > 5.5) having a maximum acidity, in terms of oleic acid, of 2.0g/100g.
   c. *Semi-fine (ordinary) — virgin olive oil*: virgin oil with good flavor and aroma (sensory score >3.5) having a maximum acidity, in terms of oleic acid, of 3.3g/100g with a margin of tolerance of 10%.
   d. *Virgin olive oil Lampante*: virgin olive oil not appropriate for consumption. This oil should undergo refining or it should be used for technical purposes. It has an off flavor or off smell (sensory score <3.5) with a maximum acidity, in terms of oleic acid, of more than 3.3g/100g.
2. **Refined olive oil**: oil obtained from virgin olive oil by a refining process that does not lead to alterations in the initial glycerol structure. This oil has a maximum acidity, in terms of oleic acid, of 0.3 g/100 g.
3. **Olive oil**: a blend of virgin oil (except Lampante) and refined olive oil, having a maximum acidity, in terms of oleic acid, of 1.5/100 g.
4. **Crude olive pomace oil**: Oil obtained by treating olive pomace with solvents.
5. **Refined olive pomace oil**: Oil obtained from crude olive pomace oil by a refining process, having a maximum acidity, in terms of oleic acid, of 0.3 g/100 g.
6. **Olive pomace oil**: A mixture of refined olive pomace oil and virgin olive oil (except Lampante). This blend should not be called olive oil.

Nowadays, oil with the indication **biological** or **organic**[43] appears in the marketplace. This oil is considered superior to virgin olive oil. The superiority of biological olive oil is attributed not only to the absence of agrochemical residues, but also to the conditions applied in the olive oil mill to get the oil from the olive fruit (e.g., low temperatures).

VIII. EFFECT OF QUALITY ON NUTRITION AND HEALTH

The quality characteristics of fats and oils contribute to nutrition and health. Thus, olive oil of good aroma and taste (containing volatile compounds such as aldeydes, ketones, esters, saturated and unsaturated alcohols, and others responsible for the good aroma) is easily digested and assimilated by the human body. This results in the absorption of the important constituents (phenols, vitamin E, etc.), present in the oil and generally in food, increasing its nutritional and health benefits.

As Table 10 shows, virgin olive oil has a higher concentration of non-glycerol constituents than refined olive oil. Some of the non-glycerol constituents are of important nutritional value, therefore virgin olive oil has higher nutritional and health benefits than refined oil.

TABLE 10

Some Non-Glycerol Constituents of Virgin Olive Oil and Refined Olive Oil[44]

Non Glycerol Constituents (ppm)	Virgin Olive Oil	Refined Olive Oil
Squalene	1500	150
β-Carotene	300	120
Aldehydes and ketones	40	10
Tocopherols	150	100
Phenols and related substances	350	80
Fatty alcohols	200	100
Sterol alcohols	2500	1500

Good quality biological or organic olive oil also has a positive effect on human health. Flavor and aroma compounds and phenols make a great contribution to nutrition and health.

IX. CONCLUSIONS

Fats and oils are an important caloric and nutritional source that contribute to a high extent to human nutrition and health. People from northern Europe, America, and Asia prefer polyunsaturated vegetable oils (seed oils). In the cattle-raising areas, butter and lard are more frequently consumed. Widespread consumption of olive oil, which is a main constituent of the Mediterranean Diet, has traditionally been limited to the countries of its production. In the rest of the world, olive oil is consumed in small quantities. However, there has recently been an increase in olive oil consumption internationally, due to greater availability and recognition of its high nutritive and health benefits.

The composition of the unsaponifiable fraction of fats and oils is very important. Some of the unsaponifiable constituents (non-glycerol), such as vitamin E, carotenoides, phenols, etc., are natural antioxidants, protecting lipid tissues from oxidation and therefore from free radicals. The latter may cause damage to DNA, facilitate the aging process, and even lead to cancer.

Polyunsaturated vegetable oils (seed oils) and monounsaturated oils (olive oil) contribute to the reduction of blood cholesterol levels. Olive oil, due to the presence of natural antioxidants, protects LDL cholesterol from oxidation and therefore may prevent atherosclerosis.

REFERENCES

1. Lanstraat, A., Characteristics and composition of vegetable-oil-bearing materials, *J. Am. Oil Chem. Soc.*, 53, 241, 1976.
2. Sonntag, N.O.V., Utilization and classification of oils and fats, in *Bailey's Industrial Oil and Fat Products*, Swern, D., Ed., New York, Wiley-Interscience Publication, 1979, pp. 352–362.
3. Bockisch, M., *Fats and Oils Handbook*, AOCS Press, Champaign, IL., 1998, pp. 1–52.
4. Mielke, T., Current world supply, demand and price outlook for oils and fats, in *Edible Fats and Oils Processing-Basic Principles and Modern Practices*, Erickson. D., Ed., AOCS Press, Champaign, IL., 1990, pp.1-9.
5. Anonymous, U.S. Department of Agriculture, Foreign Agriculture Service Oilseeds and Products, 1986, 1990, 1998.
6. Kiritsakis, A., *Olive Oil Second Edition — From the Tree to the Table*, Food and Nutrition Press, Inc., Trumbull, CT, 1998, pp.1–18,113–154, 237–259.
7. ICAP, *Oilseeds — Margarines*, Financial & Management Consultants Economic & Market Research, Business & Credit Information Publications, Athens, 1996.
8. Kiritsakis, A., *Olive Oil*, AOCS Press, Champaign, IL.,1990, pp. 5, 6, 104–127.
9. Sharpe, D., The yin and yang of economics and politics affecting the world fats and oils situation, in *Edible Fats and Oils Processing-Basic Principles and Modern Practices*, Erickson D.R., Ed. American Oil Chemists Society, Champaign IL., 1990, pp. 10–14.
10. O'Brien, R., *Fats and Oils Formulating and Processing for Applications*, Technomic Publishing Co. Inc., 1998, pp.1–46.
11. Kiritsakis, A. and William, C., Analysis of edible oils, in *Handbook of Olive Oil: Analysis and Properties*, Harwood, J. and Aparicio, R., Eds.,Aspen Publishers, Inc., Gaithersburg, MD, 2000, pp. 129-151.
12. Sonntag, N.O.V., Structure and Composition of Fats and Oils, in *Bailey's Industrial Oil and Fat Products*, Swern, D., Ed., New York, Wiley-Interscience Publication, 1979, pp. 3-4.
13. Fedeli, E., Lipids of olives. *Prog . Chem. Fats and Other Lipids*, 15, 57, 1977.

14. Jacini,G., Fedeli, E., and Lanzani, A., Research on the nonglyceride substances of vegetable oils, *J. Assoc. Offic. Anal . Chem.*, 50, 84, 1967.
15. Kiritsakis, A., The effect of olive oil constituents on the nutrition and human health, 8th Congreso Latinoamericana and AOCS, Santiago, Chile, Oct 24–27, 1999 (Abstract).
16. Mehlenbacher, V.C., *The Analysis of Fats and Oils,* The Gerrard Press Publ., Champaign, IL., 1960, pp. 242–244.
17. Boskou, D. and Morton, D., Changes in the sterol composition of olive oil on heating, *J. Sci. Food Agric.*, 26, 1149, 1975.
18. Itoh, T., Yoshita, K., Yatsu, T., Tamura, T., and Matsumoto, T., Triterpene alcohols and sterols of Spanish olive oil, *J. Am. Oil Chem. Soc.*, 58, 545, 1981.
19. Interesse, F.S., Ruggiero, P., and Vitagliano, M., Autoxidation of olive oil. Effects of chlorophyll pigments, *Ind. Agrarie*, 9, 318, 1971.
20. Anon., Programme for olive oil's consumption, EC 1992/93, *Katanalotika Vimata,* N 1,1993.
21. Montedoro, G., Bertuccioli, M., and Anichini, F., Aroma analysis of virgin olive oil by head space volatiles and extraction techniques, in *Flavor of Foods and Beverages, Chemistry and Technology,* Charalampous, G. and Inglett, G., Eds., Academic Press, New York, 1978.
22. Kiritsakis, A. and Min, D., Flavor chemistry of olive oil, *in Flavor Chemistry of Lipid foods,* Min, D., and Smouse, T., Eds., Am. Oil Chem. Soc., Champaign, IL., 1989, pp. 196-221.
23. Vazquez, R., A study of the polar compounds in olive oil by gas chromatography, *Grasas y Aceites,* 30, 309, 1980.
24. Sonitas, M. and Cichelli, A., Determination of phenolic substances in olive oil, *Riv. Soc. Ital. Scien. dell Alimen,* 10, 359, 1981.
25. Vazquez, R., Del Valle, A.J., and Del Valle, J.L.M., Phenolic compounds in olive fruits. Polyphenols in olive oils. *Grasas y Aceites,* 27, 185, 1970 .
26. Montedoro, G. and Cantarelli, C., Phenolic compounds in olive oils, *Riv. Ital. delle Sost.Grasse,* 46, 115, 1961.
27. Gutfinger, J. and Letan, A., Studies of unsaponifiables in several vegetable oils, *Lipids,* 9, 658, 1974.
28. Kinsella, E., Food lipids and fatty acids: Importance in food quality, nutrition and health, *Food Technol.*, 42, 124, 1988.
29. Tracatelis, A., *Biochemistry,* Kyriakidis Brothers Publishing Company, Thessaloniki, Greece, 1991.
30. Harwood, J., Cryer, A., and Gurr, M., Medical and agricultural aspects of lipids, in *The Lipid Handbook,* Chapman and Hall, 1986.
31. Lambert, J.P., Meat, dietary importance, in *Encyclopaedia of Food Science, Food Technology and Nutrition,* Academic Press, London, 1993, p. 2949.
32. Seher, A., Der Cholesterin-gehalt von Pflanzenolen, *Fat Sci.,Technol.*, 87,27, 1987.
33. Willet, W. and Ascherio, A., Trans fatty acids: Are the effects only marginal? *Am. J. Public Health,* 722, 1994.
34. Kiritsakis, A., Aspris, P., and Markakis, P., Trans isomerization of certain vegetable oils during frying, in *Flavors and Off Flavors, Proc. 6th Int. Flavor Conf.,* Rethymnon, Crete, Greece, July 5–7, Charalambous, G., Ed. Elsevier Science Publ. B.V., Amsterdam, 1989, pp. 883–896.
35. Mataix, J., Recent findings in olive oil research, *Eur. J. Clin. Nutr., 47, 82,* 1993.
36. Kiritsakis, A., The role of natural antioxidants to the health, in *Proc. 4th Macedonian Congr. on Nutrition and Dietary,* May 28–29, Thessaloniki, Greece, 1999, pp. 60–69.

37. Dugan, L.R., Development and inhibition of oxidative rancidity of foods, *Food Technol.,* 15, 10, 1961.
38. Viola, P., Olive oil and health. International Olive Oil Council, Madrid, Spain, 1997, pp. 26–27.
39. Kafatos, A., Olive oil consumption in Crete. One of the main characteristics of the Mediterranean–Cretan diet, *Olivae,* 56, 22, 1995.
40. Lenart, E.B., Willett, W., and Kiritsakis, A., Nutritional and health aspects of olive oil, in *Olive Oil- Second Edition, From the Tree to the Table*, Food and Nutrition Press, Inc., Trumbull, CT, 1998, pp. 299–322.
41. Trichopoulou, A., Katsoyanni K., and Gnardellis, C., The traditional Greek Diet. *Europ. J. Clin. Nutr.* (Suppl 1)*,* 47, 76, 1993.
42. International Olive Oil Council (IOOC), International trade standard applying to olive oil and olive pomace oil. COI /T., 15/NC No. 2 Rev. 6., Madrid,1997.
43. Kabourakis, E., Biocultivation of olive, *Agric. Technol.*, 1, 196, 1995.
44. Fedeli, E., The behaviour of olive oil during cooking and frying, in *Frying of Food,* Varela, G., Render, A.E., and Morton, J.D., Eds.,Ellis Horwood Ltd., Chichester, England, 1988.

5 Fruits, Vegetables, Legumes, and Grains

George D. Nanos and Dimitrios G. Gerasopoulos

CONTENTS

I. INTRODUCTION

The Mediterranean Diet is characterized by high consumption of grain products, legumes, and horticultural products (fruits and vegetables), while dairy products and alcohol (mainly wine) are consumed in moderate amounts, and meat and fish only rarely. The sustainable agriculture practiced for centuries in the semiarid Mediterranean region could not afford the high input for animal and dairy production, although sheep, goats, mules, horses, and donkeys were always part of the family operation for subsistence agriculture. These animals helped maintain soil fertility and facilitate diverse agricultural production, since this region has an appropriate climate for the low-cost production of a large variety of plant species, which, in turn, offers a complete and healthy diet to its inhabitants. In light of large expansion of horticultural product cultivation in recent decades, this chapter will discuss the importance of plant products in the economies of the region, including production, economic significance, and total availability of particular products.

The availability of plant products in the Mediterranean region will be thoroughly discussed mainly in comparison with the U.S. and European Union (EU) consumption. The nutritional importance and effect of post-harvest handling and processing on nutritional quality and the contribution to daily requirements for a healthy life and low disease risk will also be discussed.

II. PRODUCTION OF PLANT PRODUCTS

A. POPULATION

During the last decade, world population showed about a 1.5% yearly increase, a bit lower than the 1.8% increase of the two previous decades (Food and Agriculture Organization [FAO] databases). The yearly population growth of European Mediterranean countries is very low, with levels similar to the EU (<0.4%) but with a decreasing trend in the last decade. On the other hand, the yearly population growth of non-European Mediterranean countries is around 2%, also with a decreasing trend. This growth puts pressure on these countries to increase food production for local consumption, but also for more quantities to be exported for hard currency. Finally, the U.S. population growth has remained stable at 1% for the past three decades.

It should also be mentioned that the population of the major Mediterranean countries (including the ones shown in our tables plus Syria and Tunisia) adds up to 280 million inhabitants (Greece, 10.5 million) and accounts for 4.9% of the world population, a bit higher than the U.S. (around 4.7%). European Union population sums up to 6.6% of world population. It makes up a major high-buying-capacity market and is a producer of a wide array of high-quality plant products.

B. PRODUCTION TRENDS

1. Fruit and Vegetable Production Trends

World production of fruits and vegetables has increased faster than population growth over the past three decades and even faster during the last decade (Table 1). This trend results from factors such as improvements in long-distance transport, longer and larger storage capacity, reductions in post-harvest losses, and increased affluence around the world. On the other hand, fruit and vegetable production has consequences in the environment, viz., irrigation water availability and quality, fertilizer use and losses, and plant protection agents and their residues in the food chain.

TABLE 1
World Total Fruit and Vegetable plus Melon Production (*1000 Tons) and Yearly Change (CY, %) over the Last Three Decades, and for the EU (15 Member Countries), the U.S. and the Major Mediterranean Countries (Means for the Periods Shown). Data Tabulated from FAO Databases.

Fruit	1961-65	1986-88	1994-96	CY 63-87	CY 63-95	CY 87-95
World	136,230	263,802	417,000	2.66	3.17	5.63
Egypt	1,042	3,055	5,696	4.09	4.32	7.54
Greece	1,221	2,322	4,002	2.59	3.33	6.64
Italy	7,040	8,623	18,088	0.84	2.75	8.86
Morocco	754	1,500	2,505	2.76	3.36	6.27
Spain	3,814	7,435	12,750	2.68	3.37	6.58
Turkey	1,571	5,268	9,995	4.50	4.55	7.74
EU (15)	51,387	58,999	54,951	0.57	0.21	−0.89
USA	17,097	24,862	29,770	1.54	1.69	2.25

Vegetables	1961-65	1986-88	1994-96	CY 63-87	CY 63-95	CY 87-95
World	226,744	422,471	577,000	2.51	2.72	3.87
Egypt	4,370	10,453	11,255	3.42	2.75	0.92
Greece	1,407	3,706	4,187	3.75	3.11	1.52
Italy	9,859	14,277	14,672	1.53	1.23	0.34
Morocco	736	1,481	3,288	2.80	3.96	9.47
Spain	6,126	9,660	11,079	1.87	1.80	1.71
Turkey	7,164	16,559	21,195	3.30	3.09	3.07
EU (15)	36,319	49,348	52,950	1.27	1.16	0.88
USA	19,154	27,341	35,233	1.47	1.85	3.15

Fruit production in the Mediterranean countries has increased very quickly, especially during the last decade (Table 1). The climate of the region is suitable for the cultivation of many species and the production of high quality fruit that is probably directed mainly toward exports and, to a lesser extent, increased domestic consumption, due to improved buying capacity. Vegetable production has slowed during the same period in most Mediterranean countries basically due to limited capacity to store and transport vegetables (Table 1). Vegetable production in Morocco increased very quickly, as this country produced more and more low-cost summer vegetables for the EU and transportation of these products by sea and land is very efficient.

The EU fruit and vegetable production changed only slightly during the last decades as a result of abandonment of many cultivated areas in the north and increased production in the south coupled with the low-cost importation of similar products from all over the world.

Production of these major plant groups, especially vegetable production, increased steadily in the U.S. in the last decades (Table 1). This increase is higher than population growth, so it may be concluded that this trend is the result of higher consumption and more opportunities for trading.

2. Cereal and Pulse Production Trends

Cereals are a main source of energy and are being consumed in the largest amounts of any other food group in the world. They also contain many nutrients and are important in supplying our nutritional needs. Roots and tubers are also a good source of energy and nutrients, and are consumed extensively in certain areas around the world, but they are more perishable than cereals and post-harvest losses are high.

World production of cereals slowed down during the past ten years, along with a similar slowdown in population growth (Table 2). However, the EU and its major Mediterranean members showed only minor changes in cereal production in the same period. The EU produced 9% and the U.S., the largest producer in the world, accounted for 17% of world cereal production. Cereal production in the non-the EU Mediterranean countries (except Turkey, which has reached a very high production since the 1980s) increased faster than population growth in an attempt to at least provide sufficient food for the domestic population.

It can be concluded that, all over the world, cereal-production growth was similar to population growth and, in general, despite better storage and transportation technology and possibly diminished waste, consumption of cereals remained just about stable.

Pulses, or legumes such as peas and beans, are staple foods around the world. In addition to the energy they provide, they are an important source of protein, although this protein is not as high quality and digestible as animal protein. This protein is produced with very low inputs via the symbiosis of nitrogen-fixing bacteria to the roots of these plants, making these foods the most convenient and cheapest source of protein to cover human and animal needs. The leguminous plants producing these seeds, with their deep rooting system and high nitrogen content, improve soil productivity and are used very often as a rotation crop for low-input sustainable agriculture.

World pulse production is low compared with that of cereals, and has been relatively stable over the last 35 years (Table 2). Its growth is far behind the population growth, resulting in a lower availability of pulses to humans. Pulses are common mainly in the diets of some Mediterranean countries and in the U.S. There is no clear trend in the production of pulses in the Mediterranean region. The production of pulses only slightly increased in the last decade in the EU (9.2% of world production), but increased substantially in the U.S., which attained 2.8% of world production.

C. SIGNIFICANCE OF PRODUCTION FOR EACH MAJOR PRODUCT

World fruit production adds up to 417 million tons, with a mean of 74 kg per capita. If melons are included (an additional 60 million tons), total fruit production is almost 85 kg.cap^{-1} (Table 3). Many of these fruits are consumed fresh, although some quantities are processed to juice, canned products, wine, and oil. The EU Mediter-

TABLE 2
Total Cereal and Pulses Production (*1000 Tons) and Yearly Change (CY, %) over the Last Three Decades in the World, the EU (15 Member Countries), the U.S., and the Major Mediterranean Countries (Means for the Periods Shown). Data Tabulated from FAO Databases.

Cereals	1961-65	1986-88	1994-96	CY 63-87	CY 63-95	CY 87-95
World	952,116	1,778,154	2,027,892	2.52	2.26	1.64
Egypt	6,076	9,321	16,501	1.76	2.89	6.95
Greece	2,522	5,464	4,810	3.07	1.95	−1.59
Italy	14,046	18,166	20,244	1.37	1.13	1.35
Morocco	3,159	6,707	8,794	3.00	2.95	3.37
Spain	8,675	20,350	19,918	3.35	2.46	−0.27
Turkey	14,831	29,845	29,847	2.80	2.10	0.00
EU (15)	103,745	184,046	188,297	2.33	1.81	0.29
USA	169,236	267,382	347,649	1.87	2.16	3.26

Pulses	1961-65	1986-88	1994-96	CY 63-87	CY 63-95	CY 87-95
World	44,576	53,577	55,848	0.76	0.70	0.52
Egypt	411	416	506	0.05	0.65	2.43
Greece	155	58	43	−3.78	−3.54	−3.78
Italy	720	234	138	−4.25	−4.24	−6.43
Morocco	243	419	265	2.21	0.27	−5.62
Spain	673	314	374	−3.03	−1.78	2.19
Turkey	592	2,135	1,720	4.72	3.05	−2.69
EU (15)	2,392	4,910	5,157	2.87	2.29	0.61
USA	1,090	1,323	1,602	0.80	1.19	2.38

ranean countries produced three to five times more fruit than their world population share. They also produced four to five times more as kg.cap^{-1} than the mean world value. In total, Mediterranean countries produce 13.3% of world fruit production, almost three times their population share. This points out the importance of fruit production for that region. The EU produces similar fruit quantities, double its population share. Finally, the U.S. produces almost half the Mediterranean fruit production although it has a similar population. The largest producer in the Mediterranean region as kg.cap^{-1} is Greece, with five times the world and almost four times the U.S. production.

The Mediterranean region is also a large producer of melons and watermelons, with 20% of world production, four times its population share (Table 3). Turkey and Greece are the major producers, as they produce, in kg.cap^{-1}, eight to nine times more than the world, the EU, and the U.S.

Citrus is the most important fruit group, with 23% of total world fruit production (Table 3). Most of the world production is processed to juice and byproducts, but most of the Mediterranean production is consumed fresh. The Mediterranean region

TABLE 3
Significance of Production (as % of World Production and kg.cap⁻¹) for Total
Fruit and Some Major Fruits or Fruit Groups in the EU (15 Member
Countries), the U.S. and the Major Mediterranean Countries Individually
and in Total (MajMed, Including Syria and Tunisia), (Means for 1994-96).
Data Tabulated from FAO Databases.

	Fruits, noMelons		Melons		Citrus		Apples	
	% World	kg.capita⁻¹	% World	kg.capita⁻¹	% World	kg.capita⁻¹	% World	kg.capita⁻¹
World		73.6		10.7		16.7		9.1
Egypt	1.4	91.5	2.8	27.4	2.4	35.9	0.7	6.2
Greece	1.0	381.5	1.3	75.2	1.3	114.2	0.7	33.4
Italy	4.3	313.7	1.8	18.5	3.1	50.6	4.0	36.1
Morocco	0.6	96.5	1.1	26.5	1.5	55.4	0.6	11.9
Spain	3.1	322.2	2.7	40.8	5.0	119.3	1.6	21.0
Turkey	2.4	163.1	9.3	92.1	1.9	29.2	4.1	34.8
MajMed	13.3	198.4	20.2	43.5	16.1	54.3	12.3	22.8
EU(15)	13.2	147.7	6.3	10.2	9.5	24.1	18.8	26.1
USA	7.1	111.5	4.8	10.9	15.4	54.7	9.5	18.4

	Peach/Nectarine		Grapes		Olives		Population
	% World	kg/capita	% World	kg/capita	% World	kg/capita	% World
World		2.0		10.1		2.4	
Egypt	0.5	1.0	1.5	13.5	1.3	28.8	1.1
Greece	7.5	80.4	2.1	115.2	14.8	191.3	0.2
Italy	14.7	28.8	16.4	161.8	18.4	43.2	1.0
Morocco	0.3	1.4	0.4	8.6	5.1	26.4	0.5
Spain	7.8	22.1	7.6	110.1	26.8	91.6	0.7
Turkey	3.4	6.2	6.3	58.8	11.7	25.8	1.1
Maj/Med	35.2	14.1	35.3	71.7	90.0	49.2	4.9
EU(15)	36.7	11.1	42.5	65.2	59.7	21.7	6.6
USA	11.4	4.8	9.0	19.3	0.8	0.4	4.7

produces 16% of world production (three times its world population share) with
quantities and kg.capita⁻¹ similar to the U.S., another major citrus producer. Spain
and Greece produce the largest per capita quantities.

Although the Mediterranean region is not the most suitable for apple production,
this region produces 12% (mainly from the European countries) of the world apple
production, with quantities produced per capita similar to the EU and the U.S. and
at least double the world value (Table 3). Apple production in the EU is almost 19%
of world production, three times its world population share. Greece produces almost
double the quantity per capita compared with the U.S., where apples are the second-
most-important fruit consumed.

Peaches and nectarines are the most important fruit group produced in the Mediterranean region, with 35% of world production (Table 3). Most of this fruit is consumed fresh. Sixty six percent of the world's exports of canned peaches comes from Greece. These figures indicate the value of this commodity to the economy of the Mediterranean countries, especially Greece, Italy, and Spain with many times higher production per capita than the world or the U.S. These countries also produce almost all the peaches and nectarines of the EU

Grape production is one of the largest in the world, but most of the grapes are used for wine production. The Mediterranean region produces 35% of world production and 72 kg.capita^{-1} (Table 3). The European Mediterranean countries are the most important producers with more than 110 kg.capita^{-1}. Grape production in Turkey is also substantial, mainly in the form of raisins and fresh grapes, because most Muslim nations do not produce or consume wine or alcoholic beverages.

The Mediterranean region produces 30% of world tree nut production, with six times higher production per capita than the world's, three times the EU's, and twice the U.S. values (data not shown).

Olives are produced in the Mediterranean region almost exclusively (90%). The EU produces 60% of world production, mainly in the three European Mediterranean countries presented in Table 3. Greece produces more olives per capita than any other nation in the world, with 4.5 times Italy's and nine times the EU's production.

World vegetable production (roots and tubers not included) is higher than fruit production (517 vs. 477 million tons, respectively), since vegetables, depending on their availability, have always been a human dietary staple (Table 4). The mean quantity of 91 kg.capita^{-1} for the world vegetable production is above the yearly 75 kg.capita^{-1} required consumption for good health, if we accept that vegetable production is evenly distributed and post-harvest losses are around 10%. It is obvious that neither of these assumptions is true and, as a result, many nations cannot cover their minimum requirements for consumption. The Mediterranean region is exceptionally variable in microclimates, where, since antiquity, a large variety of vegetable species have been gathered or cultivated. Imported species from America also became staples during the last centuries. The Mediterranean region produces 11% of world vegetable production, more than twice its population share, and more quantities than the EU or the U.S. (Table 4). Vegetable production is very high in Greece, with the highest production per capita, almost three times the U.S. values and considerably higher than the mean Mediterranean value. The U.S. production of 121 kg.capita^{-1} is sufficient to cover the minimum requirements of the American diet, if minimal losses and even distribution around the country and through the year are assumed. This may not be fully true, resulting in areas or periods of the year without adequate vegetables.

Potatoes are a staple crop, widely produced, and consumed mainly for energy, but also, due to the consumption of large quantities, a general good source of nutrition. Potatoes are produced only in certain areas of the world, while similar quantities of other roots and tubers are grown in other areas. The total root and tuber world production is around 630 million tons, more than the world vegetable production. Unfortunately, this group includes crops very susceptible to post-harvest

TABLE 4
**Significance of Production (as % of World Production and kg.capita⁻¹) for Total
Vegetables, Cereals, and Pulses and some Major Commodities of these
Groups in the EU (15 Member Countries), the U.S. and the Major
Mediterranean Countries Individually and in Total (MajMed, including Syria
and Tunisia) (means for 1994–96). Data tabulated from FAO Databases.**

	Vegetables		Potatoes		Tomatoes	
	% World	kg.capita⁻¹	% World	kg.capita⁻¹	% World	kg.capita⁻¹
World		91.2		51.5		15.5
Egypt	1.8	153.3	0.7	31.9	6.4	90.9
Greece	0.7	324.0	0.3	89.7	2.3	195.3
Italy	2.6	235.9	0.7	36.4	6.6	101.0
Morocco	0.5	100.2	0.4	43.7	1.1	38.2
Spain	1.8	239.2	1.2	91.8	3.8	84.2
Turkey	3.0	253.8	1.7	79.5	7.9	112.9
MajMed	11.0	203.5	5.3	54.9	29.3	91.8
EU (15)	9.5	132.1	16.2	127.0	15.6	37.0
USA	6.3	121.0	7.5	81.7	13.2	43.5

	Cereals		Wheat		Pulses		Beans, Dry	
	% World	kg.capita⁻¹	% World	kg.capita⁻¹	% World	kg.capita⁻¹	% World	kg.capita⁻¹
World		357.9		99.9		9.9		3.1
Egypt	0.8	264.9	1.0	87.1	0.91	8.1	0.11	0.3
Greece	0.2	458.6	0.4	203.7	0.08	4.1	0.14	2.3
Italy	1.0	351.0	1.4	141.6	0.25	2.4	0.14	0.4
Morocco	0.4	338.7	0.9	203.2	0.47	10.2	0.05	0.3
Spain	1.0	503.4	0.9	132.2	0.67	9.5	0.16	0.7
Turkey	1.5	487.1	3.4	310.2	3.08	28.1	1.24	3.5
Maj/Med	5.3	383.0	8.9	180.0	6.02	12.0	1.86	1.2
EU (15)	9.3	506.0	16.1	244.6	9.26	13.9	0.85	0.4
USA	17.1	1,302.0	11.5	242.9	2.87	6.0	7.53	4.9

losses (which in the tropics can reach up to 90%), when handling facilities are
inadequate. Potatoes are produced in large quantities in the EU with 16% of world
production, more than double the U.S. production (Table 4). Potatoes are a staple
crop in the Mediterranean region, produced mainly for domestic consumption with
limited exports.

Tomatoes are the most important vegetable, composing 17% of the total world vegetable production (Table 4). The Mediterranean region accounts for almost 30% of world production. Mean production per capita in Mediterranean countries is almost six times higher than the world's and double the U.S. production. Greece has the largest tomato production per capita, double the mean Mediterranean value. Its production is destined for domestic consumption and exports as fresh, but mainly as processed, tomato products.

Cereal production around the world totals two billion tons, with 358 kg produced per capita (Table 4). Most of the cereal production is destined for animal feed or processing for products such as beer. The Mediterranean countries produce about 5% of world cereal production, which is similar to their population share. The EU produces large quantities of cereals but the U.S. is the major producer in the world, with 17% of world cereal production — 3.5 times more than its population share.

Wheat, as processed products, is the major dietary cereal in Europe and the U.S. (Table 4). With 9% of world production, Mediterranean countries supply substantial quantities of wheat. The EU is the major wheat producer, with 16% of world production and 2.5-fold higher production per capita than the world mean. Large quantities of wheat are also produced in the U.S., with 11.5% of world production, similar to the EU production per capita.

Legumes, or pulses, are produced in only minor quantities (one-tenth of vegetable production) (Table 4). The Mediterranean region and the EU are main producers, with higher than the world's mean production per capita.

Dried peas are produced mainly in northern European countries with the EU producing 30% of world production and Mediterranean countries producing only minor quantities (data not shown). Dried-pea production is also minor in the U.S., but some production of dried beans takes place (Table 4). Dried beans are only rarely produced in the Mediterranean countries although pulses, including other species like lentils and chickpeas, are part of the wintertime Mediterranean Diet.

In conclusion, the Mediterranean countries, especially Greece, Turkey, Italy, and Spain, are major producers of fruits and vegetables and mainly subsistence producers of cereals and pulses. The EU produces substantial fruit and vegetable quantities, mainly through the Mediterranean member countries, and high quantities of cereals and pulses. The U.S. production is directed mainly toward production of cereals, and, to a lesser extent, toward production of fruits and vegetables.

D. Exports and Imports of the Major Plant Products

The major fruit and vegetable exporters of the Mediterranean region are the same countries as the major producers, namely Spain, Italy, Turkey, and Greece. These countries, together with Morocco, export 18.5 million tons, more than twice the U.S. exports of fruits and vegetables (8.3 million tons, similar in amount to Spain's exports). Spain exports 203 kg.capita[-1], Greece 158 kg.capita[-1], Italy 95 kg.capita[-1], and Turkey only 39 kg.capita[-1]. Similarly, the EU exports 100 kg.capita[-1] and the U.S. 32 kg.capita[-1]. There are substantial quantities of wheat and its products exported from the EU (especially northern European members) and the U.S., with 89 kg.capita^{-1} and 114 kg.capita^{-1}, respectively. The Mediterranean countries export less than 41 kg.capita^{-1} wheat.

Although Italy and Spain are major producers and exporters of horticultural products, they also import large quantities of these products. If the commercial balance is calculated, all Mediterranean countries are net exporters. The U.S. is a net importer of horticultural products (with 45 kg/capita), because its own production minus exports is insufficient for domestic needs. On the contrary, all Mediterranean countries import large quantities of wheat and flour, quantities much larger than their exports. Part of the imported wheat is used either to feed the population (Morocco) or to consume and process to pasta (Italy) and export the final product (Italy annually exports 1.1 million tons of pasta). The U.S. is one of the most important wheat exporters, but its imports are also significant (1.8 million tons).

E. AVAILABILITY OVER THE YEAR

Pulses are stable foods that, properly dried and stored, can be available throughout the year, or transported easily. Cereals are also stable and, stored as raw product or after processing (flour, pasta, etc.), can also be available over the year. The quantities stored are massive, calling for similarly huge numbers of storage facilities that are relatively simple compared with the more sophisticated storage facilities needed for horticultural products. Although stable, some 10-20% of cereals are lost in large quantities from mold and insects all around the world.[1] Large quantities are also transported around the world as raw product, flour, or processed products, usually without any need for refrigeration or freezing.

Some fresh fruits and vegetables can be stored for months or produced for most of the year, so they are available almost year around. This availability is more remarkable with products transported long distances (mainly from Southern Hemisphere countries) due to relatively cheap refrigerated marine transport as well as many innovations in packaging, post-harvest treatments, and storage. These imports to Europe caused major changes in Mediterranean production toward improved quality products through intense competition. These imports also increased availability of horticultural products in Europe through the year and resulted in larger variability, which, in turn, might increase total consumption wherever it is economically feasible.

There are many fresh fruits and vegetables that cannot be stored for more than a few weeks. These species are produced, whenever possible, with various cultivars and different growing periods, for as long as it is economically or biologically feasible. Imports from the Southern Hemisphere cover part of the rest of the year. There are also fruits such as cherries and apricots that are available only for short periods of the year, and their consumption period as fresh cannot be prolonged.

Processed fruits and vegetables are available throughout the year, with only minor technological requirements for storage and transport. As a trend, as income increases in Europe and the U.S., consumption of processed foods decreases, but it will always be a way to access valuable horticultural products like dried apricots and figs or canned cherries and peaches year around. Some of these methods of preservation were used for thousands of years in the Mediterranean nations to lengthen availability of their products for the enrichment of their diets during periods of low availability of fresh products.

The recent availability of household freezers increased consumption of frozen products, mainly vegetables and ready dishes containing vegetables or fruits. These products require proper handling all through the commercial chain at temperatures well below 0°C, which means substantial energy consumption.

III. AVAILABILITY OF PLANT PRODUCTS

Based on values presented elsewhere in this volume, availability for each group of commodities can be calculated. More than 20% of fresh fruits and vegetables are lost through the post-harvest chain. Raw material for processing is mainly lost during preparation and processing, but losses are minimal thereafter. Of course, during recent decades, fresh horticultural products have been consumed in continuously higher rates than processed ones with some exceptions, like tomato products and frozen vegetables and fruit juices. Wheat and its products are more stable than fresh fruits and vegetables, with only 10–20% post-harvest losses that result from improper handling and storage, and during processing.

Based on the above discussed calculations, all the EU Mediterranean countries and Turkey have much higher fruit and vegetable availability (as kg.cap^{-1}) than southern Mediterranean countries (with Morocco being the heaviest producer among these countries) and the U.S. (Table 5). Fruit and vegetable availability in Greece is at least double the U.S. supply and generally extremely high (1,400 g.capita^{-1}day^{-1}). Even when 40% losses are assumed, this supply is very high (around 1,100 g.capita^{-1}day^{-1}). It can be assumed that part of this supply is consumed by the large numbers of tourists who spend their vacations (only during few months over the year) in Greece, and these consumers are not included in the calculations. But even larger numbers of tourists visit all the other countries presented in Table 5. Similarly, all Mediterranean countries appear to have a greater availability of wheat and its products than the U.S.

Additionally, availability of fruits and vegetables for all the EU Mediterranean countries is much higher than wheat and its products (Table 5). This confirms the importance of horticultural products as food to the Mediterranean countries, especially in those whose income is relatively high.

Finally, Greece and the major Mediterranean countries studied have higher supplies of the major food groups that compose the basis of the Mediterranean Food Pyramid (see Chapter 3) than the U.S. All these products are probably available at low prices and easily distributed and accessible in the Mediterranean countries, as production areas are near (within hours) the major consumption centers. On the contrary, the U.S. major cities are, for most horticultural products, far away (within days) from the major production areas (California, Florida, and Arizona) resulting in high prices and low product availability due to increased transportation costs.

The World Health Organization recommends daily consumption of horticultural products (excluding potatoes) to 400 g.capita^{-1}day^{-1}.[2] From Table 5 (potatoes included), we can conclude that the fruit and vegetable supply is barely enough

TABLE 5
Availability (Production plus Imports minus Exports) minus 20% Losses of Total Horticultural Products and Availability minus 10% Losses of Total Wheat and Flour Products for the U.S. and the Major Mediterranean Countries (Means for 1994–96). Data Tabulated from FAO Databases.

	Fruit and Vegetables $g.cap^{-1}day^{-1}$	Wheat and Products $g.cap^{-1}day^{-1}$
Greece	1,457	566
Italy	1,166	560
Morocco	402	686
Spain	1,039	423
Turkey	1,030	796
USA	558	329

(when 170 $g.capita^{-1}day^{-1}$ potatoes are excluded) to reach the recommended level of nutrition in the U.S. This can only be true if post-harvest losses are kept to a minimum, distribution and availability are ideally uniform, and tourist consumption is not included. On the other hand, all other countries listed in Table 5 (excluding Morocco) can easily exceed the recommended 400 $g.capita^{-1}day^{-1}$ consumption of fruits and vegetables.

A. AVAILABILITY TRENDS

FAO estimates will be used for the discussion on availability (available product for consumption after product losses having being subtracted) of each product. Wheat availability showed various trends during the last three decades, depending on which country is considered (data not shown).

Vegetable availability over the last three decades increased almost everywhere. Almost all countries presented in Table 6 cover FAO security levels for good health with >75 $g.capita^{-1}year^{-1}$ vegetables (potatoes excluded). Availability of vegetables in Greece is highest among all shown, with almost 800 $g.capita^{-1}day^{-1}$ (Table 6). This substantial vegetable consumption is a result of the variety of dishes prepared in Greek cuisine with various vegetables, plus the tradition of eating fresh- or steamed-vegetable salad with main-course dishes. U.S. and EU inhabitants eat half the quantities of vegetables consumed by Greeks. Both the U.S. and the EU occupy large areas and consist of many ethnic groups that have access or traditionally consume vegetables in various degrees, possibly resulting in populations with only minor vegetable consumption. It is also important to point out that the values of vegetable availability in Table 6 include potatoes, which is a major consumption product in the U.S. and in the EU. When potatoes are subtracted, availability of vegetables to the U.S. (87.7 $kg.capita^{-1}year^{-1}$ or 240 $g.capita^{-1}day^{-1}$) and the EU

TABLE 6
Total Fruit and Total Vegetable Availability (as kg.cap⁻¹year⁻¹) and Yearly Change (CY, %) over the Last Three Decades in the EU (15 Member Countries), the U.S., and the Major Mediterranean Countries (Means for the Periods Shown). Data Tabulated from FAO Databases.

	Fruits (Including Melons)			Vegetables (Incl. Potatoes)		
	72-74	94-96	CY 73-95	72-74	94-96	CY 73-95
EU (15)	97	120	0.96	100	116	0.67
Egypt	74	99	1.31	101	128	1.07
Greece	157	206	1.23	152	235	1.95
Italy	134	144	0.33	153	170	0.48
Morocco	39	82	3.23	21	73	5.03
Spain	124	132	0.28	137	141	0.13
Turkey	141	154	0.40	101	172	2.36
the USA	99	122	0.95	93	110	0.76

consumers (77.6 kg.capita⁻¹year⁻¹ or 213 g.capita⁻¹day⁻¹) just covers FAO security levels for good health.

Fruit availability increased in all countries presented in Table 6 during recent decades. All countries shown in Table 6 consume high quantities of fruit, ranging from 220 g.capita⁻¹day⁻¹ (Morocco) up to 560 g.capita⁻¹day⁻¹ (Greece). Again, countries attracting many tourists may be shown as overconsumers, since tourists are not included in the calculations, although most of the countries presented are famous vacation destinations.

Finally, the balance between fruit and vegetable availability showed that similar quantities of the two food groups are generally consumed in most of the countries presented in Table 6. Relatively more vegetables than fruit are available to Greeks and most Mediterranean consumers, while the opposite is true for U.S. consumers.

B. Availability of Major Plant Products

Apples are a major fruit in the diet due to their storage potential. European countries, European Mediterranean countries, and Turkey are major apple producers and consumers (Table 7A). Apples constitute 22% of EU inhabitants' total fruit availability. The corresponding value for the U.S. is 17% and for Greece only 11%.

Bananas are widely available in European countries and the U.S. (Table 7A) and constitute 10% of total fruit availability. They are not regularly consumed in Greece (only 2% of total fruit availability) because of two decades of banana import restrictions and high prices and due to large availability of significantly cheaper fruits available to Greek consumers during most of the year.

Oranges and, to a lesser extent, mandarins, consumed fresh or processed to juice, are the major fruit group available in all countries presented in Table 7A except Turkey. Similar quantities of citrus are available to the Greek and U.S. populations (21% and 37% of total available fruit, respectively) and higher than anyone else

TABLE 7
Availability (as kg.cap^{-1}year^{-1}) of Fruits (A), Vegetables (B) and Other Plant Products (C) in the EU (15 Member Countries), the U.S., and the Major Mediterranean Countries (Means for 1994–96). Data Tabulated from FAO Databases.

A. Fruits	Total	Apple	Banana	Orange	Grape	Other
EU (15)	116.0	25.7	10.3	28.0	9.0	39.7
Egypt	98.7	5.0	7.0	28.3	11.3	42.6
Greece	204.0	23.3	3.7	42.0	24.7	101.0
Italy	141.3	22.7	8.0	36.0	12.3	52.3
Morocco	81.3	11.3	3.3	23.3	8.0	35.3
Spain	129.3	21.0	9.0	34.3	6.0	55.0
Turkey	152.7	29.7	0.3	17.3	35.0	66.0
USA	109.7	18.3	11.7	41.0	7.7	26.7

B. Vegetables	Total	Potato	Tomato	Onion	Other
EU (15)	158.9	81.3	30.3	7.5	39.7
Egypt	136.7	21.0	77.0	4.5	34.2
Greece	285.6	76.3	123.0	14.9	71.4
Italy	146.4	42.0	61.7	6.1	36.6
Morocco	94.4	30.0	25.0	15.8	23.6
Spain	216.8	102.7	43.3	16.6	54.2
Turkey	172.3	59.0	71.0		
USA	148.4	60.7	40.7	9.9	37.1

C. Other	Pulses	Wheat	AlcBev	Wine	Olive	Tree Nuts
EU (15)	3.7	94.3	119.7	34.7	0	4.0
Egypt	8.2	146.1	0	0	2.3	0
Greece	5.2	138.3	57.7	16.3	8.0	10.0
Italy	5.2	147.7	81.0	58.0	2.0	6.0
Morocco	6.1	189.2	6.3	0.7	4.3	1.3
Spain	7.9	91.7	109.0	39.7	1.3	6.7
Turkey			11.0	0	5.7	6.0
USA	4.1	87.4	104.3	7.0	0	2.0

shown in Table 7A. It is important to mention that oranges and their products account for one out of every three kilograms of fruit available in the U.S. Although this fruit is highly nutritious, it points out the limited variety of fruit available to most Americans.

Lemons are heavily consumed as part of many dishes — in Italy and Greece more than anywhere else (data not shown). Availability of lemons in these countries is double the U.S. and triple the EU values.

Grapes and raisins are available in Turkey and Greece (23 and 12%, respectively, of total fruit availability) in large quantities, at least double that of the rest of the Mediterranean countries, the U.S., and the EU (Table 7A).

Olives, the best-known Mediterranean fruit, are consumed as snack, appetizer, or part of fresh-vegetable salad. They are mainly available for consumption around the Mediterranean region but only in less than 0.1 kg.capita^{-1}year^{-1} in the U.S. and the EU (Table 7C). Greeks have many more olives available than the Italians or the Spanish, mainly due to the tradition of adding olives to the Greek fresh tomato-cucumber salad, and the use of olives as appetizers.

Tree nuts are high-caloric, very nutritious food. Most of the Mediterranean countries are important consumers of almonds, walnuts and pistachios. Available tree nuts to Greeks are five times more than those available to the U.S. consumers (Table 7C).

The quantities of other fruit species available per inhabitant are also shown in Table 7A. This quantity is high in Greece, with half of the total available fruit being from other than the major fruit species. This is possible because there is large variation in available fruit species during most of the year to Greek consumers. This variation also results in higher total fruit consumption in this country. The quantity of other fruit species available in Greece is almost double that of any other country and four times higher than the U.S., where these fruit species constitute only 24% of total available fruit, the lowest among the countries presented in Table 7A. This result is important because, although produce managers of U.S. supermarkets strive to increase availability of various fruit species on the shelves, U.S. consumers only rarely consume these species.

The potato is the most important vegetable in Europe and North America. It is cooked in various ways and is very nutritious. Spanish citizens have more potatoes available than any other vegetable (Table 7B). Greeks and EU citizens have similarly large quantities of potatoes available for consumption, with the U.S. availability a bit lower. Potatoes constitute 27% of total available vegetables for Greece, 51% for the EU and 40% for the U.S. This pattern again leads to the conclusion that EU and U.S. citizens base their diets on a few vegetables. Potatoes are high in calories (100-g baked potatoes contain 110 kcal) compared with other vegetables.[3] They are often fried, which adds a substantial number of calories (100 g of French fries contain 320 kcal), and possibly contribute heavily to energy intake and obesity in the U.S. In contrast, traditional Greek dishes include baking and boiling potatoes in the presence of olive oil, lemon juice, or tomato sauce and various condiments.

Tomatoes are the second-most-important vegetable in both Europe and North America. They contain very few calories (100 g fresh tomatoes contain 20 kcal), but are more nutritious (vitamins and inorganic elements) than potatoes. They are most often eaten raw in salads, less often as tomato sauce. Tomato sauce in combination with olive oil and condiments gives substantial taste to the various baked and boiled vegetables that are very often consumed in Mediterranean countries and in large quantities in Greece. Greeks have tremendous amounts of tomatoes available (three times the U.S. availability per capita) since this vegetable is used in so many traditional Greek dishes, with the most familiar being the Greek fresh tomato and cucumber salad with onions, olives, olive oil, oregano, and feta goat cheese (Table 7B). Although, during previous decades, fresh tomatoes in Greece were available in affordable prices for only a few months, in recent years, tomatoes are more and more consumed all through the year due to the large off-season greenhouse production. Many of the Mediterranean countries also have large quantities of tomatoes and their products available (Table 7B). Tomatoes constitute 43% of total vegetable availability for Greece, 27% for the U.S., and 19% for the EU. If we divide Greek tomato availability per capita in roughly equal amounts of fresh and tomato sauce, we can calculate the importance of this vegetable to the Greek diet.[3] Greeks consume daily up to 337g fresh tomatoes and tomato products covering 12% of P, 21% of Fe, 71% of vitamin A, 87% of vitamin C and 24% of dietary fiber of the Recommended Daily Allowance (RDA) for a healthy adult (if substantial losses are not considered). U.S. citizens get roughly only one-third of these amounts from tomatoes.

Onions are available in small quantities, but in Spain, Morocco, and Greece are eaten much more often than the other countries listed in Table 7B. Onions are usually consumed boiled or fried, but in Greece, onions are often consumed raw in the aforementioned tomato and cucumber salad.

The rest of the vegetables obtainable are also presented in Table 7B. Greeks have almost double the quantity of any other country. Besides the widely known peppers, squashes, cucumbers, lettuce, cabbages, etc., dark-green leafy vegetables are also included here. These are available throughout the year either cultivated or wild grown. The variability of nutritional components in these many species is also high, but some of these vegetables, such as the dark leafy ones and peppers, contain appreciable amounts of valuable nutrients such as iron, folate, antioxidants, and anti-nutritional compounds. This group of vegetables constitutes 25% of total available vegetables for Greece, the U.S., and the EU, but because vegetable availability in the U.S. and the EU is low, this quantity is also low.

Availability of legumes is similar among Mediterranean countries and a bit higher than in the EU and the U.S. (Table 7C).

Wheat and its products can be consumed in large quantities in many ways around the Mediterranean countries (Table 7C). Availability of wheat products to Spanish consumers is similar to the EU and the U.S., and about 44% lower than in the other Mediterranean countries. Breads, pitas, pizzas, and pastas are the major wheat products in the Mediterranean Diet Pyramid (Chapter 3). On the contrary, most wheat products in the U.S. are consumed in the form of cakes, cookies, pies, doughnuts, etc. with the addition of substantial amounts of sugar and shortenings, which result in high-caloric-value foods and possibly reduced wheat-product consumption.

Alcoholic beverages include spirits (consumed generally in quantities less than 5 kg.capita^{-1}year^{-1}), beer, and wine. The EU and the U.S. inhabitants have large quantities of alcoholic beverages available, while these products are barely available in Muslim countries due to religious prohibition (Table 7C). There are only moderate amounts of alcoholic beverages available to Greeks (as presented in Mediterranean Diet Pyramid), almost half of that available to EU and U.S. consumers. The major alcoholic beverage for the EU, the U.S., and Spain is beer, while in Italy, wine covers 72% of total alcoholic beverage availability. Wine constitutes 29, 36, and 28% of total alcoholic beverage availability for the EU, Spain, and Greece, respectively. Wine consumption in Greece is probably underestimated, as many inhabitants produce their own wine. U.S. consumers have very low amounts of wine available (7% of total alcoholic beverages), although, in the light of many scientific findings, wine consumed in moderate quantities is excellent for good health.[4]

C. Factors Affecting Availability and Consumption

The kinds of products and the quantities available for consumption in each area depend on many factors, including distance from major production areas, size of city, time of the year, family traditions, religion, price, etc. This is particularly true for many plant products, especially fresh fruits and vegetables, which are very perishable and often available only seasonally. These products have to be transported and efficiently distributed to retailers and also bought and consumed in a timely manner at home. Wheat products, pulses, and vegetable oils are much more durable and available during the year. Similarly, processed and frozen products are available year round.

The area of residence and time of year are of extreme importance to the kinds of products consumed by an individual. Large cities are supplied year round with many kinds of produce and are all properly handled and available in the produce departments of supermarkets. In sparsely inhabited areas, there are often fewer products available and those to be found may be of lower quality. On the contrary, if these rural areas are close to production areas, many plant species are available in the highest possible freshness and at the lowest price in local farmers' markets or from backyard gardens. These situations are common in Greece for a large number of vegetables. In many areas of Greece, wherever irrigation water is cheap, consumers themselves produce many of the plant products they consume (these quantities have not been included before in this chapter), especially fresh herbs. In addition, many small farmers produce for local farmers' markets. The result is availability of many plant species harvested just a few hours before use (highest nutritional value) at low prices to consumers. On the contrary, until recently, mountainous areas of Greece were isolated and fresh produce during the winter was scarce, which meant very few products available for consumption, including grain products, pulses, potatoes, apples, greens, dairy products, and canned or dried plant products.

The availability of time to purchase and prepare food is another issue influencing food patterns. When the capable adults of a household are all working, it is not often possible to manage a garden or shop at a farmers' market. Produce departments are the convenient solution. Consumers' available time for meal preparation is often scarce, resulting in increased consumption of simple, easily prepared foods; ready-to-eat foods; or minimally processed, mainly horticultural, products. The modern busy life-style reduces the possibility of consuming a variety of products daily, especially plant products, since this requires a substantial amount of time.

Age and gender are major factors influencing a food-consumption pattern, and a number of studies have been conducted on the subject. School children often eat fewer fruits and vegetables than recommended in Spain and Italy and lower quantities than adults.[5,6,7,8] Elderly people eat different kinds of foods for health reasons and according to the different traditions in Spain and Greece.[9,10] Men need to consume more energy daily than women. Women are more concerned about health and weight, so they tend to eat healthier foods, but still consume fewer fruits and vegetables and lower quantities of calcium and vitamins than men do in the U.S.[11]

Local traditions are the strongest driving force influencing types of food consumed. Around the Mediterranean countries, staples are prepared combining flour and milk, or flour, milk, and eggs resulting in highly nutritious material for easily prepared meals, especially when fresh products are scarce. In Greece, many meals based on vegetables or meat are prepared with the addition of tomato sauce, herbs, and onion. This red sauce is often prepared from fresh tomatoes whenever available. Another white sauce used often in Greece is prepared from fresh egg and lemon juice. Main dishes often contain highly nutritious green vegetables in combination with other vegetables, rice, or meat. Dishes with various vegetables seasonally available are also common, which means that many vegetables are consumed in addition to those eaten as salads. Also, preparation of combination dishes with meat and vegetables is the rule, or, alternatively, meat or fish will be consumed with one or two side vegetable dishes. The availability is endless, resulting in high vegetable consumption with a number of species consumed in each meal, possibly the best combination for a complete diet, if coupled with fresh or dried fruit. All the above dishes are prepared with olive oil and various, often fresh, herbs, which add delicious taste and antioxidants to foods, accompanied with bread consumption, thus increasing even further the variability in diet.[12,13]

Religious reasons can also influence food consumption. Greek Orthodox religion includes, yearly, almost 110 days of fasting (no meat or animal products consumed except some seafoods), plus all Wednesdays and Fridays, when only pulses or vegetables are usually consumed. This fasting may, in part, have resulted in all this variability of Greek cuisine without the use of animal products. Muslim religion does not include fasting, but prohibits pork meat and alcohol consumption.

Finally, the attitude of Greeks and many Mediterranean inhabitants have toward food and its preparation encourages creative and healthful menus. They prepare delicious meals and want a variety of tastes on their table. Lunch or dinner can be a social event, usually a chance for the family to gather. The meal often starts with small quantities of appetizers and strong alcoholics. This relaxes the diners so they can slowly eat the rest of the dishes accompanied with wine, very often homemade.

IV. NUTRIENT COMPOSITION AND VALUE

A. NUTRIENT CONSTITUENTS AND PROCESSING-RELATED CHANGES

1. Carbohydrates and Organic Acids

The carbohydrate content of leafy vegetables ranges from 2 to 9%, while that of starchy roots and tubers ranges from 15 to 25% (potatoes contain about 18.5% carbohydrates). Fruits also vary widely in their carbohydrate content (1.5–26%). Ripe fruits contain no starch; the main sugars are sucrose, fructose, and glucose. Their relative importance varies among commodities. Pulses provide significant amounts of carbohydrates in the form of starch, which typically composes 25–50% of the seed weight.[14] Cereal grains contain 74–78% soluble carbohydrates, 64% of which is starch, located mainly in the endosperm. Additionally, cereal grains contain about 2.5% free sugars (glucose, fructose, maltose, sucrose, and oligosaccharides). Organic acids are only minor constituents of plant food (usually below 1%) and, together with carbohydrates, contribute to energy intake from plant consumption.

It has been reported that storage and processing procedures have little effect on the carbohydrate and organic acid content of fruits and vegetables.[15]

2. Fats

Green vegetables and fruit contain low levels of fat, however, this fat should not be overlooked since it represents a good source of 18:3ω3 (linolenic acid) and 18:2ω6 (linoleic acid) for human diet. The ω-3 eicosapentaenoic acid (20:5ω3) and ω-6 docosahexanenoic acid (22:6ω3) fatty acids in animal tissues may come directly from the diet or by precursors supplied by the diet such as linolenic and linoleic acid from vegetable sources, mainly the chloroplasts of green leafy plants and seeds, respectively.[17] Commodities rich in fat are olives, containing 15–40% (on a fresh-weight basis), and tree nuts, containing 50–60% fat. Most nuts are rich in monounsaturated fatty acid (oleic acid), except walnuts, which are rich in polyunsaturated fatty acids (linoleic and linolenic). Fat content of grains is also low. The lipid content of wheat barley and rice is 1–2% and of whole oats 4–6%.

3. Proteins

Fruit protein content is 1% or less. Starchy vegetables contain 1–4% protein, while leafy and stem vegetables and sweet corn contain 4–8%. Proteins in fruit and leafy vegetables are mainly considered as non-structural constituents. They are major components of the cytoplasm of living cells and are involved as enzymes in catalyzing metabolic processes. Pulses and nuts are important sources of plant protein, providing about 15–30% and 10–25% protein by weight, respectively. Proteins of pulses are predominately globulins, which reside in protein bodies of the cotyledons. Globulins are rich in acidic amino acids and poor in sulfur-containing amino acids.

Protein of pulses is also composed of albumins (functional proteins, rich in sulfur-containing amino acids), glutelin-like and other enzyme proteins.[17] Cereal proteins in grain or in flour are composed of two protein types (totaling 6–14% protein content in flour): water soluble proteins (albumin 6–12%, globulin 5–11%), and insoluble proteins (gluten 78–85% and prolamin). Cereal protein is rich in glutamic acid and proline and poor in lysine and sulfur-containing amino acids (Table 8).[18,19]

TABLE 8
Major Amino Acid Content of Plant Protein Sources (mg/g Protein)

Plant source	Lysine	Sulfur Amino Acids	Threonine	Tryptophan
Legumes	64	25	38	12
Cereals	31	37	32	12
Nuts	45	46	36	17
Fruits	45	27	29	11
Leafy vegetables	31	9	22	9

Calculated from Food and Agriculture Organization (1985) and U.S. Department of Agriculture (Hoke, 1983) data.

Losses of essential amino acids during processing and cooking have been reported when foodstuffs are subjected to high temperatures and prolonged periods of heat.[20] Stored wheat flour loses protein value (loss of available lysine) in the presence of oxygen, thus requiring refrigeration to retain 90% of protein value after 6 months of storage. Heat and water during improper storage also result in protein and fat changes that influence flour behavior during end-product preparation.

4. Dietary Minerals

Fruits and vegetables are moderate sources of minerals, particularly potassium, magnesium, iron, and calcium.[3] As bioavailability of nutrients depends on the chemical form of the nutrient and the presence of interfering substances, the amount of minerals in fruit and vegetables may not give a good indication of their nutritive value.[21] Potassium content of fruits and vegetables ranges between 60–600 mg/100 g fresh weight, while the other minerals are present in considerably lower amounts.

Mineral content of fresh commodities cannot change with storage. Mineral losses can occur due to changes in Fe bioavailability after prolonged storage and redistribution of K and Ca from edible to non-edible parts of a food. Processing methods or cooking procedures do not destroy minerals, but in certain cases, their quantity is reduced due to leaching.[22]

5. Vitamins

One of the nutritional advantages of fruits and vegetables is that they offer high concentrations of vitamins (particularly A, in the form of β-carotene, and C), and low calorie and fat content. Carrots represent an excellent source of vitamin A, containing as high as 24,000–28,000 IU followed by spinach, beet greens, and parsley.[3] Good sources of vitamin C (ascorbic acid) are kiwifruit, citrus, pepper, strawberries, and tomatoes, which contain 0.5–4 mg vitamin C per g fresh weight. Vitamin E (tocopherol), a well-known antioxidant, is present in high concentrations in nuts, olive oil, and some vegetables. Vitamin K is found in leafy vegetables. Fruits and vegetables contain moderate or low amounts of thiamin. However, grains, legumes, and nuts are rich sources of thiamin. Green vegetables are particularly rich in riboflavin followed by cereals, nuts, starchy vegetables, and fruit. Potatoes contain 1.3–3.2 mg of niacin per 100 g, while leguminous seeds contain 3 mg per 100 g. Individual fruits and vegetables contain similar amounts of niacin. Cereals are the major source of plant-derived niacin in the human diet. Folate is also an essential important vitamin that is present in most green vegetables.

Vitamin C and A contents differ among fruit and vegetable varieties.[23,24] It was also found that ascorbic acid and vitamin A increase during maturation, and decrease during handling, depending on the conditions during storage, transportation, and marketing.[25,26,27] Vitamin E content of fruits and vegetables is also reduced during post-harvest handling. Fruit stored at modified or controlled atmosphere storage tend to retain more ascorbic acid and other vitamins at low O_2, but not in elevated CO_2 concentrations.[28] The vitamin C in fruits and vegetables is destroyed during extended storage, due to inappropriate temperatures and relative humidity, or physical damage and chilling injury.[29] Starchy vegetables lose 75–80% of ascorbic acid over 9 months of storage. Leafy vegetables lose ascorbic acid during storage mainly due to wilting stress at high temperatures. Ascorbic acid may also be lost through bruising and mechanical damage.

Processing of many fresh commodities is used for extended storage and availability. Processing of grain is necessary for almost all its uses by humans. The nutritional quality of food is diminished with processing, because of nutrient sensitivity to heat, pH, light, and O_2, or a combination of these factors.[30] Minimally processed fruits and vegetables can be expected to contain lower values of ascorbic acid and vitamin A than those that are intact.[31] Heat (blanching or pasteurization) is a major processing procedure to stabilize foods for extended storage by inactivating enzymes and microorganism spores. Green leafy, root vegetables, and high-starch-content or other vegetables and fruits subjected to heat treatment retain about 75% of their ascorbic acid due to oxidative reduction, and show little decrease in riboflavin, β-carotene, vitamin E, vitamin K, thiamin, or niacin.[30,32] In canned juices or fruits and concentrated foods such as tomato paste or citrus marmalade, vitamin C is a major nutrient despite the losses during processing. These products continue to lose vitamin C during storage, so that refrigerated storage is necessary for more than a few months' storage. Vitamin A is much more stable during storage. In general, water-soluble vitamins (vitamin C and the B complex) are much more susceptible to losses following harvest or post-harvest handling and processing methods than fat-soluble vitamins (A, D, E, and K). Vitamin losses during cooking are also attributed to leaching into the cooking water.

Freezing at temperatures $< -18°C$ of blanched (in steam or water) horticultural products results in usually minor losses during storage, especially in vitamin C, although blanching causes some losses.

All these methods of storage result in nutrient losses that depend on duration and temperature of processing and duration and temperature of storage thereafter. Finally, heat processing of fresh or processed products also takes place at home just before consumption with further nutrient losses.

6. Dietary Fiber

The definition of dietary fiber includes all plant non-starch, non-digestible carbohydrates including cellulose, hemicellulose, pectin, gums, and lignin. The composition of dietary fiber is related to parenchymatous flesh, lignified vascular tissues, and cutinized epidermal tissues included in edible plant parts.[33] The composition of dietary fiber is related to its physical properties and results in various physiological effects on humans, such as water-holding capacity/viscosity, adsorption/ion exchange, and interaction with the intestinal flora.

All green land plants contain dietary fiber. The dietary fiber content of fruits, vegetables, tree nuts, and pulses is given in Table 9. Pectic substances, in combination with cellulose, are responsible for the structural properties of fruits and vegetables, while they contribute to diet 0.5–3.1 g of dietary fiber per 100 g fresh weight. Leguminous seeds and some grain products contain as high as 1.2–13.5 g of dietary fiber per 100 g.[34]

Heat treatment causes insoluble dietary fiber content to increase as a result of the complexing of its components with protein and amino acids.[35]

7. Other Health-Related Constituents

Recently, antioxidants have become important food constituents for the health-conscious and -educated public. The level of antioxidants differs within the cultivars, the stage of harvest maturity, and storage length.[36] The Mediterranean Diet is characterized by high consumption of vegetables high in flavonoid content, one of the most important categories of antioxidants in the human diet.[13] Major plant flavonoids include flavonols (myricetin, quercetin, kaempferol) and flavones (luteolin, apigenin). Analysis of raw vegetables collected from the wild, commonly used in traditional Mediterranean Diet, such as fennel, chives, poppy, and sorrel, reveal that they contain higher quantities of flavonoids than other cultivated vegetables or fruits. In particular, the quercetin content of some wild vegetables is even higher than that of red wine.[37] Grape juice contains 86 mg.L^{-1} quercetin and 82 mg.L^{-1} rutin (the glycoside of quercetin). Additionally, red wine contains resveratrol, salicylic acid, and other flavonoids such as catechin and epicatechin.

TABLE 9
Dietary Fiber (DF) Content of Edible Parts of Fruits, Vegetables, Tree Nuts, and Pulses. (Modified from Englyst et al.[33])

Fruits	DF (%)	Vegetables	DF (%)	Tree Nuts and Pulses	DF (%)
Apple, fresh	1.6	Asparagus, cooked	1.7	Almonds, kernel	7.4
Apricot, fresh	2.3	Beans, frozen, cooked	3.1	Hazelnuts, kernel	6.5
Apricot, dry	12.0	Broccoli, cooked	3.0	Walnuts, kernel	3.5
Banana, yellow	1.1	Cabbage, raw	4.0	Chestnuts	4.3
Blackberries, raw	3.1	Carrot, fresh, raw	2.4	Broadbeans, cooked	5.4
Cherries, sweet, raw	1.2	Cauliflower, cooked	1.6	Red kidney beans, dried, cooked	6.7
Figs, dry	7.5	Celery, raw	3.7	Chick peas, cooked	4.8
Grapes, fresh	0.7	Cucumber, raw	0.5	Lentils, cooked	1.9
Kiwifruit, raw	1.7	Leeks, cooked	2.3		
Nectarines	1.2	Lettuce, raw	1.2		
Olives, canned	2.9	Okra, cooked	4.8		
Orange, fresh	2.1	Onion, raw	2.0		
Peach, fresh	1.5	Peas, frozen, cooked	5.2		
Pear, with skin	2.0	Pepper, green, raw	1.6		
Plums, fresh	1.6	Potato, flesh, cooked	1.1		
Prunes, dry	6.9	Spinach, cooked	1.6		
Strawberries, fresh	1.4	Tomato, fresh, raw	1.1		

Bioavailability of the nutrients within the total pool will depend on a number of factors before and after harvest and, to a large extent, on antinutritional compounds. Antinutritional factors or compounds are those that, when consumed in the diet, reduce the nutrient value of food to less than predicted from its proximate analysis. A classical example is protein digestibility in pulses, which is known to be lower than that of the cereal or the animal-derived protein. Antinutritional compounds are derived from food of mainly vegetable origin such as potatoes (glycoalkaloids, protease inhibitors, lectins), beans (glucopyrimidonones, protease inhibitors, lectins, tannins), and brassicas (glucosinolates, tannins, erucic acid). However, the loss of nutritive value due to antinutritional compounds in vegetable-based diets is minor compared with the benefits of such a diet. Glycoalkaloid content is very low in potato flesh, which is the edible part of the tuber.[38] Lectins are carbohydrate-binding cell-aglutinatory proteins, which can bind to the gut wall and disrupt its function, while protease inhibitors bind and inhibit the action of digestive enzymes. Tannins bind proteins and interfere with digestion, while phytate exhibits inhibitory effects on digestive enzymes. Liener and Kakade[39] reported that most plant protease inhibitors are destroyed by heat (cooking), leading to an enhancement of nutritional value of the protein. Polyphenol-condensed tannins accumulate in seeds, fruit, and leaves of a wide range of commercially important crops and, unlike protease inhibitors, tannins and phytate are heat stable.

B. Contribution to the Diet

To estimate the contribution of fruits, vegetables, pulses, grains, and other plant products in the diet, the availability data from Table 7 and published nutrient composition tables for ready-for-consumption products were used.[3]

A 40% loss from the total available quantities in Table 7 was subtracted to account for other than processing losses, mainly mishandling of products before preparation for consumption and throwaway parts. After that, individual fruit availability values were multiplied by nutrient composition of apples (raw, peeled), oranges (raw, whole, no seeds, no peel), lemons (juice, raw), banana (raw, peeled) and grapes (raw, var. Thompson seedless).[3] The authors also made the arbitrary assumption that the contribution of the "other" fruits (Table 7A) in nutrients could be represented by the average nutrient composition of apricots, cherries, nectarines, peaches, plums, kiwifruit, pears, melons, strawberries, and watermelon. Similarly, the contribution of potatoes (baked), tomatoes (raw), and onions (raw, chopped) in nutrients was estimated. Once more, the authors arbitrarily assumed that the contribution of the other vegetables (Table 7B) could be represented by the average of nutrient composition of root, fruit, and leafy vegetables. For pulses, the average of beans (dry, cooked, drained), lentils (cooked, drained) and chickpeas (dry, cooked); and for tree nuts, the average of almonds (shelled, whole), filberts (shelled), walnuts (shelled, whole), and pistachio nuts (dried, shelled) were used. The contribution of grains on nutrient content in diet was based on wheat flour (sifted) and rice (raw, white, enriched), of wine, both red and white wine; and of olives, both green and black ripe olives. The values obtained represented the annual nutrient contribution of plant products and each plant group in diet and were divided by 365 to obtain the daily availability. These values were used to construct Tables 10 and 11, which are discussed below.

The daily intake of energy from fruits, vegetables, nuts, grains, wine, and olives for the EU countries or the U.S. does not exceed 1000 calories per capita mainly due to low availability values. Such consumption provides less than 50% of the total calories required according to the U.S. Department of Agriculture RDAs. However, Mediterranean consumers average more than 1300 calories daily from plant-derived food sources. Spanish nutrient availability data reveal that the Spanish diet is quite far from the Mediterranean Diet consumed by Greek, Italian, Moroccan, and Egyptian consumers; often it is only slightly different from EU and U.S. consumer diets.

A large portion of protein RDAs (>60% for males and 80% for females) is supplied from plants, mainly cereals, and, to a lesser extent, vegetables, in the Mediterranean Diet. Consumers from the EU and the U.S. derive less than 50% of their protein needs from plant consumption.

Consumers from all countries in Table 10 derive barely 25% of calcium RDAs and about 50% of phosphorus RDAs from available edible plants. Plants also cover almost all consumer needs in iron, and Mediterranean inhabitants have >50% higher iron quantities available from plants than EU and U.S. inhabitants. Most of the minerals available to consumers come from cereals, vegetables, and, to a lesser extent, fruits.

TABLE 10
Total Daily Contribution Per Capita of Calories and Nutrients Based on Fruits, Vegetables, Pulses, Nuts, and Grains Availability in EU, Mediterranean Countries and the USA

		Calories Kcal	Protein g	Ca mg	P mg	Fe mg	Vit. A IU	Thiamin mg	Riboflavin mg	Niacin mg	Ascorbic Acid mg
Total (fruits vegetables,	EU	911	25.3	152	343	10.2	1513	1.3	0.9	11.3	62
nuts, pulses, grains)	Egypt	1352	36.2	149	407	15.4	2341	2.1	1.2	17.9	92
	Greece	1399	39.2	262	541	16.0	4250	2.1	1.4	17.9	162
	Italy	1334	35.4	185	433	14.3	2274	2.0	1.3	16.7	114
	Morocco	1378	39.2	148	399	16.3	1231	2.3	1.5	19.0	74
	Spain	1016	28.9	214	425	11.2	2151	1.5	1.0	12.3	104
	USA	810	23.0	136	298	9.3	1583	1.3	0.8	10.6	73
Adult male RDA		2700	56	800	800	10	5000	1.4	1.6	18	60
Adult female RDA		2000	44	800	800	18	4000	1.0	1.2	13	60

TABLE 11
Comparative Daily Contribution per Capita of Calories and Nutrients Based on Fruits, Vegetables, Pulses, Nuts and Grains Availability in the EU, Greece, and the USA

		Calories Kcal	Protein g	Ca mg	P mg	Fe mg	Vit. A IU	Thiamin mg	Riboflavin mg	Niacin mg	Ascorbic Acid mg
Fruit	EU	88	0.8	12.5	20.7	0.3	394	0.1	0.1	0.6	23.2
	Greece	170	2.1	46.6	46.6	0.6	1040	0.2	0.2	1.5	79.9
	USA	84	0.8	21.4	20.4	0.3	336	0.1	0.1	0.5	34.2
Vegetables	EU	104	5.1	93.8	125.0	1.8	1112	0.2	0.2	1.5	38.7
	Greece	152	7.2	130.7	180.0	3.2	3165	0.3	0.4	2.7	82.0
	USA	90	4.4	80.2	107.3	1.7	1243	0.2	0.2	1.4	38.4
Pulses	EU	9	0.6	2.2	9.1	0.1	1	0.0	0.0	0.1	0.2
	Greece	12	0.8	3.0	12.7	0.2	1	0.0	0.0	0.1	0.0
	USA	10	0.6	2.4	10.1	0.1	1	0.0	0.0	0.1	0.0
Nuts	EU	42	1.3	10.7	30.1	0.3	6	0.0	0.0	0.3	0.1
	Greece	105	3.4	26.7	75.0	0.6	15	0.1	0.1	0.8	0.2
	USA	21	0.7	5.3	15.0	0.1	3	0.0	0.0	0.1	0.0
Cereals	EU	623	17.5	27.3	148.8	7.4	0	1.1	0.7	8.9	0.0
	Greece	919	25.8	40.5	219.7	10.9	0	1.5	1.3	13.1	0.0
	USA	596	16.5	26.6	142.9	7.1	0	1.0	0.7	8.4	0.0
Wine+Olives	EU	46	0.0	5.0	9.4	0.2	0	0.0	0.0	0.1	0.0
	Greece	41	0.0	14.3	7.0	0.4	29	0.0	0.0	0.0	0.0
	USA	10	0.0	1.1	2.1	0.1	0	0.0	0.0	0.0	0.0
Adult male RDA		2700	56	800	800	10	5000	1.4	1.6	18	60
Adult female RDA		2000	44	800	800	18	4000	1.0	1.2	13	60

Mediterranean inhabitants derive almost all their needs for thiamin, riboflavin, and niacin from cereal and vegetable consumption, but EU and U.S. inhabitants gain only a portion of their RDAs. Mediterranean inhabitants also cover around half of their vitamin A (in the form of β-carotene) RDAs from plants, while this value is even lower for EU and U.S. consumers. Actually, Greek consumers cover almost all their vitamin A needs from plants, mainly due to high tomato availability and consumption. Inhabitants of non-Mediterranean countries just cover their ascorbic acid RDAs, but all Mediterranean consumers, especially Greeks, have available quantities of ascorbic acid well above the 60 mg RDA. In conclusion, vitamins A and C are supplied to the human diet by fruits and vegetables.

Dietary fiber availability was estimated from total fruit and vegetable availability and a mean dietary fiber content for each group calculated from the content of various major commodities. Dietary fiber availability for Greeks was 26 g.capita^{-1}day^{-1} from fruits and vegetables and for the EU and the U.S. consumers 14g.capita^{-1}day^{-1} (the U.S. National Cancer Institute recommends 20–30 g dietary fiber daily intake). Additional quantities of dietary fiber must be added, especially to the Greek diet, by tree nuts, olives, pulses, and whole-wheat products.

Increased consumption of fruits, vegetables, grains, and nuts in the Mediterranean Diet provides around 50% of the daily energy required for humans as well as a large part of the essential vitamins and, to a lesser extent, minerals, and the entire quantity of dietary fiber and other health-related constituents. Correspondingly, EU and U.S. consumers have much lower quantities of the above constituents available and do not satisfy their dietary fiber needs, because of consumption of limited quantities of, mainly, fruits and vegetables.

V. CONCLUSIONS

The Mediterranean region countries produce significant amounts of fruits and vegetables, while northern European countries focus their production on cereals and pulses. U.S. agricultural production is mainly focused on cereals, with only half the Mediterranean region's fruit and vegetable production, although their populations are of similar size. This results in low horticultural product availability for U.S. consumers that barely covers the recommended daily consumption of 400 g.capita^{-1}day^{-1} (potatoes excluded) for good health.

Production and availability of horticultural products to Greek consumers is much higher per capita than in the U.S. Greeks also have a wide variety of fruits and vegetables available and integrated into their everyday life with various means for preparation and use. They also consume substantial quantities of cereals, but in forms that do not include the addition of high-calorie shortenings and sugar. These habits result in a large intake of nutrients from horticultural commodities and cereals, and in only minor dependence on meat and meat products.

REFERENCES

1. Williams, P.C., Maintaining nutritional and processing quality in grain crops during handling, storage and transportation, in *Postharvest Physiology and Crop Preservation*, Lieberman, M., Ed., NATO Advanced Study Inst., Series A, Vol. 46, Plenum Press, New York, 1983, 425.

2. Schmidtbauer, L., Nicht Nutritive Inhaltsstoffe in Obst und Gemuse, *Ernahrungsumschau/ Ernahrungsiehre und Praxis*, 2, B5, 1995.

3. Gebhardt, S.E. and Matthews, R.H., *Nutritive Value of Foods*, USDA, Human Nutrition Information Serv., Bull. No. 72, 1981.

4. Watkins, T.R., Wine: Nutritional and Therapeutic Benefits, *Amer. Chem. Soc.*, Washington, 1997.

5. Perez-Llamas, F., Garaulet, M., Nieto, M., Baraza, J.C., and Zamora, S., Estimates of food intake and dietary habits in a random sample of adolescents in southeast Spain, *J. Human Nutr. Diet.*, 9, 463, 1996.

6. Garaulet, M., Perez-Llamas, F., Rueda, C.M., and Zamora, S., Trends in the Mediterranean Diet in children from southeast Spain, *Nutr. Res.*, 18, 979, 1998.

7. Carcassi, A.M., Curidori, C., and Licheri, D., Food consumption and nutritional knowledge of a sample of secondary school children, *Riv. Soc. Italiana Scienza Alimentazione*, 17, 243, 1988.

8. Gabriele, D., Nardozi, C., Giovannone, E., Elia, D., and Martinelli, S., Breakfast and between-meal snack consumption in preschool and school children, *Clin. Dietolog.*, 18, 159, 1991.

9. Fernandez-Ballart, J., Gordillo, B.J., Arija, V., and Marti-Henneberg, C., Food consumption, feeding habits and nutritional state in the community of Reus: Diet and nutritional balance in subjects over 60 years old, *Rev. Clinica Espanola*, 185, 282, 1989.

10. Kouris, A., Wahlqvist, M.L., Trichopoulos, A., and Polychronopoulos, E., Use of combined methodologies in assessing food beliefs and habits of elderly Greeks in Greece, *Food Nutr. Bull.* 13, 139, 1991.

11. U.S. Department of Agriculture, Agricultural Research Service, Data Tables: Food and Nutrient Intakes by Region, 1994-96, USDA, Washington, D.C., 1998.

12. Lionis, C., Faresjo, A., Skoula, M., Kapsokefalou, M., and Faresjo, T., Antioxidant effects of herbs in Crete, *Lancet*, 352, 1987, 1998.

13. Trichopoulou, A., Vasilopoulou, E., and Lagiou, A., Mediterranean Diet and coronary heart disease: Are antioxidants critical?, *Nutr. Rev.*, 57, 253, 1999.

14. Salunkhe, D.K., Kadam, S.S., and Chavan, J.K., *Postharvest Biotechnology of Food Legumes*, CRC Press, Boca Raton, FL, 1985.

15. Bender, A.E., Nutritional effects of food processing, *J. Food Tech.*, 1, 261, 1966.

16. Simopoulos, A., Terrestrial sources of omega-3 fatty acids: purslane, in *Horticulture and Human Health*, Quebedeaux, B. and Bliss, F.A., Eds., Prentice-Hall, Englewood Cliffs, NJ, 1988, 93.

17. Norton, G., Bliss, F.A., and Bressani, R., Biochemical and nutritional attributes of grain legumes, in *Grain Legume Crops*, Summerfield, R.J. and Roberts, E.H., Eds., W. Collins and sons, London, 1985, 73.

18. Food and Agriculture Organization, Amino Acid Content of Foods and Biological Data on Proteins, Nutritional Studies No 24, FAO, Rome, 1985.

19. Hoke, I.M., Table of Amino Acids in Fruits and Vegetables, the USDA, Human Nutr. Inform. Serv., Nutrient Data Res. Branch, 1983.

20. Dudek, J.A., Influence of food processing on nutritional composition of fruits and vegetables, in *Horticulture and Human Health*, Quebedeaux, B. and Bliss, F.A., Eds., Prentice-Hall, Englewood Cliffs, N.J., 1988, 33.

21. Godber, J.S., Nutrient bioavailability in humans and experimental animals, *J. Food Qual.*, 13, 21, 1990.

22. Odland, D. and Eheart, M.S., Ascorbic acid, mineral, and quality retention in frozen broccoli blanched in water, steam and ammonia steam, *J. Food Sci.*, 40, 1004, 1975.

23. Brecht, P.E., Keng, L., Bisoni, C.A., and Munger, H.M., Effect of fruit portion, stage of ripeness and growth habit on chemical composition of fresh tomatoes, *J. Food Sci.*, 41, 945, 1976.

24. Watada, A.E., Aulenbach, B.B., and Worthington, J.T., Vitamins A and C in ripe tomatoes as affected by stage of ripeness at harvest and by supplementary ethylene, *J. Food Sci.*, 41, 856, 1976.

25. Kader, A.A., Heintz, C.M., and Chordas, A., Postharvest quality of fresh and canned clingstone peaches as influenced by genotypes and maturity at harvest, *J. Amer. Soc. Hort. Sci.*, 107, 947, 1982.

26. Matthews, R.F., Crill, P., and Locasio, S.F., Beta-carotene and ascorbic acid contents of tomatoes as affected by maturity, *Proc. Florida State Hort. Soc.*, 87, 214, 1974.

27. Nagy, S, Vitamin C content of citrus fruit and their products: a review, *J. Agric. Food Chem.*, 28, 8, 1980.

28. Weichmann, J., The effect of controlled-atmosphere storage on the sensory and nutritional quality of fruits and vegetables, *Hort. Rev.*, 8, 101, 1986.

29. Kader, A.A., Influence of pre-harvest and post-harvest environment on nutritional composition of fruit and vegetables, in *Horticulture and Human Health*, Quebedeaux, B. and Bliss, F.A., Eds., Prentice-Hall, Englewood Cliffs, N.J., 1988, 18.

30. Kramer, A., Effect of storage on nutritive value of food, *J. Food Qual.*, 1, 23, 1977.

31. McCarthy, M.A. and Matthews, R.H., Nutritional quality of fruit and vegetables subject to minimal process, in *Minimally Processed Refrigerated Fruits and Vegetables,* Wiley, R.C., Ed., Chapman & Hall, London, 1994, 313.

32. Salunkhe, D.K., Bolin, H.R., and Reddy, N.R., *Storage, Processing and Nutritional Quality of Fruits and Vegetables*, Vol. II, Processed Fruits and Vegetables, 2nd Ed., C.R.C. Press, Boca Raton, FL., 1991, 162.

33. Englyst, H.N., Bingham, S.A., Runswick, S.A., Collinson, E., and Cummings, J.H., Dietary fiber (non-starch polysaccharides) in fruit, vegetables and nuts, *J. Human Nutr. Diet.*, 1, 247, 1988.

34. Englyst, H.N. and Cummings, J.H., Improved method of measurement of dietary fiber as non-starch polysaccharides in plant foods, *J. Assoc. Off. Anal. Chem.*, 71, 808, 1988.

35. Phillips, R.D., Starchy legumes in human nutrition, health and culture, *Plant Foods Human Nutr.*, 44, 195, 1993.

36. Curry, E.A., Effect of post-harvest handling and storage on apple nutritional status using antioxidants as a model, *HortScience,* 7, 240, 1997.

37. Hertog, M.G.L., Flavonols and flavones in foods and their relation with cancer and coronary heart disease, Ph.D. thesis, Agricultural University Wageningen, The Netherlands, 1994.

38. Wood, F.A. and Yang, D.A., TGA in Potatoes, Canada Dept. of Agric., Publ. no. 1533, 1974.

39. Liener, I.E. and Kakade, M.L., Protease inhibitors, in *Toxic Constituents of Plant Foodstuffs*, 2nd ed., Liener, I.E., Ed., Academic Press, New York, 1980, 169.

6 Milk and Dairy Products

Antonios J. Mantis

CONTENTS

I. INTRODUCTION

Milk is secreted by mammals for the nourishment of their young, but for countless generations, it has formed an important part of man's diet, not only for the infant but, in many societies, as part of everyday diet throughout life. Milk from domesticated animals has been used as a food for man since prehistoric times. Some sources mention that as early as 3000 BC. in Mesopotamia, where the Sumerians developed a profound civilization, there are the earliest signs of milking an animal and processing the milk to prepare other dairy products. In the Hebrew Bible, milk, butter, and cheese are mentioned incidentally, which implies their existence for extended periods of time in the past. Homer (1184 BC) mentions that Cyclops Polyphemus was in his cave, preparing cheese from sheep's and goat's milk, which may have been the ancestor of today's traditional feta cheese in Greece. Later on, Pliny (23–79 AD) wrote about "sour milk cheeses" that may have been the ancestors of today's Domiati and Akawi, two popular white-brined cheeses produced in Egypt and other Middle East countries.[1,2]

From these ancient times, civilizations that occurred around the Mediterranean basin (Egyptians, Phoenicians, Hebrew, Greeks, Romans, etc.) incorporated milk and dairy products into their everyday diets.

Sheep's and goat's milk made up the predominant milk produced in the Mediterranean area in ancient times, but today, cow's milk constitutes more than 85% of the total milk produced. However, the milk of sheep and goats is produced in all Mediterranean countries — in some of them, in quantities that represent 20% to 60% of the countries' total milk production.

Milk is a complex biological fluid often described as a complete food because it contains proteins of a high biological value, carbohydrates in the form of lactose, (the milk sugar), fat, vitamins, and minerals.

Raw milk may contain various pathogenic microorganisms or chemical contaminants that could have an adverse effect on human health. It is important, therefore, for raw milk to be produced, maintained, and processed under conditions that will prevent microbiological and chemical hazards, preserve the nutritive value, and ensure its safety as food.

II. PRODUCTION OF MILK AND DAIRY PRODUCTS

Milk production in the Mediterranean countries, in comparison with other areas of the world, can be considered satisfactory. Analytical data concerning production by

TABLE 1
Milk Production in the Mediterranean Countries for 1997
(MT x 1000)[3]

Country	Cow	Sheep	Goat	Buffalo	Camel	Total	Per capita kg/year
			Non EU Members				
Albania	707	68	85	0	0	860	270
Algeria	850	175	145	0	6	1,176	42
Bosnia Herzegovina	202	3	0	0	0	205	61
Croatia	622	6	0	0	0	628	140
Cyprus	133	19	25	0	0	177	238
Egypt	1,324	91	15	1,890	0	3,320	53
Israel	1,124	18	12	0	0	1,154	207
Lebanon	158	31	37	0	0	226	75
Libya	98	39	14	2		153	30
Malta	41	2	3	0	0	46	122
Morocco	979	27	34	0	4	1,044	40
Slovenia	568	0	0	0	0	568	285
Syria	1,009	524	77	796	0	2,406	113
Tunisia	613	15	11	0	1	640	72
Turkey	8,914	826	249	87	0	10,076	164
Yugoslavia	2,081	46	0	0	0	2,127	201
Sub-total	**19,423**	**1,890**	**707**	**2,775**	**11**	**24,806**	**108**
			EU Members				
France	24,917	243	486	0	0	25,646	442
Greece	755	650	460	0	0	1,865	177
Italy	10,876	758	150	144	0	11,928	208
Spain	6,108	284	325	0	0	6,716	169
Sub-total	**42,656**	**1,935**	**1,421**	**144**	**0**	**46,156**	**279**
Total	**62,079**	**3,825**	**2,128**	**2,919**	**11**	**70,962**	**179**
EU (15)	120,997	2,033	1,500	144	0	124,674	355
USA	70,801	0	0	0	0	70,801	260

animal species and country are given in Tables 1 and 2, using data obtained from the FAO database and referring to the year 1997.[3,4] From the evaluation of these data it is evident that milk production in all 20 Mediterranean countries (total population 393 million) totals 70,962,000 metric tonnes (MT) (179 kg/capita/year), which equals the production of milk in the U.S. The latter, with a smaller population, has a per capita production of 260 kg. However, the comparison of production indices in individual Mediterranean countries reveals great differences. Thus, France is the leading country in the group, with a total milk production of 25,646,000 MT, which is more than a third of the total production. France, Greece, Italy, and Spain, all members of the European Union (EU), produce a total of more than two thirds of the whole quantity. This production averages to 279 kg/capita/year for these countries, while the remaining 16 Mediterranean countries, non-members of the EU,

TABLE 2
Production of Dairy Products in the Mediterranean Countries for 1997
(MT x 1000)[4]

Country	Cheese All Kinds	Butter & Ghee	Evaporated Milk	Whole Milk Powder	Skim Milk Powder	Whey Powder
Non EU Members						
Albania	11.2	1.5	0	0	0	0
Algeria	1	1.7	0	0	0	0
Bosnia Herzegovina	13.5	0.05	0	0	0	0
Croatia	1.9	2.4	0.3	3.8	0.1	2.8
Cyprus	5.6	0	0	0	0	0
Egypt	402	91	0	0	0	0
Israel	93	4.5	0	0	0	0
Lebanon	21	0	4	0	15	0
Libya	0	0	0	0	0	0
Malta	0.3	0	0	0	0	0
Morocco	7.4	16	0	0	0	0
Slovenia	18	2.2	0.4	1.7	3	0
Syria	86	14	0	0	0	0
Tunisia	6.4	1.8	0	0	0	0
Turkey	133	120	0.04	0	0	0
Yugoslavia	18	0	0.05	2.3	0	0
Sub-total	**818.3**	**255.2**	**4.79**	**7.8**	**18.1**	**2.8**
EU Members						
France	1,625	465	43	270	380	520
Greece	224	5	0	0	0	0
Italy	918	90	50	0.8	0	5.2
Spain	160	24	68	10	14.5	0
Sub-total	**2.927**	**584**	**161**	**280.8**	**394.9**	**525.2**
Total	**3,745.3**	**807.9**	**165.79**	**288.6**	**412.6**	**528**
EU (15)	6,454	1,771	1,397	923	1,176	1,106
U.S.A.	3,644	522	918	55	577	515

produce less than a third of the total quantity with an average production of 108 kg/capita/year. The above differences become more distinct if the comparison is done within smaller groups of countries —within the North African group, the per capita production is less than 50 kg. Milk production in Albania appears most satisfactory, as a production figure of 270 kg/year is recorded. The highest per capita production is found in France (442 kg/year), whereas the lowest is in Libya (30 kg/year).

A. COW'S MILK

Cow's milk is the main milk produced in the majority of the Mediterranean countries, accounting for 87% of the total milk quantity. There is an exception for Greece, where sheep's and goat's milk production is greater than that of cow's milk, and for Egypt, where buffalo milk comes first, with 57% of the total milk production.

B. Sheep's and Goat's Milk

From ancient times, the Mediterranean area, and especially the Middle East and Balkan area, was the place where sheep and goats were raised and their milk was probably the main kind produced. This tradition, along with the mountainous nature of many countries, was the main reason that sheep's and goat's milk played an important role in the agricultural economy and, consequently, in the diet of many Mediterranean countries such as Greece, Syria, and Algeria. It is important to note that, although the total sheep's and goat's milk production in the Mediterranean countries amounts to only 5,953,000 MT (8.4%), this is almost twice the quantity produced in the whole EU. In the U.S., production of such milk has not been tabulated.

C. Dairy Products

Cheese is the principal dairy product traditionally prepared in all Mediterranean countries. Today, with the exception of Libya, all countries contribute to a total cheese production of 3,746,300 MT, a quantity that equals that of the U.S. Some countries process a large portion of their milk production into cheese. Greece and Egypt, for instance, process more than 50% of their total milk production while France, Italy, and Greece process more than 70% of their sheep's and goat's milk into cheese. In addition, France is the main cheese producer, with a total quantity of 1,625,000 MT, while the four EU countries account for 77% of the total quantity produced in all Mediterranean countries. The same pattern applies also for butter, where France contributes 65% of the total production. From the countries outside the EU, only Turkey appears as a butter-producing country, with 15% of the total quantity produced.

As far as fermented milks are concerned, there are no concrete data in individual countries because these products are usually listed as "liquid milk." However, yogurt is a popular product from ancient times in the Eastern Mediterranean countries (Turkey, Lebanon, Syria) and also in Greece, Italy, and Spain. It is calculated that, in these countries, 10–15% of the liquid milk represents yogurt or different types of cultured milk (e.g., xynogala, ayran, leban).

III. AVAILABILITY STATISTICS

Availability of milk and dairy products in the Mediterranean countries varies according to the milk production in each, and the import–export balance, which is affected by the economic situation of each country as well as tradition. Availability data for dairy products (with the exception of butter) obtained from FAO databases, are given in Tables 3 and 4. These data give an idea of the per capita availability for each Mediterranean country, as well as the change in availability from 1970 to 1977. From Table 3, it is evident that an increase in availability is recorded in all Mediterranean countries

TABLE 3
Per Capita Availability of Milk Equivalent in the Mediterranean Countries[5]

Country	1970	1980	1990	1997	% change 1997/1970
		kg/capita/year			
		Non EU Members			
Albania	90	132	158	278	208
Algeria	50	82	106	94	88
Cyprus	130	132	199	195	50
Egypt	34	37	39	42	23
Israel	179	195	207	186	3
Lebanon	82	115	97	93	13
Libya	61	102	103	82	34
Malta	162	188	176	196	21
Morocco	28	33	34	32	14
Syria	54	86	95	96	77
Tunisia	48	67	71	79	64
Turkey	161	173	139	129	-20
		EU Members			
France	236	267	268	251	6
Greece	159	198	224	248	56
Italy	182	249	254	251	38
Spain	121	164	149	164	35
USA	206	232	255	251	22

between 1970 and 1977, except in Turkey, where a decrease of 20% is recorded. Countries with a low figure in availability of milk equivalent during 1970 managed to achieve an increase of more than 50% by 1997, and in the case of Albania, an increase of 208% is recorded. Thus, for 1997, Albania comes first with 274 kg/capita/year, followed by France with 251 kg/capita/year. Greece and Slovenia follow with 248 kg and 213 kg per capita, respectively.

Another group of countries (Malta, Israel, Cyprus, Spain, Yugoslavia, Croatia, and Turkey) have an availability that falls between 100 and 200 kg/capita/year, while the remaining countries have an availability of less than 100 kg/capita/year. The lowest availability figures are recorded for the North African Mediterranean countries and this is in agreement with the low production figures in these countries. All Mediterranean countries, except France, have a negative balance between production and availability. This means that they consume more milk products than they produce. France is the only country with a surplus in the dairy sector, with an availability of only 251 kg/capita/year of milk equivalent, while it produces almost twice this quantity (443 kg of milk/capita/year).

Some Mediterranean countries import large quantities of dairy products, which, in some cases, equal their national production (e.g. Libya, Lebanon), or represent a

TABLE 4
Per Capita Availability of Milk Equivalent and Energy Supply in the Mediterranean Countries for 1997[5]

Country	Per Year (Kg)	Per day: Protein (g)	Fat (g)	kcal	% of Total kcal
	Non EU Members				
Albania	278	26	29	447	16.0
Algeria	94	9	7	144	5.0
Bosnia Herzegovina	67	5	6	85	3.7
Croatia	139	12	12	204	8.3
Cyprus	195	19	25	398	12.0
Egypt	42	4	4	61	2.0
Israel	186	16	10	195	6.0
Lebanon	93	9	9	139	4.0
Libya	82	8	7	143	4.0
Malta	196	19	22	328	10.0
Morocco	32	3	2	41	1.5
Slovenia	213	19	16	294	9.4
Syria	96	10	12	181	5.4
Tunisia	79	7	6	125	3.8
Turkey	129	12	11	205	5.8
Yugoslavia	178	16	16	285	9.4
	EU Members				
France	251	24	23	361	10.0
Greece	248	23	24	354	10.0
Italy	251	16	17	260	7.4
Spain	164	15	15	260	7.8
EU 15	244	21	19	318	9.3
USA	251	22	22	377	10.1

fraction up to 40–50% of their production (e.g. Greece, Italy). We must also mention that a substantial portion of the total milk production, equal to 5,426,000 MT, is not used as human food, but for other purposes, mainly animal feeding. Concerning the energy supply, it is observed (Table 4) that, in some Mediterranean countries with a high availability in milk equivalent, the energy supply (capita/day) represents more than 10% of the total energy supplied from animal and vegetable sources. However the energy supplied by milk products in some Mediterranean countries is still very low (e.g. Bosnia, Algeria, Morocco, Libya, Tunisia) representing less than 5% of the total food energy. Cheese is the main dairy product consumed in the Mediterranean area. However, from Table 5, it is evident that there are great differences among countries in per capita availability. Thus, Greece is on the top of the list with 25.5 kg/capita/year, followed closely by France, with 22.2 kg/capita/year. Those two countries are also on the top of the world list of cheese consumers. Italy, Israel, and

TABLE 5
Cheese Availability and Energy Supply in the Mediterranean
Countries for 1997[5]

Country	Total (MT × 1000)	kg/year	Per capita Per day Protein (g)	Fat (g)	kcal
		Non EU Members			
Albania	13	4.1	2.9	3.3	45
Algeria	15	0.5	0.3	0.3	4
Bosnia Herzegovina	19	5.3	3.6	4.5	56
Croatia	21	4.6	3.1	3.8	48
Cyprus	5	6.5	3.2	4.2	52
Egypt	383	5.9	2.1	2.0	29
Israel	94	16.1	10.3	5.6	100
Lebanon	32	10.3	5.0	5.3	69
Libya	7	1.3	0.7	1.1	13
Malta	5	14.1	9.9	11.8	150
Morocco	9	0.4	0.2	0.2	3
Slovenia	18	9.0	6.1	7.4	93
Syria	85	5.7	2.6	3.3	41
Tunisia	9	0.9	0.6	0.7	9
Turkey	129	2.0	1.6	0.5	12
Yugoslavia	19	1.8	1.2	1.5	19
		EU Members			
France	1,297	22.2	15.6	17.7	221
Greece	268	25.3	16.0	17.2	227
Italy	1,119	19.5	9.8	12.5	158
Spain	226	5.7	4.0	3.9	53
EU (15)	6,139	18.8	10.1	10.5	142
USA	3,780	13.9	8.9	11.0	137

Malta follow with 19.5, 16.1 and 14.1 kg/capita/year, respectively. However, cheese availability in the majority of the Mediterranean countries falls below 10 kg/capita/year. The lowest availability is found in the North African Mediterranean countries (less than 1.0 kg/capita/year), and only Egypt scores a 5.9 kg/capita/year. Total availability of cheese in all Mediterranean countries adds up to 3,780,409 MT (9.6 kg/capita/year), which is almost satisfactory, but only as an average figure, because if we group up the non-EU member countries, we observe an availability of only 3.8 kg/capita/year, while in the four Mediterranean countries that are members of the EU (Table 5) the figure is up to 17.6 kg/capita/year. This is higher than that of the U.S. and almost equals the average cheese availability in the EU.

TABLE 6
Butter Availability and Energy Supply in the Mediterranean Countries[5]

Country	Total (MT × 1000)	kg/year	Per capita Per day Protein (g)	Fat (g)	kcal
Non EU Members					
Albania	2	0.7	0	1.5	13
Algeria	1.6	0.4	0.1	0.9	8
Bosnia Herzegovina	0.8	0.2	0.1	0.5	5
Croatia	2.5	0.5	0	1.2	11
Cyprus	0.9	1.2	0	2.6	23
Egypt	132	2	0	4.5	40
Israel	3	0.5	0	1.1	10
Lebanon	4	1.3	0	3	26
Libya	3	0.5	0	1.2	10
Malta	0.2	0.7	0	1.5	13
Morocco	32	1.2	0	2.6	23
Slovenia	2	0.9	0	2.1	18
Syria	21	1.4	0	3.2	28
Tunisia	7	0.8	0	1.7	15
Turkey	123	1.9	0	4.3	38
Yugoslavia	4	0.3	0.1	0.8	7
EU Members					
France	531	9.1	0.2	20.2	179
Greece	12	1.1	0	2.5	22
Italy	123	2.1	0.1	4.7	42
Spain	14	0.3	0.1	0.8	7
EU (15)	1,667	4.5	0.3	9.9	86
USA	501	1.8	0	4.1	36

In conclusion, cheese, which is a concentrated, nutrient-rich food, contributes greatly to the human diet in some Mediterranean countries like Greece, France, Italy, and Israel, and, to a lesser degree, in some others (Lebanon, Malta, Spain, Cyprus, Slovenia, and Croatia). For the rest of the Mediterranean countries, cheese does not play an important role as a food.

Finally, the available data for butter (Table 6) reveal that France is not only a big butter producer but has also an availability of 9.1 kg/capita/year. In all other Mediterranean countries, availability falls below 2 kg/capita/year. Data for the availability of other dairy products are not presented because their contribution to the diet has been calculated as "milk equivalent" and it is given in Table 3.

IV. CHEMICAL COMPOSITION OF MILK AND DAIRY PRODUCTS

The term milk is used, in the legislation of most countries, for cow's milk only. The milk of all other species is labeled specifically (e.g. goat's milk, sheep's milk, buffalo milk, and others).

Milk contains the nutrients required for the growth and development of the neonate. All milks contain specific proteins, fats that are easily digested, lactose, minerals, vitamins, and other components that may have important role in the development of the young of the relevant species. The above milk components, however, may differ quantitatively from species to species. Some milks, such as human milk, are rich in lactose, others such as cow's or sheep's milk are rich in caseins, whereas human and donkey milk are rich in serum proteins. Table 7 presents the chemical composition of cow's, sheep's and goat's milk, which are the main milks produced in the Mediterranean area. Since cow's milk represents the vast quantity of total milk and it is the most studied, it will be the basis for the analysis that follows.

A. MILK COMPOSITION

The average gross composition of cow's milk is: water 87%, fat 3.5%, proteins 3.4% (caseins 2.8%, serum proteins 0.6%), lactose 4.9%, and ash 0.8%.[6,7] This composition fluctuates significantly according to the animal breed, lactation period, the animal's feed, and season of the year. The milk of the Mediterranean indigenous goat has almost the same gross composition as cow's milk, with the fat content being a little higher. However, sheep's milk is richer in all main constituents (7% fat, 5.5% protein) except in lactose. Thus, the total solid content of cow's and goat's milk averages to 12.5%, while that of sheep's milk is up to 18%.[8]

1. Fat

Milk fat is excreted in the form of small droplets, which in cow's milk range in size from 1 to 12 μm. During the excretion from the mammary secretory cells, fat globules are encapsulated with a "fat globule membrane," which maintains the integrity of the globule and renders it compatible with the aqueous environment. A fat globule consists mainly of triglycerides (95–96%, w/w), diglycerides (1–2%) and monoglycerides (0.1–0.3%). Furthermore, other important constituents like phospholipids (0.8–1.0%), sterols and, especially, cholesterol (0.2-0.4%), fat-soluble vitamins (A, D, E) and carotenes, are in minor quantities.[9,10] In the overall picture fatty acids constitute 85% of the total lipid fraction of milk. More than 80 different fatty acids, which are of simple, double, or multiple chain, saturated or unsaturated, have been identified in milk fat. The most important among them and their percentage distribution in a 100-g total fatty acid fraction are presented in Table 12. The non-volatile saturated palmitic, steatic, and myristic acids represent the major part of the saturated fraction (40–42% of total fatty acids), while oleic and linolenic acids constitute the unsaturated fraction, which represents about 30–32% of the total fatty acids. The composition of the milk fat globule membrane is quite different from that of the rest of the globule, consisting of proteins (40% w/w of dry membrane), phospholipids

TABLE 7
Chemical Composition of Milk of the
Main Milk-Producing Animals[7]

| Component | Unit | Fresh Whole Milk | | |
		Cow	Sheep	Goat
			Per 100 g	
Energy	kcal	64	104	70
Water	g	88.0	82.0	87.2
Fat	g	3.5	7.0	4.5
Protein	g	3.3	5.5	3.5
Lactose	g	4.8	4.7	4.4
Oleic acid	g	1.1	1.6	1.2
Linoleic acid	g	0.2	0.2	0.1
Calcium	mg	120	190	130
Phosphorus	mg	100	140	100
Potassium	mg	150	180	170
Sodium	mg	50	50	40
Chloride	mg	100	80	130
Magnesium	mg	12	18	15
Iron	μg	50	90	70
Zinc	μg	360	500	350
Cholesterol	mg	13	11	10
Pant. acid	mg	0.3	0.4	0.3
Vit. C	mg	1.0	4.5	1.5
Vit. E	mg	0.1	0.2	0.1
Vitamin A	μg	40	70	50
Carotene	μg	20	10	0
Thiamin	μg	40	80	50
Riboflavin	μg	170	360	150
Vit. B_6	μg	50	80	50
Vit. B_{12}	μg	0.5	0.6	0.0
Biotin	μg	3.5	9.0	4.0
Vit. D	μg	0.1	0.2	0.2

(27%), neutral lipids (14%), and traces of some other constituents like cerebrocides, gangliosides, protein carbohydrates, and lipid bound carbohydrates.[11,12] A fat constituent with great importance in today's diet is cholesterol, which makes up the 0.2–0.4% of the total lipid fraction, 70% of which is located in the nucleus and 10% in the membrane of the fat globule. The rest is dispersed in the aqueous phase of the milk.

2. Proteins

Milk proteins are classified as either caseins or whey proteins. All the caseins exist with calcium phosphate in unique hydrated, spherical complexes known as micelles, which are formed by association of nearly spherical sub-units, the submicelles. Micelles have a diameter of 10–20 nm and are dispersed in the aqueous phase of the milk.

Caseins form the major part of milk proteins in the majority of milks with the exception of human milk, which is richer in whey proteins than in caseins. Cow's milk contains 3.2–3.6 g of protein per 100 ml, 75–80% of which are caseins that exist in four different forms designated as α_{s1}-casein, α_{s2}-casein, ß-casein, and κ-casein. Each one of these proteins exhibits genetic polymorphism and thus appears in more than one genetic variant. The α_{s1}-casein constitutes about 34%, the α_{s2}-casein about 8%, and ß-casein 25% of the total protein fraction. The κ-casein constitutes 9% of the total milk proteins and it is the only casein with a carbohydrate complex in its molecule. The carbohydrate moiety is positioned in the outer surface of the almost spherical casein micelle, stabilizing its size and keeping it dispersed in the aqueous phase of the milk.[13-18]

The above four forms of casein are bound together with calcium phosphate bonds to form submicelles, which are combined further to form micelles.[19]

Whey proteins are the proteins that remain in the milk serum after the acid precipitation of caseins. The most significant of them are the α-lactalbumin, β-lactoglobulin, serum albumin, proteose-peptones, and the immunoglobulins. Together they make up 20% of the total protein fraction of the milk. The most important whey protein is β-lactoglobulin, which represents about 10% of the total protein of the milk, followed by α-lactalbumin (4%) and proteose-peptones (4%).[20,21]

3. Carbohydrates

Lactose is the predominant carbohydrate of the milk of all animal species and its concentration varies between 4.5 and 4.9 g/100 ml in the milk of cows, sheep and goats, while human milk is rich in lactose, averaging 7.0 g/100 ml. Lactose is the sugar of milk and does not exist, in significant amounts, elsewhere in nature.[22] Apart from lactose, milk contains in small quantities some monosaccharides such as glucose and galoctose in quantities 10–20 mg/100ml, oligosaccharides or glycoproteins containing fucose, N-acetyl-neuraminic acid, or N-acetyl-galactosamine, which is part of the κ-casein molecule.[23]

4. Minerals and Trace Elements

The major mineral constituents of milk consist of calcium, phosphate, sodium, potassium, magnesium, and chloride. The monovalent ions such as Na^+, K^+ and Cl^- are present almost entirely as free ions. The multivalent ions Ca^{++}, Mg^{++} exist principally in complexes that include large amounts of Ca-citrate and Mg-citrate and lesser quantities of CaH_2PO_4.[24] In cow's milk, 50% of calcium exists in inorganic colloidal form, 20% is bound to caseins together with phosphorus, and 30% is found in ionic form.[25] The average concentration of minerals in the milk of cows, sheep, and goats is presented in Table 3.

Apart from the above minerals, which play an important role in nutrition, other elements that are essential to the diet of humans and other animal species are also present in very small quantities (μg/ml). These elements are characterized as trace elements or microminerals, and the most important of them are iron, zinc, manganese, copper, cobalt, selenium, iodine, and fluorine.

5. Vitamins

Milk contains almost all the vitamins — some in satisfactory quantities, others only in traces.

Table 3 gives the concentration of the principle fat- and water-soluble vitamins of the milk of cows, sheep and goats. Among the fat-soluble ones, vitamin A exists mainly in the form of its palmitic acid ester, vitamin D as a mixture of D_2 and D_3, and vitamin E as α-tocopherol. There are only traces of vitamin K.

Among the water-soluble vitamins, those of the B complex and especially thiamin, riboflavin, B_6, pantothenic acid, niacin and biotin, are always present in milk.[7,26]

6. Enzymes

Milk contains many enzymes, some of which (lactoperoxidase, xanthine oxidase, proteinases, lipase, lysozyme, phosphatase) play an important role in retaining the quality of milk or dairy products. Some (e.g., phosphatase, xanthine oxidase) are useful indicators of correct processing. However, they do not appear to play any significant role as nutrients.[27,28]

B. COMPOSITION OF DAIRY PRODUCTS

1. Cheese

Cheese is the result of rennet coagulation of milk and the removal of whey. The degree of whey removal, the amount of salt added, the time required for ripening, as well as the environmental conditions of the ripening room, are the critical factors that regulate the degree of water retention as well as the concentration of caseins and other constituents of milk. The technology involved for the production of each variety of cheese may lead to a special product with distinct organoleptic qualities, but all cheeses are characterized by:

a. The high percentages of proteins, ranging usually between 18 and 26 g/100 g. The proteins are mainly caseins because whey proteins are removed with the whey and only small amounts are trapped in the aqueous phase of the cheese.
b. High percentage of fat ranging between 15 and 30 g/100 g of cheese.
c. Low levels of lactose in all ripened cheeses, because most lactose is removed with the whey and the remaining is fermented to lactic acid and other metabolic products.
d. High levels of some salts including those of calcium, phosphorus, sodium, and chloride.

Table 8 presents the gross chemical composition of some varieties of cheese produced in the Mediterranean area, while Table 9 gives a more detailed chemical composition of representative samples of cheese varieties ranging from soft (feta) to very hard (Parmesan).

TABLE 8

Gross Chemical Composition of Some Representative Varieties of Cheese Produced in the Mediterranean Area[2,29–31]

Cheese Variety	Country of Origin	Kind of Milk	Type of Cheese	Moisture	Fat	Protein	Ash	Salt
						g/100g		
Akawi	Egypt	Cow/Sheep	Semi-hard	51	22	22	5.0	3.8
Anthotiros	Greece	Cow (Whey)	Soft	64	18	15	3.0	1.5
Brinzza	Israel	Sheep	Soft	56	20	18	6.0	2.2
Camembert	France	Cow	Soft	52	22	24	4.0	2.0
Domiati	Egypt	Cow	Soft	56	20	18	6.0	4.0
Feta	Greece	Sheep	Soft	54	22	20	4.0	2.8
Haloumi	Cyprus	Sheep/Goat	Semi-hard	45	25	24.5	5.5	3.5
Kaseri	Greece	Sheep/Goat	Semi-hard	39	28	28	5.0	2.2
Kefalotyri	Greece	Sheep/Goat	Hard	35	32	27	6.0	4.0
Manchego	Spain	Sheep	Hard	40	28	27	5.0	2.7
Manouri	Greece	Sheep (Whey)	Soft	45	35	15	5.0	1.4
Mizithra (fresh)	Greece	Cow (Whey)	Soft	70	11	15	4.0	1.4
Mozzarella	Italy	Buffalo/Cow	Soft	56	16	23	5.0	2.8
Parmesan	Italy	Cow	Very hard	32	20	34	5.0	3.0
Pecorino Romano	Italy	Sheep	Hard	36	32	26	5.0	3.7
Roquefort	France	Sheep	Soft	40	31	24	5.0	3.5
String Cheese	Syria	Cow	Soft	49	20	25	6.0	4.8
Telemes	Greece	Cow/Sheep	Soft	55	22	19	4.0	3.0

2. Yogurt

The chemical composition of natural yogurt is based on the composition of milk from which it is made and on the changes occurring during the heat treatment and also during lactic acid fermentation. The chemical composition of all other types of yogurt depends not only on the composition of the relevant milk used for fermentation but also on the degree of adding or subtracting milk constituents (e.g. fat, protein concentrate etc.) or other permitted additives like fruits, carbohydrates, stabilizers etc. The chemical changes of milk constituents during fermentation result in the reduction of lactose (about 15-20% of lactose is fermented to lactic acid), the appearance of lactic acid and the increase in the content of free peptides, free amino

TABLE 9
Chemical Composition of Cheese Varieties Representative of Some Mediterranean Countries[7]

Component	Unit	Feta (50% Fat in Dry Matter)	Goat Semi-Soft Cheese (45% Fat in Dry Matter)	Roquefort (52% Fat in Dry Matter)	Mozzarella	Provolone	Parmesan
				per 100 g			
Energy	kcal	295	281	374	255	351	358
Water	g	52	54	40	57	41	33
Fat	g	22	21	32	20	27	22
Protein	g	20	22	21	18	25	38
Lactic acid	g	0.4	0.4	0.6	0.8	0.8	0.4
Oleic acid	g	4.3	6.1	7.3	5.9	8.1	6.8
Linoleic acid	g	0.5	0.6	0.8	0.8	0.3	0.9
Calcium	g	0.5	0.5	0.6	0.4	0.7	1.4
Phosphorus	g	0.4	0.4	0.4	0.3	0.5	0.9
Potassium	g	0.2	0.2	0.1	0.1	0.1	0.1
Sodium	g	1.3	0.8	1.6	0.5	0.9	1.0
Chloride	g	1.9	1.2	2.4	0.7	0.9	1.4
Magnesium	mg	25	25	40	20	24	44
Iron	mg	0.3	0.4	0.5	0.3	0.4	0.6
Zinc	mg	2	3	2.5	1.7	2.6	3.6
Cholesterol	mg	48	36	72	46	123	53
Vitamin A	mg	0.2	0.2	0.3	0.2	0.1	0.3
Pant. acid	mg	0.5	1.2	0.5	0.4	0.2	1.2
Niacin	mg	0.2	3.5	0.7	0.3	0.1	0.2
Vit. E	mg	0.5	0.6	0.6	0.6	0.4	0.7
Carotene	µg	10	10	50	120	50	140
Thiamin	µg	40	50	40	40	10	30
Riboflavin	µg	300	500	60	350	200	500
Vit. B_6	µg	100	200	200	100	100	100
Vit. B_{12}	µg	1.5	2.8	1.0	2.0	1.5	2.0
Biotin	µg	2.4	10	2.3	2.2	1.5	2.8

acids and free fatty acids. Changes also occur in the vitamin content due either to the effect of heat treatment or to the bacterial metabolism. Finally in the natural yogurt a slight decrease in the caloric value (3-4%) is observed in comparison to the relevant milk, due to the fermentation of lactose to lactic acid.[32]

Table 10 gives the detailed chemical composition of some types of yogurt that usually appear in the market.

TABLE 10
Chemical Composition of Cultured Dairy Products[7]

| Component | Unit | Cow's Milk | | | | Whole Sheep's Milk Yogurt |
| | | Whole Milk | Strained Yogurt | Fruit Yogurt | Buttermilk | |
				per 100 g		
Energy	kcal	64	133	95	34	94
Water	g	88	78	79	91	82
Fat	g	3.5	10	3	0.5	6
Protein	g	3.3	6	2.9	3.2	5.5
Lactose	g	4	4	3.5	3.5	3.8
Other Carboh.	g	0	0	9.8	0	0
Lactic acid	g	0.8	0.8	0.7	0.7	0.8
Oleic acid	g	1.1	3	0.9	0.2	1.4
Linoleic acid	g	0.1	0.4	0.1	0.6	0.2
Calcium	g	0.1	0.1	0.1	0.1	0.2
Phosphorus	g	0.1	0.2	0.1	0.1	0.1
Potassium	g	0.2	0.1	0.1	0.1	0.2
Sodium	mg	50	40	50	60	50
Chloride	mg	100	80	90	110	80
Magnesium	mg	12	9	11	13	18
Iron	μg	50	80	160	100	90
Zinc	mg	0.36	0.40	0.38	0.50	0.50
Cholosterol	mg	13	37	11	2	9
Vitamin A	μg	40	110	30	10	60
Carotene	μg	20	60	20	0	10
Thiamin	μg	20	20	20	30	40
Riboflavin	μg	170	230	180	160	360
Vit. B_6	μg	50	40	40	40	80
Vit. B_{12}	μg	0.5	0.7	0.4	0.2	0.6
Pant. acid	μg	360	520	300	350	440
Niacin	μg	100	80	90	100	480
Biotin	μg	3.5	5.0	3.0	3.4	9.0
Vit. C	μg	100	100	100	100	450

V. NUTRITIONAL EVALUATION OF MILK AND DAIRY PRODUCTS

A. MILK

Milk is the only complete food for the newborn of mammals. This applies to human newborns also, but after the first few months of life, milk is no longer enough to satisfy the nutritional needs of a child. However, milk continues to be an excellent food, not only for children but for every age, because it is a source of proteins of high biological value, of calcium and phosphorus and of certain vitamins. Furthermore, its fat and carbohydrate contributes in a satisfactory degree to the daily caloric requirements. Thus, 1 l of milk can satisfy 50% of the daily protein needs, 100%

of calcium and phosphorus, 40% of vitamin A, and 60% of riboflavin.[25] The coverage is far better for a 5-year-old child, who can find 70% of needed protein and 60–100% of needed vitamins, thiamin, and riboflavin in 1 l of milk.[33]

1. Proteins

Milk proteins correspond very well to human requirements and therefore are regarded as high quality. The biological value of proteins in raw milk is 0.9, based on a value of 1.0 for whole-egg protein. The biological value of a protein is related to its amino-acid composition, as well to the availability of these amino acids. In this respect, milk proteins have a high content in essential amino acids (Table 11). Thus, milk proteins are very often used, as are egg proteins, in the evaluation of the nutritive value of food proteins. Milk proteins are slightly deficient in the sulfur amino acids methionine and cysteine, in respect to caseins, while whey proteins contain satisfactory quantities of sulfur amino acids.

TABLE 11
Essential Amino Acids in Cow's Milk Protein (g/100g Protein)[25,33,35]

Amino Acid	Total Protein	Casein	Total Whey Protein	Lactalbumin
Cystine	0.9	0.34	0.9	3.4
Isoleucine	6.4	6.10	6.4	6.2
Leucine	10.4	9.20	10.4	12.3
Lysine	8.3	8.20	8.3	9.1
Methionine	2.7	2.80	2.7	2.3
Phenylalanine	5.2	5.00	5.2	4.4
Threonine	5.1	4.90	5.1	5.2
Tryptophan	1.4	1.70	1.4	2.2
Tyrosine	5.3	6.30	5.3	3.8
Valine	6.8	–	6.8	5.7

Table 4 gives the milk protein intake in the Mediterranean countries. This table reveals great differences among countries. Albania heads the list with 25.7 g of milk protein/capita/day, followed by France and Greece with 24.1 g and 22.8 g/capita/day, respectively. The majority of Mediterranean countries fall between 14 and 20 g/cap/day, while in some countries (e.g., Egypt, Morocco), daily milk protein intake is less than 5 g/capita.

2. Fat

Milk fat is regarded as the most digestible of the various dietary fats and oils. The reason for this is found in the state of dispersion of milk fat globules and the composition of milk fat in fatty acids. The state of dispersion refers to the milk fat globules that are absorbed without a previous enzymatic breakdown, due to their state of emulsion. Furthermore, if milk is homogenized, the size of the fat globules is reduced by 15 to 20 times, and this increases the rate of absorption and, therefore, the digestibility of milk fat. In addition, the melting point of milk fat lies below the human body temperature and it is known that the digestibility of fats with a melting point below 45°C (e.g., butter) is 95% or higher.

On the other hand, the fatty acid composition of milk fat favors digestibility because it contains high levels of short- and medium-chain fatty acids, which are more easily absorbed than the long-chain ones (Table 12). The unsaturated portion of the fatty acids of milk represents about 32–35% of the total fatty acids, with oleic being the dominant (29%) unsaturated fatty acid. Linoleic (≈3%) and arachidonic acids (0.5%) are essential fatty acids that play an important role in the diet. However, milk fat cannot be regarded as a food rich in essential fatty acids.[25,34]

TABLE 12
Fatty Acid Composition of Milks Used as Food[9,10]

| Fatty Acid | Animal Species | | | |
| | Cow | Sheep | Goat | Buffalo |
	(g/100 g of total fatty acids)			
Butyric	3.3	4	2.6	3.6
Caproic	1.6	2.8	2.9	1.6
Caprylic	1.3	2.7	2.7	1.1
Capric	3	9	8.4	1.9
Lauric	3.1	5.4	3.3	2
Myristic	9.5	11.8	10.3	8.7
Palmitic	26.3	25.4	24.6	30.4
Palmitoleic	2.3	3.4	2.2	3.4
Stearic	14.3	9	12.5	10.1
Oleic	29.8	20.0	28.5	28.7
Linoleic	2.4	2.1	2.2	2.5
Arachidonic	4.1	1	4	0

Milk fat also contains phospholipids, which constitute the 0.2–1.0% of the total lipids. Phospholipids consist of more fractions, the main ones being cephalin and sphingomyelin. Phospholipids play a vital and important role in the body (cell membrane function, blood clotting, central neural system, etc.) and, in this respect, milk fat is important in the human diet — especially for children.

Milk fat also contains cholesterol, a substance with a vital role in the body metabolism but causing great controversy as one of the factors responsible for atherosclerosis. The average cholesterol of milk is 13–15 mg/100ml and this corresponds to 3 mg/g of milk fat. Thus, milk contains less cholesterol than other animal foods (e.g., meat, egg yolk, liver, brains, or shrimp). The cholesterol content of milk products depends on their fat content. The milk of sheep and goats contains about equal amounts of cholesterol. Furthermore, as it is evident from Table 12, that these milks do not differ significantly in their fatty acid composition.[10]

Considering the data of tables 3, 4, 5, and 6, it becomes obvious that the contribution of milk fat to the diet of people around the Mediterranean Sea differs greatly. In some countries, availability of milk fat is higher than 20 g/capita/day (France, Greece, Albania, Cyprus, Yugoslavia, Malta), in others, the supply of fat falls between 10 and 20 g/capita/day, and, in a few others, the availability falls below 10 g/capita/day.

3. Lactose

Lactose represents one third of the calories supplied by milk, but with just 4.8 g/100 ml, milk is not regarded as an important carbohydrate food. Apart from supplying net calories in the body, lactose also improves calcium absorption and supplies energy for the intestinal flora. Because of its relatively slow absorption, lactose acts as a slight laxative, which becomes more apparent in larger doses or when a lactose-intolerance syndrome is present. Furthermore, lactose helps in the metabolism of magnesium.[35]

4. Minerals

Sodium, potassium, and chloride are present in cow's milk mainly as free ions and in concentrations higher than that in human milk (Table 3). Cow's milk is a good source of dietary calcium and phosphorus. In many European countries and in North America, milk and dairy products contribute to the human diet 50–70% of the total calcium intake.[37] The same applies for some of the Mediterranean countries with a high per capita availability of milk or cheese (e.g., France, Albania, Greece, and Italy). Phosphorus also exists in satisfactory amounts in milk and it is calculated that 30–35% of the daily intake comes from milk or dairy products.

From the trace element group, only zinc exists in concentrations worth mentioning and it is calculated that 15–25% of the daily human needs are satisfied with milk or dairy products.

5. Vitamins

Milk is a good source of vitamin A, riboflavin and thiamin (Table 3) and thus 1 l of milk can cover 30–60% of an adult's daily needs.[7,25,38]

B. Dairy Products

1. Butter

The fat content of butter is usually 84-85% (the rest being water), while that of cream varies according to the type of cream, ranging from 18 to 48%. This affects the nutritional and caloric value of cream. The rest of the constituents of cream are the same as in milk, which means that, in the water phase of the cream (80–50% of total weight), proteins, lactose, water-soluble vitamins, and minerals are dispersed or dissolved. Thus, the nutritive value of cream is quite different from that of butter. Butter retains only the fat-soluble vitamins, while cream has all the nutrients of milk. However, during the storage of cream, and especially of butter, vitamin A and carotenes may decrease due to oxidation phenomena, while triglycerides may be hydrolyzed due to the residual lipolytic effect after processing, or to bacterial activity (lipolysis).

Table 6 portrays the profile of butter availability in the Mediterranean countries as well as the energy supply from butter. It is obvious that, with the exception of France, where large quantities of butter (20.2 g/capita/day) are consumed, the Mediterranean countries exhibit an availability of less than 5.0 g/capita/day, and almost half have an availability of less than 2.0 g/capita/day. In comparison, we observe that the average availability in the EU is 9.9 g/capita/day, while, in the U.S., the availability falls to half of that quantity (4.1 g/capita/day). These data suggest that, in the majority of Mediterranean countries, butter does not contribute too much to milk-fat intake. However, this figure changes when we take into consideration the availability of cheese, a dairy product rich in milk fat.

2. Cheese

Cheese is a vitamin-rich, fermented food with a high content of protein, fat, calcium, and phosphorus. Its caloric and nutritive value is far greater than milk, and better than many other foods. Furthermore, because of the fermentation process and the technology of production, the water-insoluble constituents of milk (caseins and fat) are concentrated by up to 6–8 times. The degree and selection of concentration depend on the type of cheese, the kind of milk used, and the type of coagulation (enzymatic or acidic). Milk components are concentrated through the removal of the whey.

Fermentation also creates significant changes in the constituents of milk. Proteins are coagulated and split to peptones and peptides. Fat also is hydrolyzed to some degree and the fraction of free amino acids is increased. The fraction that is free fatty acids contains mainly short chain ones (butyric, capric, caprilic), which contribute to the flavor of cheese. The water-soluble components are drained with the whey and only small amounts remain in the cheese trapped in the water phase. Thus, cheese is rich in fat-soluble vitamins, but retains smaller amounts of water-soluble vitamins of the B complex and is practically deficient in lactose because what remains in the cheese is further fermented to lactic acid and other products (aldehydes, ketones) that contribute to the aroma and taste of the cheese.

Cheese is a concentrated source of proteins of high biological value. The protein fraction consists almost entirely of caseins and only small amounts of whey proteins are present. The content of caseins in essential amino acids is presented in Table 11. From the minerals, calcium and phosphorus are concentrated in cheese because they are associated in a high percentage with the caseins, while potassium, sodium, and magnesium are removed with the whey. Only chloride is present (as sodium chloride) at concentrations of up to 2–4%, because of the addition of salt.

From Table 5, it is evident that cheese contributes to the diets of Mediterranean people in a different degree depending on the country. Thus, the energy supplied with cheese varies from less than 20 kcal/capita/day in lower consumers (e.g,. Algeria, Morocco, Tunisia, Turkey, Yugoslavia, Libya) to more than 200 kcal/capita/day in the higher consumers (e.g., Greece, France). All the other countries fall between these values according to their cheese-consumption patterns.

3. Yogurt

The nutritive value of natural yogurt is based on the chemical composition of the milk from which it is produced, but with some changes in the constituents of the milk due to the fermentation process and the action of yogurt's lactic acid bacteria (*Streptococcus thermophilus* and *Lactobacillus delbrueckii* subsp. *bulgaricus*). For the other types of yogurt that cannot be described as "natural," the nutritive as well as the caloric value of the product depends on what amounts of milk protein, fat, whole-milk powder, carbohydrates, fruits, and other additives such as stabilizers, jelling ingredients, aroma-giving substances, or colorants are added. However, the numerical values of the constituents of yogurt tell only part of the story, because there are some aspects of the behavior of yogurt in the human body that are not revealed by chemical analysis. Yogurt proteins are of high biological value, higher than that of cheese proteins, not only because they contain the sulfur-rich amino acid whey proteins, but also because of the coagulation and fermentation process, which increases their digestibility.[39,40] The only carbohydrate in natural (plain) yogurt is lactose, which is fermented to lactic acid. When yogurt is ready for consumption, 15–20% of the lactose has been fermented. Yogurt also contains all the minerals of milk, but its calcium is absorbed better from the intestine and in a shorter time. Generally, yogurt is digested in half the time required for milk.[41]

In yogurt, the vitamins of the B complex are partially used by the lactic acid bacteria. Thus folic acid, pantothenic acid, B_{12} and biotin are decreased (> 50%), while folic acid and choline are increased (> 100%) due to bacterial metabolism. However, 100% of vitamin C and 10–20% of thiamine are inactivated by the heat process involved in yogurt production.[29,42,43]

4. Therapeutic Properties of Yogurt and other Fermented Milks

Yogurt and other fermented milks undoubtedly have a beneficial effect on the function of the intestine and they are considered foods that promote human health. Many authors[44-46] have reported the beneficial properties of fermented milk, especially:

- The antimicrobial activity of lactic acid bacteria of yogurt and other fermented milks against pathogenic bacteria such as *Salmonella, Shigella, Escherichia coli,* etc.[44-48]
- The better function (increased motility) of the intestine because of the lactic acid and the action of lactic acid bacteria
- The regeneration of the natural gut flora after antibiotic treatment with lactic acid strains such as *Lactobacillus acidophilus* and *L. bifidus*[49,50]

- The possible lowering effect on blood cholesterol level[51,52]
- The antitumor effect of yogurt bacteria on certain types of tumors in mice and rats[53-56]

C. The Effect of Heating on Milk Nutrients

Milk destined for human consumption either as liquid milk or as dairy products is subjected, for technological and hygienic purposes, to different heating processes. The temperatures involved in milk heating usually fall into three heating zones: (1) Pasteurization involving heating at 72°C for 15–20 seconds, (2) Ultra-High Temperature (UHT) heating in the zone of 135–140°C for 1–2 seconds and (3) in-bottle or -can sterilization, which involves a time–temperature combination of 110–120°C for 15 to 30 minutes. The above processing methods have different effects on milk nutrients.

1. Pasteurization

Time-temperature combination for HTST (High-Temperature-Short-Time) pasteurization involves heating at 72°C at least for 15 seconds at least or equally effective combinations.

The above time-temperature effect on milk nutrients can be considered as negligible. Only a slight reduction in vitamin C is observed, along with the inactivation of phosphatase, the enzyme used as an index of effective pasteurization.[57]

2. UHT and In-Bottle Sterilization

Both methods destroy almost all bacterial forms, or at least inactivate bacterial spores for the time required for the product to be marketed at ambient temperatures (commercial sterility). The effect of heating involved in both methods on milk nutrients can be summarized as follows:

- Proteins, especially β-lactoglobulin, denature up to 60–80%, but this affects the nutritional value of the proteins to a lesser degree. It is observed that sulfur amino acids are destroyed by 10% in UHT milk and up to 30% in sterilized milk.[58] Caseins are more resistant to heat, but both groups of proteins suffer from the losses of the amino acid lysine, which is destroyed at a rate of 2-10% in UHT milk and up to 30% in bottle sterilized milk. In prolonged heating (>20 minutes) there is always the chance of lysinoalanine (LAL) formation, which is nephrotoxic for rats.[25]
- Fat is affected only when milk is sterilized in bottles or cans, when there is a high degree of destruction of the unsaturated nature of the polyunsaturated fatty acids (60–80%). In the UHT milk, this loss is much lower (<30%).[59,60]
- Vitamins are affected to a different degree. Vitamin A, riboflavin, pantothenic acid, biotin, and vitamin D are almost unaffected. There is a complete destruction of vitamin C and a considerable destruction

(20–60%) of thiamin, B_6, B_{12}, and folic acid in evaporated milk, while, in UHT milk, the destruction is limited to 5–20%.[59-62]
- Calcium is precipitated to a certain percentage, but this does not affect the absorbability of calcium from the intestine.[63]

3. Drying

Today's technological methods for the production of milk powder used for human consumption do not involve high temperature, which is always kept around the pasteurization zone. Spray drying is the usual method and the whole process results in only a slight reduction of thiamine (10–20%) and a greater one in vitamin C (50%).[64,65] However, the storage conditions of milk powder can result in significant changes in fatty acids (oxidation), and discoloration (Maillard reaction), which involves reaction of lactose with the proteins and destruction of the amino acid lysine.[66]

VI. SAFETY OF MILK AND DAIRY PRODUCTS

Milk as a highly nutritious food represents an ideal substrate for the growth and multiplication of pathogenic or spoilage microorganisms. Pathogenic microorganisms in milk are derived from either the animal, from the human handlers, or from the environment during the collection, storage, and transportation of milk to the processing plant. Dairy products can be further contaminated during processing. Some pathogenic bacteria (*Mycobacterium tuberculosis, Brucella*) do not multiply freely in milk, while viruses do not multiply at all. If the temperature of storage is favorable for growth, most pathogenic bacteria can multiply, and some may produce toxins and thus increase the risk for the consumer. Furthermore, in milk, a risk for the consumer can arise from the presence of different chemical substances that might have an adverse effect to human health.

A. PATHOGENIC MICROORGANISMS

Outbreaks of milk-borne illness can be traced back to the beginning of the 20th century. It is reasonable to believe that such diseases always existed, but their study became a public health concern during the last century and especially after World War II. The most important diseases transmitted to man through milk and the causative agents are presented in Table 13.[67-70]

Historically, the profile of the most important milk-borne diseases changed profoundly in the second half of the century. Diseases like diphtheria, scarlet fever, tuberculosis, and typhoid fever, which predominated during the years up to 1950, declined dramatically and today appear to have mainly historical interest. At the same time, other diseases such as brucellosis, salmonellosis, and staphylococcal poisoning, along with newly emerged ones like listeriosis, yersiniosis, campylobacteriosis and *E. coli* O157:H7 colitis became important as milk-borne zoonoses. However, after the legally prescribed heat treatment of milk in the majority of countries after 1950, milk-borne outbreaks have continued to decrease, and today,

TABLE 13
Pathogenic Microorganisms of Public Health Importance
Transmitted from Milk or Dairy Products[67-70]

Microorganism	Disease
A. Mainly of historical importance	
Corynebacterium diphtheriae	Diphtheria
Streptococcus pyogenes	Scarlet fever, septic sore throat
Salmonella typhi	Typhoid fever
Mycobacterium tuberculosis	Tuberculosis
Mycobacterium bovis	
B. Current public health concern	
Brucella spp.	Brucellosis
Listeria monocytogenes	Listeriosis
Salmonella (other than typhi)	Salmonellosis
Campylobacter jejuni	Campylobacteriosis
Yersinia enterocolitica	Yersiniosis
Enteropathogenic *E. coli*	
(Verotoxic E. coli O157:H7)	Hemorrhagic colitis
Staphylococcus aureus	Food intoxication
Bacillus cereus	B. cereus, food poisoning
Clostridium	Botulism
C. Uncommon and/or suspected	
Shigella spp.	Shigellosis
Strept. zooepidemicus	Pneumonia, systemic infections
Mycobacterium paratuberculosis	John's/Crohn's disease
Toxoplasma gondii	Toxoplasmosis
Coxiella burnetii	Q fever
Viruses	
• Foot and Mouth Disease Virus	• Foot and mouth disease
• Poliovirus	• Poliomelitis
• Hepatitis A	• Hepatitis
• Tic-born encephalitis complex	• Encephalitis
• Norwalk and Norwalk-like virus	• Gastroenteritis

represent only a small percentage of the total food-borne outbreaks. Thus, in Europe, milk and dairy products have been incriminated in only 4.6% of the total food-borne cases during the years 1991–1993[71,72], while, for the same period, the figure was 4.2% for USA;[73] from 1975–1984, the figure was 5.6% for Canada.[74]

According to the report on the trends and sources of zoonotic agents in animals, feedstuffs, food, and man in the EU for 1997[75,] it is evident that brucellosis, campylobacteriosis, listeriosis, yersiniosis and hemorrhagic colitis due to *E. coli* O157:H7, are the main food-borne diseases in which milk and dairy products can be implicated.

Salmonellosis, although presenting a high incidence of human cases in the EU (average 73 cases/100,000 inhabitants) is due mainly to the consumption of eggs and poultry, with no references to milk or dairy products. The same report[75] mentions that, during 1977, according to the report of the member states of the EU, there were registered 3068 human cases of brucellosis (1/100,000), 205,556 cases of salmonellosis (73/100,000), 85,753 cases of campylobacteriosis (30/100,000), 5683 cases of yersiniosis (2/100,000), 614 cases of listeriosis (2/1,000,000), and 1912 cases of VTEC (Verotoxin *E. coli* O157:H7). Except for the salmonella infection, in which milk and dairy products are not implicated, in all other infections there was a non-defined percentage of cases credited to the consumption of raw milk or unpasteurized non-fermented dairy products. The epidemiological situation in the Mediterranean countries cannot be assessed correctly because of the lack of a reporting system in many of them. However, no Mediterranean country is recognized as brucellosis-free, and, although all of them legally prescribe pasteurization of milk, cases of human brucellosis due to the consumption of raw milk or unripened cheese are common.

Data published by the WHO[71,72] indicate that, in France during the years 1990–1992, milk and dairy products were responsible for 5.8% of the total food-borne cases, and in Israel, almost all cases (26.5%) were blamed on cheese consumption. In Spain, during the period of 1985–1992 on average, 3.8% of cases, and in Turkey during 1991, 12.9% of cases were attributed to cheese. In Malta, the main cause of human brucellosis was the consumption of cheese prepared at home.

B. RESIDUES AND CONTAMINANTS

The hygienic status of milk and dairy products can be affected by the presence of chemical hazards such as residues of antimicrobials, anthelminthics, pesticides, and hormones or the presence of chemical or physical hazards such as mycotoxins, polychlorinated biphenyls (PCB's), dioxins and furans, heavy metals, and finally radioactive elements.[76]

However, the existing data suggest that the levels of contaminants in milk in all countries applying a monitoring system for substances like heavy metals, pesticides, and persistent polychlorinated environmental chemicals like PCB's and dioxins, are declining and are always below the permissible levels.[76] Thus biological hazards play the most important role in determining the safety of milk and dairy products with the chemical hazards representing a small percentage of the total health risk.

C. INCREASING THE SAFETY OF MILK AND DAIRY PRODUCTS

The production of dairy foods of high quality and safety is based on a number of independent measures taken at different levels of production (farm, processing plant, retailer). At the farm, measures are relevant to the health of the animal and the protection of milk from contamination during collection, storage, and transportation to the processing plant. Processors apply methods to ensure microbiological quality (e.g. pasteurization, UHT treatment, fermentation, etc.). Finally, pasteurized milk or other dairy products are distributed under refrigerated conditions.

Many of the above measures have been put in place by government regulations, along with standards and end-product testing for microbiological or chemical parameters and adulterations. Today, there is a growing awareness that end-product testing cannot by itself ensure the safety of a food. To be able to prevent the different hazards that might enter food and reach the consumer, it is necessary to take preventive measures in all the steps of production and marketing from stable to table. The critical points in the production chains in which a hazard might occur must be identified and the relevant hazards must be monitored. The hazards that must be controlled are biological (microorganisms or their toxins), chemical (residues or contaminants), and physical, such as radioactivity, foreign bodies, etc.[77,78] To identify and enforce these standards, the Hazard Analysis Critical Control Point (HACCP) system came into use. An HACCP system identifies hazards and applies measures for their control to ensure the safety of a food. It should be applied all the way from the primary production at the farm to the consumer's table. In 1996, the USDA/FSIS[79] published the proposed rule Pathogen Reduction Hazard Analysis and Critical Control Point (HACCP) systems for meat and poultry inspection in the U.S., which gradually became effective starting July 25, 1996. The EU, in Directive 93/43, advised the industry to apply procedures for the management of food safety based on the principles of the HACCP system in the different sectors of the food industry, and published useful guidelines for such programs.[82] The application of an HACCP system does not imply that the measures concerning the concept of good hygiene practice (GHP) and good manufacturing practice (GMP) such as prescribed by Directive 92/46[80] for milk and 93/43[81] for food hygiene are not necessary. On the contrary, they are the basis on which the HACCP system will rely for effective critical control point monitoring. Today, dairy industries are among the first to recognize the necessity and to apply HACCP systems. This ensures the safety of dairy products and continues to decrease their implication in food-borne diseases.

VII. CONCLUSIONS

Milk production in the Mediterranean countries varies greatly, since there are countries with a production of more than 200 kg/capita/year and others with a production of less than 100 kg/capita/year. Thus, the availability, which is governed by the production and import–export balance, varies accordingly.

- Countries with a high production of milk have also a satisfactory availability in milk equivalent, which falls between 250–300 kg/capita/year. The relevant energy supply in these countries coming from milk and dairy products is significant, representing 10–15% of the total energy supplied by the diet, and 30–50% of the energy supplied by foods of animal origin.
- In some Mediterranean countries with a moderate production of milk, the availability of milk equivalent falls between 100 and 200 kg/capita/year. In these countries, the contribution of milk and dairy products to the diet can be characterized as inadequate.
- Finally, there are Mediterranean countries (mainly the North African ones) with a very low availability in milk equivalent (less than 5 g of milk protein intake per capita/day) and thus milk and dairy products have an insignificant contribution to the diet of their people.

REFERENCES

1. Tamine, A. Y., Dalgleish, D., and Banks, W., Introduction, in *Feta and Related Cheeses*, Robinson, P.K. and Tamine, A. Y., Eds., Ellis Horwood, London, 1991.
2. Scott, R., *Cheesemaking Practice*, 2nd. ed. Elsevier Appl. Sci. Publ., London, 1986.
3. FAO, Faostat Databases, http://apps.fao.org/lim500/nph-wrap.pl? Production. Livestock. Primary, 1999.
4. FAO, Faostat Database, http://apps.fao.org/lim500/nph-wrap.pl? Production. Livestock. Derived, 1999.
5. FAO, Faostat Database, http://apps.fao.org/lim500/nph-wrap.pl? Food. Balance Sheet.
6. Lee, F.A., *Basic Food Chemistry*, AVI Publ. Co. Westport, Conn., 1975.
7. Renner, E., Renz-Schauen, A., and Drathen, M., *Nutrition Composition Tables of Milk and Dairy Products*, Drathen, V. M., Ed. Giessen, 1996.
8. Johnson, A. H., The composition of milk, in *Fundamentals of Dairy Chemistry*, 2nd ed. Webb, B.H., Johnson, A.H., and Alford, J.A., Eds., AVi Publ. Co. Westport Connecticut, 1974, Chap. 1
9. Kurtz, F. E., The lipids of milk. Composition and properties, in *Fundamentals of Dairy Chemistry* 2nd ed., Webb, B. H., Johnson, A. H., and Alford, J. A., Eds. AVI Publ. Co. Westport Conn., 1978, Chap. 4
10. Christie, W. W., The composition and structure of milk lipids, in *Developments in Dairy Chemistry*, Vol. 2, *Lipids,* Fox, P.F. ed., Appl. Sci. Publs, London, 1983, Chap. 1
11. Keenan, T. W., Dylewski, D. P., and Woodford, J. A., Origin of milk fat globules and the nature of the milk fat globule membrane, in *Developments in Dairy Chemistry, Vol. 2 Lipids*, Fox. P. F., ed. Appl. Sci. Publ. London, 1983, Chap. 3.
12. Mulder, H. and Walstra, P. *The Milk Fat Globule*, Commonwealth Agriculture Bureau, England, 1974.
13. Mercier, J. C., Brignon, G., and Ribadeau-Dumas, B., Structure primaire de la casein αs_2 bovine, *Eur. J. Biochem.* 23, 41, 1971.
14. Eigel, W. N., Buttler, J. E., Ernstrom, C. A., Farrel, H. M. Jr., Harwalker, V. R., Jenness, A., and Whitney, R. McL. Nomenclature of proteins of cow's milk. 5th revision, *J. Dairy Sci.* 67, 1599, 1984.
15. Swaisgood, H. E., Characteristics of milk, in *Food Chemistry*, 3rd ed., Fennema, O. R., Ed. Marcell Dekker, Inc. New York, 1996, Chap. 14.
16. Brignon, G., Ribadeau-Dumas, B., Mercier, J. C., Pelisier, J. P., and Das, B. C., Complet amino acid sequence of bovine αs_2 casein, *FEBS Lett.* 76, 277, 1977.
17. Swaisgood, H. E. Chemistry of milk proteins, in *Developments in Dairy Chemistry*, Vol. 1, *Proteins*, Fox, P. F. ed. Appl. Sci. Publs. London, 1982, Chap. 1.
18. Walstra, P., On the stability of casein micelles. *J. Dairy Sci.* 73, 1975, 1990.
19. Slattery, C. W., Review: Casein micelle structure. An examination of models. *J. Dairy Sci.* 59, 1547, 1976.
20. Brew, K., Kastellino, F. G., Vanaman, T. C., and Hill, R. L., The complete amino acid sequences of bovine α-lactablumin, *J. Biol. Chem.* 245, 4570, 1970.
21. Bell, K. M., McKentzie, H. A., Murphy, W. H., and Show, C., β-Lactoglobulin (Droughtmaster). A unique protein varient, *Bioch. Bioph. Acta*. 214, 427, 1970.
22. Nickerson, T. A., Lactose, in *Fundamentals of Dairy Chemistry*, 2nd ed. Webb, B.H., Johnson, A.H., and Alford, J.A., Eds. AVI. Publ. Co. Westport, Conn., 1978, Chap. 6.
23. Jenness, R., The composition of milk, in *Lactation,* Vol. III., Carson, L., and Smith V.R., Eds., Acad. Press. London, 1974, Chap. 1.

24. Holt, C., The milk salts: Their secretion, concentration and physical chemistry, in *Developments in Dairy Chemistry*, Vol. 3, *Lactose and Minor Constituents*, Fox, P. F., Ed., Elsvier Appl. Sci., London, 1985, Chap. 6.

25. Renner, E., *Milk and Dairy Products in Human Nutrition*, W-Gmbh, Verlang, Munchen, 1983.

26. Jensen, R.G. and Water, B. Fat-soluble vitamins in bovine milk, in *Handbook of Milk Composition*, Jensen, R. G., Ed., Acad. Press, New York, 1995, Chap. 8.

27. Shahani, K. M., Harper, W. J., Jensen, R. G., Perry, R. M., and Zittle, C. A., Enzymes in bovine milk, *J. Dairy Sci.* 56, 531, 1975.

28. Fakye, N. Y., Other enzymes, in *Advanced Dairy Chemistry,* I. *Proteins*, Fox P.F., Ed., Elsvier Appl. Sci. London, 1992.

29. Wilster, G. H., *Practical Cheesemaking*, O.S.U. Book Stores, Corvallis, Oregon, 1980.

30. Kosikowski, F.K. and Mistry, V.V., *Cheese and Fermented Milk Foods*, Vol. I; Origins and Principles, Kosikowski, F. V., Publ. Westport Conn., 1997.

31. FAO/WHO, Recommended International Standards for Cheese and Government Acceptances, FAO, CAC/ C_1-C_{25}, Rome, 1972.

32. Rasic, J. Lj. and Kurmann, J. A., *Yogurt: Scientific Grounds, Technology, Manufacture and Preparations*, Technical Dairy Publ. House, Copenhagen, 1978.

33. Alais, C., *Science du Lait. Principles de Techniques Laitieres*, 3ème ed. Sep. Paris, 1974.

34. Gurr, M. I., The nutritional significance of lipids, in *Developments in Dairy Chemistry*, Vol. 2, Fox, P. F., Ed. Appl. Sci. Publs, London, 1983, Chap. 8.

35. Gordon, W. G. and Kalan, E. B., Proteins of milk, in *Fundamentals of Dairy Chemistry*, Webb, B. H., Johnson, A. H., and Alford J. A., Eds., The AVI Publ. Comp. Inc., Westeport, Connecticut, 1978 Chap. 3.

36. Featherstone, W. R., Morris, M. L., and Phillips, P. H., Influence of lactose and dried skim milk upon the magnesium deficiency syndrome in the dog. I. Growth and biochemical data, *J. Nutr.*, 79, 431, 1963.

37. Schaafsma, G., The significance of milk as a source of dietary calcium, in *Int. Dairy Federation Bull.,* No 166,1982.

38. Causeret, J., Lhuissier, M., and Hugo, D., Les vitamins dans les proteins laitieres, *Ann Nutr. Aliment.* 24B, 169, 1970.

39. Kon, S.K., *Milk and Milk Products in Human Nutrition*, FAO Nutritional Series No 27, Rome, 1972.

40. Stojsavljevic, T. and Curic, R., A study on the amino acids of yogurt. I. Amino acid content and biological value of the proteins of different kinds of milk, *Milchwissenschaft*, 26, 147, 1971.

41. Helferich, W. and Westhoff, D., *All About Yogurt,* Prentice Hall Inc., Englewood, NJ, 1980.

42. Reddy, K. P., Sahani, K. M., and Kulkarni, S. M., B-Complex vitamins in cultured and acidified yogurt, *J. Dairy Sci.*, 59, 19, 1976.

43. Tamine, A. Y. and Robinson, R.K., *Yogurt, Science and Technology*, Pergamon Press, Oxford, 1985.

44. Racic, J. Lj. and Mitic. S., Contribution a l' étude de l' activité antibiotique des souches des culture du yogurt, *Le Lait* 43, 489, 1964.

45. Singh, J. and Lexmimarayana, H., Antibacterial activity of *Lactobacilli*, *Indian Dairy Sci.* 26, 135, 1973.

46. Spillmann, H., Puhan, Z., and Bonhegyi, M., Antimicrobielle activitat thermophiler *lactobazillen*, *Milchwissenschaft*, 339, 148, 1978.

47. Singh, J., Khanna, A., and Chandez, H., Antibacterial activity of yogurt starter in cow and buffalo milk, *J. Food Prot.* 42, 664, 1979.

48. Gilliland, S. E. and Speck, M. L., Antagonistic action of *Lactobacillus acidophilus*, toward intestinal and food-borne pathogens associative culture, *J. Food Protect.*, 40, 820, 1977.

49. Bianchi-Salvatori, B., Camaschella, P., and Bazigaluppi, E., Distribution and adherence of *Lactobacillus bulgaricus* in the gastroenteric tract of germ-free animals, *Milchwissenschaft*, 39, 387, 1984.

50. Hargrove, R. E. and Alford, J. A., Growth rate and feed efficiency of rats fed yogurt and other fermented milks, *J. Dairy Sci.,* 61, 1, 1978.

51. Speck, M. L., Interaction among lactobacilli and man, *J. Dairy Sci.,* 59, 338, 1976.

52. Mann, G. V., A factor in yogurt which lowers cholostrol in man, *Atherosclerosis*, 26, 335, 1997.

53. Reddy, G. V., Shahani, K. M., and Banerjee, M. R., Inhibitory effect of yogurt on Ehrlich ascites tumor cell proliferation, *J. Natl. Cancer. Inst.,* 50, 815, 1973.

54. Farmier, R. E., Shahani, K. M., and Reddy G. V., Inhibition effect of yogurt components, *J. Dairy Sci.,* 58, 787, 1975.

55. Reddy, G. V., Frient, B. A., Shahani, K. M., and Farmier, R. E., Antitumor activity of yogurt components, *J. Food Prot.* 46, 8, 1983.

56. Shahani, K. M., Friend, B. A., and Bailey, P. J., Antitumor activity of fermented colostrums and milk, *J. Food Prot.* 46, 385, 1983.

57. Lewis, M. J., Advances in heat treatment of milk, in *Modern Dairy Technology,* Vol. 1, *Advances in Milk Processing,* Robinson, R. K., Ed. Elsvier Appl. Sci. London, 1986, Chap. 1.

58. Aboshama, K. and Hansen, A. P., Effect of ultra high temperature steam injection processing on sulfur containing amino acids, *J. Dairy Sci.,* 60, 1374, 1977.

59. Van Eekelen, M., Heijne, J.J.I.G., Nutritive value of sterilized milk, in *Milk Sterilization,* FAO Agr. Studies No 65, Rome, 1965.

60. Metha, R. S., Milk processed in ultra-high temperature. A review, *J. Food Prot.*, 43, 312, 1980.

61. Burton, H., Ford, J. E., Perkin, A. G., Potter, J. W. G., Scott, K. J., Thompson, S. V., Toothill, T., and Edwards-Webb, J. D., Comparison of milks processed by the direct and indirect methods of ultra-high temperature sterilization. IV. The vitamin composition of milks sterilized by different processes. *J. Dairy Research*, 37, 529, 1970.

62. Görner, F., and Uherova, R., Retention von einigen Vitaminen während der Ultrachocherhitzung von Milch, *Nachrung* 24, 713, 1980.

63. Pelet, B. and Donath, A., Effect of utilization of homogenized cow's milk on nitrogen balance, phosphorus, calcium and potassium in new-born infants. *Helvetica Pediatrica Acta,* 29, 35, 1974.

64. Kon, S. K., *Milk and Milk Products in Human Nutrition*, FAO, Nutritional Series No 27, Rome, 1972.

65. Harris, R. S. and Karmas, E., *Nutritional Evaluation of Food Processing,* AVI Publ. Co. Westport Conn., 1975.

66. Moller, A. B., Andrews, A. T., and Cheeseman, G. C., Chemical changes in ultra-heat-treated milk during storage, II. Lactuloselysine and fructoselysine formation by the Maillard reaction, *J. Dairy Res.* 44, 267, 1977.

67. Kaplan, M. M., Abdussalam, M., and Bilega, G., Diseases transmitted through milk, in *Milk Hygiene*, WHO monograph series No 48, Geneva, 1962. pp. 11–74.

68. Heeschen, W. H., Introduction, in *The Significance of Pathogenic Microorganisms in Milk*, International Dairy Federation (IDF) No S.I. 9405, Brussels, 1994.

69. Boor, K. J., Pathogenic microorganisms of concern to the dairy industry, *Dairy Food and Envir. San.*, 17, 714, 1997.

70. Ryser, E. T., Public health concerns, in *Applied Dairy Microbiology*, Marth, E. H. and Steele, J. L., Eds, Marcell Dekker Inc., New York, 1998, Chap. 11.

71. WHO. Surveillance programme for the control of food-borne infections and intoxications in Europe, 4th Report 1983/1984. Institute of Veterinary Medicine, Berlin, 1990.

72. WHO. Surveillance programme for the control of food-borne infections and intoxications in Europe, 5th Report 1985/1989. Institute of Veterinary Medicine, Berlin, 1992.

73. Bean, N. H., Goulding, J. S., Daniels, M. T., and Angulo, F. J., Surveillance for food-borne disease outbreaks. U.S. 1988–1992. *J. Food Prot.* 60, 1265, 1997.

74. Todd, E. E. D., Food-borne disease in Canada-a 10-year summary from 1975–1984. *J. Food Prot.* 55, 123, 1992.

75. European Commission. Trends and Sources of Zoonotic Agents in Animals, Feedstuffs, Food and Man in the EU in 1997, Document VI/8495/98EN-Rev-2, 1998.

76. International Dairy Federation (IDF). *Monograph on Residues and Contaminants in Milk and Milk Products*. Special Issue 9701, Brussels, 1997.

77. Pierson, M. D. and Corlett, D. A., *HACCP Principles and Applications*, Chapman & Hall, London, 1992.

78. International Commission on Microbiological Specifications for Foods (ICMSF). *Microorganisms in Foods*. 4. Application of Hazard Analysis Critical Control Point (HACCP) system to ensure microbiological safety and quality. Blackwell Scientific Publ. London, 1988.

79. USDA/FSIS, Pathogen Reduction. Hazard Analysis and Critical Control Point (HACCP) Systems. Final Rule. Federal Register Vol. 61, No 144, pp. 38806-38898, 1996.

80. European Commission Council Directive 92/46/EEC of 16 June 1992, Laying down the health rules for the production and placing on the market of raw milk and milk-based products. Official Journal Of the European Communities. No L. 268, 14.09.1992, p.1.

81. European Commission Council Directive 93/43/EEC of 14 June 1993, on hygiene of foodstuffs. Official Journal Of the European Communities. No L.175, 14.06.1993, p.1.

82. European Commission Principles for the development of risk assessment of microbiological hazard under Directive 93/43/EEC, concerning the hygiene of foodstuffs. European Communities. Publ. Office, Luxemburg, 1998.

7 Meat and Meat Products

Spyros A. Georgakis

CONTENTS

I. INTRODUCTION

Throughout time, nations of the world have developed their own distinctive dietary habits. Locally grown and produced foodstuffs, national customs, and traditions, as well as contact with neighboring people, all contribute to the making of a regional diet. One such regional diet is the so-called Mediterranean Diet, which has deservedly attracted considerable attention from scientists and connoisseurs on a global level.

Greece is the exemplary case study for the Mediterranean Diet, since Greek dietary habits have remained largely unaffected through the ages. Countless historical sources and archaeological findings bear witness to the parallel of today's eating habits with those of Ancient Greece. The lean, muscular appearance of Greek youths of old portrayed in sculpture and pottery are reflected in today's new generations – although today, Greeks are much taller, partly due to the increased consumption of protein.

0-8493-0110-6/01/$0.00+$.50
© 2001 by CRC Press LLC

Rising living standards may have led to increased consumption of meat and dairy products, but essentially the same species of plant and animal life have remained central to nutrition since the time of Homer.

For centuries, Greeks have relied on their home-grown produce. Although largely mountainous and lacking in great plains, this part of the world is blessed with a remarkably mild climate that supports great biodiversity. In addition to mainland produce, the Mediterranean generously offers its people a wealth of fish and seafoods.

Meat and its products feature strongly in the Mediterranean Diet. Despite the pressures of modern life, many Greeks are deeply religious people and adhere to strict fasting according to the Orthodox Christian calendar, which limits consumption of red meat. For many centuries, meat has been a festive food, reserved for the great holidays and celebrations such as weddings, and it has therefore enjoyed a privileged position within the culture of the eastern Mediterranean.

The example of meat demonstrates that changing lifestyles and the erosion of traditional cultures will not only alter the identity of the Mediterranean people, but will ultimately affect the harmony of their diet — ironically, at a time when the benefits of that particular way of eating have become recognized worldwide.

II. MEAT AND MEAT PRODUCTS

A. MEAT

1. What is Meat?

To the average person, meat is the linear muscle tissue of warm-blooded animals (mammals, fowl) that humans consume. This definition of meat includes the small blood vessels, the muscle peritoneum and pieces of tendons that belong to them as well as intramuscular fat.

According to Judge,[1] meat is defined as "those animal tissues which are suitable to use as food."

To be suitable for human consumption, meat should possess certain recognizable qualities or characteristics, the combination of which results in the total meat quality.[2] These features are classified in the following four categories:

1. **Sensory features**. Color, smell, taste, tenderness, and juiciness are those qualities that man judges through the senses.
2. **Nutritional value**. Can be judged on the basis of meat's content of:
   - Nutritional components such as the quantity and quality of proteins and fats and the quantity of carbohydrates.
   - Components with no nutritional value themselves, but which facilitate a more efficient usage of nutritional elements and help in various body functions. These are vitamins, minerals, and trace elements.
   - Elements that define the taste of meat, such as organic acids, non-protein nitrogenous extracts, etc.

- Digestive ability, biological value, and, finally, the method of processing the meat.

3. **Hygienic and toxicological condition**. The hygiene of meat depends on the existence or absence of a variety of pathogenic microrganisms, and on the existence of metabolic products of these pathogens. The toxicological condition depends on the existence and concentration of residues of organic and inorganic substances (chemicals), regardless of how these substances came to be present in the meat.
4. **Technological qualities**.

2. Postmortem Physiological Changes in Meat

A series of changes must take place before a slaughtered animal can be offered as meat for consumption. These changes are of vital importance to human nutrition and the quality of the product, and they start immediately after the animal is slaughtered. They form a chain of complex biochemical and physiochemical reactions in which the meat's enzymes play a pivotal role. The end results of these processes are two natural and desirable conditions: First, rigor mortis, and second, the maturation of the meat.[3,4] Mature meat is tender, chewable, juicy, digestible, and full of aroma and flavor.[5] Its color depends on animal species, age, type of feeding, and also on its fat content. Younger animals tend to have light red meat. A small quantity of fat between the muscle tissue — what is commonly referred to as marbling — is desirable and denotes meat of excellent nutritional value.

The time period required for the maturation process depends on many factors. Of great importance is the temperature of the environment in which the meat is kept, the species of animal, and its condition before slaughter.[6] In chilled cabinets, bovine meat matures in 13–14 days, pork in 3 days, and poultry in 36 hours.[4,7,8]

During the maturation process, important transformations take place in the structure of muscle tissue that combine to give meat its desirable characteristics. Thus, changes in collagen, the destruction of the Z line in the muscle tissue due to the action of calpaine, the hydrolysis of Tronin-T, Nebulin, Aktin and a-Aktinin, all contribute to the tenderness of the meat.[7]

However, diversions from the expected maturation processes can occur, and these result in abnormal maturation, and, therefore, tough meat that is difficult to chew, watery, sticky, and too dark or too light in color. Water retention can be too great, in which case, we have DFD (dark, firm, dry) meat and the DCB condition (dark cutting beef); or it can be too little, which results in PSE (pale, soft, exudative) meat. Quick freezing of the carcass in very low temperatures before the onset of rigor mortis can result in the shortening of the tissue length (cold shortening) which makes meat tough and difficult to chew even after maturation.[3,8,9] In all of these cases, meat is still suitable for consumption, but is of inferior quality and consumers will reject it.

Following maturation, if meat is not consumed and if it is not packaged, stored, and protected accordingly, bacteria will start to grow that will ultimately lead to rotting, and the final stages of decomposition and destruction.[10,11]

B. Meat Products

All foodstuffs that are mainly meat or in which meat is included are considered meat products. This category does not include frozen meat, but does include minced or ground meat.

This is the largest food group there is. The range of products is extremely varied, partly because essentially the same product may take different names in different parts of the world or may be labeled under a variety of brand names, depending on the manufacturer. Lerche's study of 1972[12] listed no fewer than 1127 kinds of sausages in West Berlin and West Germany alone. The preferred method for classification of meat products is according to the technology of processing.[13,14]

Many products that fall under diverse classification categories play an important part in the Mediterranean Diet. Currently, these include minced and some processed canned meat such as corned beef, chopped meat, and luncheon meat; some boiled sausages, especially of the frankfurter type; a great variety of dry-cured traditional Greek sausages such as those originating in the regions of Lefkas and Thasos, and the semi-dry Serres sausages; and, finally, freshly made meat burgers (*soutzoukakia*). Very widely consumed are beefburgers (hamburgers), and the traditional Greek meat delicacies called gyros and souvlaki.

III. PRODUCTION, IMPORT, EXPORT, AND AVAILABILITY OF MEAT AND MEAT PRODUCTS

A. Production of Meat

To respond to the necessary dietary requirements for protein of high biological value, modern man rears various animals, usually in an industrial manner.

On a global level, animal husbandry represents a considerable percentage of world economies — the exact monetary value of which is difficult to calculate. The national economy of certain countries is almost entirely dependent on the production of meat (such as New Zealand), while others lacking in this sector are obliged to import large amounts. In Greece, the expenditure for meat imports is very high, following that of petroleum imports. According to statistics obtained from the Bank of Greece,[15,16] the following amounts were spent for imports of meat and by-products: 1985 —$522,181,000; 1990 — $880,391,000; 1997 — $874,697,000.

In 1998, on a global level, there were 1.3 billion cattle, 160 million buffalos, 19 million camels, 1.05 billion sheep, 675 million goats, 956.5 million pigs and 13.6 billion chickens.[17,18] The largest farms are to be found in the U.S. and the European Community (EU,)[15] in Australia, and in China, where more than 360 million pigs are reared. The number of animals shows a small but steady yearly increase.

During the past few decades, certain states have placed great emphasis on the development of bovine meat production and, from the mid-1980s onward, a trend has developed for the production of "organic" meat, especially in France. This trend has spread to Italy, Germany, Sweden, the U.S., and Japan. Greece joined these efforts to produce organic meat a few years back. The term organic is used to classify meat that derives from animals that were bred under natural conditions, with organic feeds, i.e., feeds that were free of additives, growth promoters, and meat meal, and raised in natural surroundings with plenty of space. These animals are normally slaughtered when they are less than 24 months old (usually 16–17 months); transport and slaughtering procedures are planned so as to avoid stress for the animal. This meat's pH_{24} should amount to less than 6.0. The meat is offered to the consumer only after the maturation process is complete, which for bovine meat means at least 7 days in refrigeration.

Total meat and meat-product production in some Mediterranean countries, as compared with the U.S., is presented in Table 1.[21] The comparison yields two conclusions:

1. Overall meat production is on the increase.
2. The percentage of growth is steadily decreasing.

Meat production in Greece is steadily decreasing, with an average factor of 3.7% between 1990 and 1997. At the same time, the growth rate of meat production, which, according to FAO, reached 21% during the same period, is increasing in the U.S. Similarly, in Israel, the increase rate reached 37%.[22] The decrease in meat production in Greece can be attributed to unchanging levels of consumption in addition to deterrent factors for farming such as high production costs, lack of manual labor, and reluctance on the part of younger generations to take up farming.

TABLE 1
Meat (M) and Meat Product (MP) Production (metric tons) in the USA and some Mediterranean Countries[21,23]

Year	Product	USA	Greece	Albania	Cyprus	Egypt	Israel	Italy	Spain	Turkey
1961	M	16,513,030	155,846	25,410	11,404	295,960	62,550	1,470,650	659,863	477,924
	MP	21,000	6,935	*	711	*	*	1,528	*	*
1970	M	21.330,296	308,520	31,180	33,331	369,175	105,545	2,495,800	1,489,427	571,695
	MP	42,630	150	*	1,779	*	*	2,331	*	*
1980	M	24,450,200	531,201	41,800	33,635	435,441	184,790	3,563,737	2,643,842	687,683
	MP	16,142	29,525	*	1,893	*	280	3,762	100	*
1990	M	28,638,768	528,541	54,000	67.038	780,405	233,645	3,947,563	3,466,616	1,160,869
	MP	15,570	32,231	*	3,451	*	1,240	4,507	*	614
1997	M	34,889,000	509,105	61,800	94,240	120,074	321,900	4,059,242	4,276,658	1,254,923
	MP	17,380	35,263	400	4,730	*	1,300	11,200	3,200	*

* There are no statistics available.

Furthermore, red meat has suffered from serious incidents such as bovine spongiform encephalopathy, or BSE (mad cow) disease, and cases of substances such as dioxins (1998), which have all played their part in the creation of a negative climate toward the consumption of red meat. In addition, in some countries such as Turkey, consumers suffer economic difficulties, which explain low levels of meat production.

Despite falling meat production, there is a noteworthy increase in certain sausage meats and other meat products (Table 1).

B. IMPORTATION OF MEAT AND MEAT PRODUCTS

Table 2 shows meat and meat products imports[23] that took place during the years 1961 to 1967 in eight Mediterranean countries, as well as the U.S. With the exception of Turkey, Cyprus, and the U.S., meat imports increased during the last decade. Again, the same trend for a diminishing growth rate during the years 1990 to 1997 is apparent.

TABLE 2
Meat (M) and Meat Products (MP) Imports (metric tons)[21–23]

Year	Product	USA	Greece	Albania	Cyprus	Egypt	Israel	Italy	Spain	Turkey
1961	M	525,078	28,159	0	5,013	12,458	3,925	81,786	12,241	13
	MP	159,168	3,019	*	3,550	2,145	1,520	10,998	3,303	*
1970	M	1,046,836	130,887	0	5,746	9,251	37,634	428,594	109,726	*
	MP	328,406	6,082	*	3,760	5,328	2,086	19,103	11,647	*
1980	M	1,153,891	126,327	0	7,423	136,256	28,063	771,946	59,249	*
	MP	229,501	6,464	*	2,397	12,059	–	32,792	18,411	*
1990	M	1,411,779	242,436	4,500	6,337	124,740	28,264	1,099,438	236,910	10,295
	MP	257,360	12,366	*	1,673	9,881	10	37,391	25,189	123
1997	M	1,335,282	361,377	13,311	4,843	135,569	58,851	1,155,092	261,307	975
	MP	191,425	13,563	1,677	1,481	1,965	240	33,715	32,170	45

* There are no statistics available.

Imports of meat products follow an upward trend, apart from the period 1990–1997 when a slowdown is observed. Imports into the U.S., Egypt, and Israel, especially, have been curbed dramatically.

C. EXPORT OF MEAT AND MEAT PRODUCTS

Apart from the U.S., the countries under discussion are not self-sufficient in meat production. Certain kinds of meat however, such as pork, exceed demand within these countries and are therefore exported (Table 3).

Exports from Central and Northern Europe usually target the Mediterranean countries as well as Russia. A significant quantity of pork is exported from Denmark to Korea and Japan, countries that pose extremely high standards for meat imports. Meat exports from the EU (924,353 MT) during 1997 were very significant, since there were 2,200,000 MT more than the imports for the same year (1997) while the EU exported 5,200,000 MT more than the U.S.

Exports of meat products (Table 3) were limited by comparison with imports. The exceptions to this trend are in the U.S., Italy, and Spain, where exports of meat

TABLE 3
Exports of Meat (M) and Meat Products (MP) from the USA and some Mediterranean Countries (metric tons)[21,22]

Year	Pro-duct	USA	Greece	Albania	Cyprus	Egypt	Israel	Italy	Spain	Turkey
1961	M	170,972	8	0	*	80	462	7800	1575	34
	MP	20,998	5	0	17	30	0	12,621	902	11
1970	M	122,925	48	0	864	43	248	22,251	5219	3880
	MP	18,118	26	0	0	0	0	25,972	632	14
1980	M	582,129	3334	90	221	81	18,453	104,352	19,854	8016
	MP	16,485	23	0	35	2	1,826	52,589	7683	0
1990	M	1.206,672	5203	5	750	5586	7,212	161,913	83,683	8606
	MP	68,966	2454	0	70	111	3,048	49,741	5136	150
1997	M	4,004,012	18,571	238	3717	1378	7,019	346,801	437,238	10,253
	MP	387,330	10,273	0	125	140	3,110	85,918	85,744	1,468

* There are no statistics available.

products during the year 1997 were double the imports. The kinds of meat products that are more likely to be exported are local traditional products.

D. AVAILABILITY OF MEAT AND MEAT PRODUCTS

A closer look at imports and exports can indicate the total meat consumption of a region. Table 4 shows meat consumption (including consumption of meat products) per person per year. To calculate the figures for meat products, we assume that the amount of lean meat represents 30% or less of the average weight of meat products. The yearly increase in the amount of meat consumption is steady in the U.S., while it varies for other countries (Figure 1).

TABLE 4
Total Availability of Meat (kg/year/person) in the U.S. and some Mediterranean Countries[28]

Year	USA	Greece	Albania	Cyprus	Egypt	Israel	Italy	Spain	Turkey
1961	88.7	21.7	15.3	28.3	10.8	30	30.5	20.1	17.37
1970	105.7	49.0	14.6	56.8	10.7	48.1	53.9	46.2	16.9
1980	108.2	64.9	15.6	60.8	13.1	50.2	75.2	70.3	15.3
1990	112.9	71.5	17.8	95.9	16.4	54.6	85.2	92.2	71.0
1997	117.6	78.7	24.1	111.8	20.1	63.3	85	102.6	19.6

It is important to consider the amount of protein of both vegetable and animal origin consumed in Mediterranean countries and the U.S. Table 5 shows such a

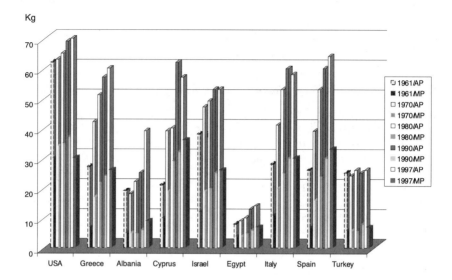

FIGURE 1   Animal (AP) and meat (MP) protein availability (kg/yr/person) in the USA and some Mediterranean countries.

comparison. Figure 1, based on the data of Table 5, shows the correlation between meat protein availability and vegetable protein availability. There is an evident trend for reduction in meat protein availability in the U.S., Greece, and Italy.

To make this transition clearer, we used the Animal Protein Availability (APA) Index, which defines the ratio of consumed vegetable protein to animal protein (Figure 2).

The ideal index is 1.0. That means that the animal protein should represent about 50–55% of the total protein. Obviously, a negative indication for the APA would reflect a low percentage of consumption of meat from animal sources (Table 6).

Figure 2 demonstrates how consumption patterns in the listed countries diverge from the suggested ideal. The figures prove that, in the majority of countries in question, APA is negative, which means that, despite the increase in meat consumption, consumption of vegetable protein dominates.

In some countries, the consumption of meat protein is far from the ideal, even in countries with more advanced economies. In the U.S., the APA index remained stable from 1961 to 1997, with values around 0.5, which is far from the ideal (Table 6). This simply means that protein consumption from animal sources in the U.S. is higher than from vegetable sources. However, even in other countries such as Greece, consumption of proteins from animal sources between 1961 and 1997 increased, with a parallel decrease in consumption of protein of vegetable origin. Consumption of animal protein in 1961 was 27.3 g/day/person, while that of vegetable protein was 56.2 g/day/cap. The ratio was completely altered in 1997, when consumption of animal protein increased to 60.7 g/day/person vegetable protein (APA: 0.89).

Regarding the consumption pattern of the type of fat consumed in the Mediterranean countries, the ratio of animal to vegetable fat consumption is fairly homo-

TABLE 5
Total Availability of Vegetable and Meat Proteins and Fats (kg/year/person)[22,28]

Year	USA	Greece	Albania	Cyprus	Egypt	Israel	Italy	Spain	Turkey
1961									
Vegetable proteins	32.3	56.2	47.5	44.9	50.5	51.0	52.7	52.7	65.3
Animal proteins	62.8	27.3	19.0	21.7	8.3	38.2	28.6	26.4	25.9
Meat proteins	30.6	7.3	5.7	10.4	4.0	12.0	11.2	7.5	6.2
Vegetable fats	40.8	61.1	15.1	59.7	27.9	54.1	43.3	45.6	45.8
Animal fats		25.3	30.1	21.8	11.6	31.7	32.8	22.3	30.9
1970									
Vegetable proteins	31.4	57.1	51.1	46.8	55.5	49.6	55.4	43.6	66.7
Animal proteins	63.5	42.0	18.6	39.0	8.5	47.5	41.8	39.8	24.7
Meat proteins	34.6	17.4	5.3	19.8	4.0	19.3	20.2	16.5	5.9
Vegetable fats	54.3	70.1	21.4	64.0	70.1	58.6	64.5	54.6	44.3
Animal fats	62.1	37.8	30.9	40.8	12.3	40.0	46.8	34.3	28.4
1980									
Vegetable proteins	31.8	51.1	56.0	39.8	62.2	47.9	53.9	43.5	71.2
Animal proteins	65.5	51.7	22.1	40.1	10.5	49.9	53.7	53.8	26.8
Meat proteins	35.7	22.4	22.1	40.1	10.5	49.9	53.7	53.8	26.8
Vegetable fat	63.4	79.4	32.6	67.8	47.1	64.9	67.3	65.9	59.8
Animal fats	63.6	45.2	27.5	42.4	17.6	38.0	61.5	46.3	28.6
1990									
Vegetable proteins	38.4	53.4	56.3	40.7	71.1	50.9	49.8	43.5	76.4
Animal proteins	69.0	57.9	25.2	62.4	13.3	53.1	60.0	60.4	25.7
Meat proteins	37.4	24.3	6.5	32.2	6.2	25.1	30.6	30.5	
Vegetable fats	74.5	89.3	30.4	72.0	41.0	75.8	80.3	80.6	67.4
Animal fats	64.0	51.0	33.5	55.0	17.0	40.2	70.0	56.4	25.8
1997									
Vegetable proteins	41.8	54.2	59.1	41.9	74.2	51.8	50.1	42.6	71.3
Animal proteins	70.5	60.7	39.1	57.4	14.8	53.0	58.5	64.2	26.5
Meat proteins	38.9	26.4	9.3	36.8	7.5	26.0	30.1	33.4	7.4
Vegetable fats	75.7	97.9	33.7	71.5	41.1	77.0	77.0	88.6	75.4
Animal fats	67.1	55.4	45.1	75.1	16.5	36.2	67.8	58.0	25.5

geneous. With the exception of Albania and Cyprus, the consumption of vegetable fat is dominant.

In a study of fat consumption in the years 1961 to 1997, there is an initial rise in the total amount consumed that continues to the mid-1960s. This rise can be attributed to the unusual nutritional conditions that followed World War II. During that time, average citizens were interested only in covering their own daily needs. The most accessible and economical source of energy is fat and, therefore, high

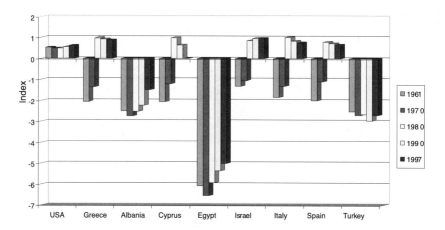

FIGURE 2   Index APA in the USA and some Mediterranean countries. (APA: animal protein availability defines the ratio of vegetable protein consumed to animal protein consumed.)

TABLE 6
Index of Animal Protein Availability (APA)*

Year	USA	Greece	Albania	Cyprus	Egypt	Israel	Italy	Spain	Turkey
1961	0.52	−2.05	−2.53	−2.06	−6.08	−1.33	−1.85	−1.99	−2.52
1970	0.49	0.8	−2.74	−1.2	−6.53	−1.33	−1.32	−1.09	−2.69
1980	0.48	0.8	−2.53	0.9	−6.50	0.96	1.00	0.8	−2.65
1990	0.56	1.0	−2.74	0.7	−5.46	−1.04	0.83	0.72	−2.97
1997	0.63	0.6	−2.73	0.7	−4.89	−0.99	0.86	0.66	−2.68

*Defines the ratio of vegetable to animal protein consumed.

consumption of fat during that period is understandable. When the situation improved, and average citizens were in a position to choose the foods that appealed most in the desired quantities, the range of consumed foods became wider and more discerning.

In terms of assessing nutrition, it is important to study the energy value of daily consumed foods as well as their origin. Judging from the data shown in Table 7, we can conclude that, in all countries, the provision of nutritional energy is an issue. Taking into account the suggestion that the required energy for a moderately active adult male is approximately 2400 calories and up to 4200 for intense physically active males, while for women, 2000 up to 3200 cal per day[24,27,30,31] is considered appropriate, then it appears that an average of 2500 calories/day/person is a realistic expectation. More important, however, is the source of this energy. Carbohydrates are burned to produce about 4.0 cal/g, fats 9.0 cal/g, and proteins 4.0 cal/g. Muscle tissue is very poor in carbohydrates, and the energy generated derives from the fat and proteins it contains. The current trend, however, is for consumption of low-fat

TABLE 7
Energy Consumption(cal/day/person)[22]

Year	USA	Greece	Albania	Cyprus	Egypt	Israel	Italy	Spain	Turkey
1961									
Vegetable	1,877	2,448	1,850	2,159	1,979	2,359	2,462	2,277	2,433
Animal	1,006	374	385	320	144	497	452	355	465
Meat	335	93	87	134	49	139	145	90	65.3
1970									
Vegetable	2,041	2,581	2,031	2,483	2,203	2,401	2,779	2,192	2,626
Animal	924	556	393	578	153	613	643	541	427
Meat	366	195	88	289	50	233	257	180	86
1980									
Vegetable	2,217	2,537	2,275	2,206	2,903	2,350	2,749	2,340	2,936
Animal	943	578	391	510	211	602	832	772	443
Meat	388	248	92	276	59	224	347	282	74
1990									
Vegetable	2,520	2,786	2,187	2,313	2,958	2,527	2,639	2,449	3,167
Animal	966	745	470	951	217	636	932	819	399
Meat	407	277	108	420	75	247	395	378	359
1997									
Vegetable	2,705	2,581	2,279	2,375	3,066	2,689	2,605	2,450	3,128
Animal	994	798	582	1,054	220	589	902	860	397
Meat	424	313	123	487	86	256	389	416	87

meat. While meat has a very high concentration of proteins, it offers relatively low caloric value to the human body.

IV. NUTRITIONAL EVALUATION OF MEAT AND MEAT PRODUCTS

The chemical composition of muscle tissue that is utilized for human consumption varies slightly from species to species.[24–26] These variations, which do not normally exceed 2%, can be attributed, apart from the species of the animal, to age, sex (steer, cow, ox, etc.), and the animal's nutrition and care before slaughter as well as the commercial classification to which it belongs.

The main constituents of muscle tissue are water, proteins, fats, carbohydrates, and minerals, as well as other trace amounts that do not play an important role in nutrition.

The main contents of muscle tissue are water 65–80% (average 75%),[27] protein 16–22% (average 19.5%),[1,27,28] fat and carbohydrates about 1%, vitamins and minerals. Other constituents are found in trace amounts and do not play an important role in nutrition.

Meat's proteins (sarcoplasma and stromal)[1,27,28] are of high biological value as they contain significant quantities of all the necessary amino acids.[50]

Amino acids are absolute necessities for the human body, and the nervous system in particular. One should not overlook the fact that the neuropeptides contain 50–80% of essential amino acids.[50] Consumption of lower-quality proteins, those that contain a lower percentage of essential amino acids, may result in the diminishing of amino acids in blood.[50] The body's proteins are made up of 20 different amino acids. This is related to the nature of our genetic code, the codons of which contain only these 20 amino acids.[37] Those that the human body can synthesize are called "non-essential." The rest, the essential amino acids, must be obtained through food.

Nitrogenous extractives (0.8–1.8%) represent another group of non-protein nitrogenous substances that are related to proteins. They are important because they provide much of the aroma and flavor of cooked meat and stimulate excretion of gastric juices. When protein analysis is performed in meat by the Kjeldahl method, these substances are estimated as total protein.

The main carbohydrates of meat are glycogen, glucose, and their intermediates. All together, they average 1.0% of total meat weight. The main organ in which carbohydrates first deposit is the liver.

Many organizations in the U.S. and Europe, such as the Food and Nutrition Board of the (U.S.) National Academy of Sciences (NAS), the American Dietetic Association (ADA), and the Deutsche Gesellschaf für Ernahrung (DGE) have not established RDAs for fat in the diet. Recent recommendations in other guidelines from the NAS suggest limiting fat consumption to no more than 30% of total calories in the diet.

Fats are important components of a balanced diet. They add flavor and appetite appeal to foods. They are a concentrated source of calories, providing 9 calories per gram, while carbohydrates and protein provide only 4 calories per gram. They supply essential fatty acids and aid in the absorption of the fat-soluble vitamins A, D, E, and K.

Animal fats and vegetable oils contain mixtures of saturated and unsaturated fatty acids. It is the proportion of saturated to unsaturated fatty acids contained in the glycerides that gives fats and oils their individual physical properties.

According to the instruction of the U.S. Department of Agriculture,[46] the energy supplied to the adult organism from dietary fat must originate at a percentage of 10% or less from saturated fatty acids, 10% or less from polyunsaturated fatty acids, and 15% or less from monounsaturated acids.

Fats of animal origin have been blamed during the past few decades for inducing hypercholesterolemia, and therefore have been deemed responsible for the onset of coronary disease. This link has neither been convincingly proved nor disproved. The content of fat in lean meat (the part of the meat that humans consume) is relatively low and does not exceed 3–5%.[31] This quantity varies depending on the species of animal, and is mainly relevant to its nutrition and degree of fattening.

Fats found in the meat of mammals used for human consumption include saturated (such as C_{12}, C_{14}, C_{16}, C_{18} and C_{20}) monounsaturated (C_{14}, C_{16}, C_{18}) and polyunsaturated (C_{16}, C_{18}, C_{20}) fatty acids in variable quantities that mainly depend on the animal's nutrition.

Unsaturated fatty acids are to be found in a percentage ranging from 39.9– 58.5% and the saturates in a percentage ranging from 41.5–60.1% of the meat's total content of fatty acids.[31,35]

The consumption of lamb meat in Greece is relatively high, making the content of fatty acids of this kind of meat very important. According to Arsenos,[47] fat from carcasses of Greek lambs studied had a high proportion of palmitic (22.7%), stearic (15.8%), and oleic acids (40.9%) and a low proportion of palmitoleic (3.7%), linoleic (4.9%), and linolenic acids (1.8%). There is a significant effect of level of nutrition on the fatty acid composition of carcass fat. Unsaturated fatty acids were higher in lambs fed on higher levels of concentrate than in those fed on lower levels.

Meat contains a range of vitamins in significant quantities. Special attention should be paid to the quantities of vitamin E, which acts as an antioxidant.

A comparison of the average person's needs in vitamins with those found in meat yields the following:

- 100 g of beef provides an adult with 23% of daily allowances in thiamine, 17% in riboflavin, 140% in B_{12}, and 20% in B_6.
- 100 g of pork provides an adult with 53% of daily allowances in thiamine, 24% in riboflavin, 35% of B_1, 35% in B_{12}, 28.8% in niacin, and 17% in B_6.

Meat also contains minerals and trace elements in considerable quantities[23,24,52,53] in the following amounts (mg/100g meat):

- Major elements, calcium (13 mg) , phosphate (200 mg), magnesium (22 mg), potassium (350 mg)
- Trace elements, copper (0.068–0.42 mg), manganese (20 mg), fluorine (0.16 mg), cobalt (0.032-0.110 mg), iron (0.41–360 mg), zinc (0.3 mg)

The chemical compositions of edible offals are shown in Table 8. They provide variable amounts of protein and fat as compared with muscles. The variety meats are less costly sources of proteins and vitamins than normal skeletal muscles. Liver, for example, contains large quantities of iron, niacin, riboflavin, and vitamin A. However, it also contains more cholesterol than muscle tissue.

Apart from the above-mentioned components, meat also contains various enzymes, hormones, and organic acids in small quantities. Sometimes, other organic or chemical substances may be traced in meat that might have been absorbed through the food chain, the water, the air, or the administration of pharmaceutical substances. These do not constitute natural meat ingredients and should not be present in meat destined for consumption.

According to the instruction of the U.S. Department of Agriculture's (USDA), nationwide food consumption survey of 1985,[46] the energy supplied to the adult organism from dietary fat must originate at a percentage of no more than 10% calories from saturated fatty acids, 10% or less from polyunsaturated fatty acids, and 15% or less from monounsaturated acids.

TABLE 8
Chemical Composition of the Principal Organ Meats (Offals) (% W/W)[25,45,49,51]

	Proteins g	Fat g	Fatty Acids g	Polyunsaturated* Fatty Acids	Cholesterol mg	Fe mg	Zn mg	Cu mg	P mg	Vitamin C mg	Folic Acid mg	Thiamin mg	Riboflavin mg	Vitamin B₁₂ mg
Liver														
Beef	20.2	7.8	5.8	28.0	270	7.8	4.3	2.3	280	15	290	0.18	3.6	110
Sheep	20.1	10.3	7.6	18.0	430	10.0	4.4	9.9	400	12	240	0.26	4.4	81
Pork	21.3	6.8	5.0	36.9	200	17.0	8.2	2.5	390	9	110	0.21	3.1	26
Kidney														
Beef	15.7	2.6	5.8	28.0	270	8.0	3.0	0.7	300	10	75	0.25	2.3	31
Sheep	16.5	2.7	7.6	18.0	430	12.0	4.1	0.6	360	9	79	0.56	2.1	79
Pork	16.3	2.7	5.0	36.0	200	6.4	4.7	0.8	330	11	43	0.19	2.1	15
Heart														
Beef	17.1	3.6	2.8		140	7.7	3.5	0.7	270	6	2	0.21	1.1	15
Sheep	17.1	5.6	4.4		140	8.1			390	11	4	0.45	1.5	14
Pork	18.9					7.7	3.5	0.7	270	4	1	0.23	1.0	10
Tongue														
Beef	15.7	17.5			768	4.9			230	2	5	0.06	0.29	4
Sheep														
Pork	15.7	17.5			78	4.9						0.06	0.29	4
Brain														
Sheep	10.3	7.6		10.8	2.200	1.4	0.2		320	17	6			

*Of the total of fatty acids.

V. CHOLESTEROL AND MEAT

It is known that cholesterol is an essential component of the membrane in animal and human cells. Neural cells, in particular, have more cholesterol than the rest,[38] probably because the cellular membrane extends to a greater surface. Cholesterol is produced daily by the human body. Meat, like other foods of animal origin, contains varying amounts of cholesterol according to the percentage of fat, which is significant for consumers who are concerned about their cholesterol levels (Table 9).

TABLE 9
Content of Fat and Cholesterol in Various Kinds of Meat[39,44,53]

Kind of Meat	Fat %	Cholesterol mg/100g
Pork		
Pork loin	7.0	53.4
Filet	1.6	54.9
Neck	11.9	62.2
Pork belly	27.1	43.4
Beef		
Loin	2.6	49.3
Shoulder	2.9	56.7
Filet	3.7	50.8
Roast beef	6.3	48.5
Goat		
Loin	0.6	75.1
Chicken		
Brisket	0.7	43.4
Chicken legs with skin	15.1	84.6
Chicken legs without skin	6.45	84.0

It is important to note that cholesterol content in meat does not correspond directly to fat content, as is the case in other foods.[40–42] The average cholesterol content in the most widely consumed meats is between 45 and 95 mg/100 g. On the basis of this data and in combination with the information presented in Table 4, during the year 1980, Greeks consumed, on average, about 120 mg cholesterol daily, and 127 mg in 1997. Opinion is divided over the desired amount of cholesterol an adult should consume per day. Perhaps a more realistic expectation would be nearly 300 mg per day.[40,41] Daily consumption of half an egg, 180 g of meat and 500 ml of milk or its equivalent in dairy products does not result in more than 300 mg/day/person.

In terms of health concerns, the critical factor is the oxidation of cholesterol, because the by-products of oxidation seem to have a negative effect on the normal biological functions of cholesterol. Oxidation of cholesterol might inhibit biosynthesis, which may lead to senility, atherosclerosis, carcinogenic phenomena, etc.[43,58] The superoxides that form during the oxidation of fat act on the oxidation of cholesterol. The addition of vitamin E to animal feeds has been found to lessen the oxidation of cholesterol.

VI. THE ROLE OF MEAT IN THE NUTRITION OF MEDITERRANEAN PEOPLE

In order to maintain the various systems in the body in a good working order, man must consume foods of both vegetable and animal origin in ideal quantities. It is also known that providing the body with proteins of high biological value, in combination with vitamins and trace elements, aids mental activity to a greater extent than carbohydrates. Meat is the perfect food to fulfill such needs. If we compare these findings with the data in Tables 5, 7–10 it is easy to conclude that meat is a vital and irreplaceable ingredient.

Modern man's needs in nutritional ingredients are influenced by lifestyle occupation, gender, age, and the general state of one's health. The issue is so complicated that a generic nutritional plan could never be devised. Nutritional programs can only apply to groups of individuals who share age group, general state of health, etc.

There is no consensus among researchers in diet and nutrition regarding the quantity of meat that should be consumed daily.[48]

An adult male of 45–50 years of age with a primarily sedentary lifestyle, needs at least 2,400 calories daily. A balanced diet requires that 38 g of protein, at least, should be provided for meeting nitrogen and essential amino-acid requirements. The consumption of a portion of 230 g of lean fresh meat will cover the recommended amount of protein, while the calories provided will not exceed 10–12% of the recommended amount. Fat is in very low levels and the cholesterol provided does not reach beyond 120–130 mg. At the same time, trace-element needs are met to a satisfactory degree.

Special mention should be made of the provision of iron through meat. In the form found in meat, iron is absorbed by the human body in quantities between 22% and 28%, while iron in vegetables is less concentrated (2–5%).[54] Regarding vitamins, those of the B complex existing in meat will cover a significant portion of the recommended daily intake.

The importance of meat for a balanced diet and the general well-being of societies has become clear. For people who do not adhere to a low-calorie diet and require proteins of high quality, meat is ideal. A thorough look at all types of recommended diets, apart from those that exclude meat for non-nutritional reasons, will reveal meat's central importance. In nutritional terms, many claim meat is irreplaceable. A dividing argument among scientists is how much of it we should consume. The claim is that 50% of our daily needs in protein must be of animal origin and 65–70% of these must come from meat and its products.

The increase of meat consumption is not the same in all Mediterranean countries. Albania and Egypt showed a very sharp increase over the last decade, while overall consumption remains low (Tables 4 and 5). In the U.S., total meat consumption is very high, probably the highest in the world.[59] After a curb in the growth rate between

1971 and 1975, the rate of growth increased in the years between 1991 and 1997 — but by a small margin.

On the other hand, Cyprus, Italy, Spain, and Greece have seen a negative pattern of meat consumption (Table 10 and Figure 1). This shows that meat consumption for the period in question increased by a lesser degree than it had increased in the period before. In Greece, after a serious reduction in the increase rate during the years 1970 to 1980, there is only a slight decrease in the rate of consumption increase, which indicates a relative stabilization of consumption. Turkey remains unclassifiable, since the unstabilized pattern of consumption between 1961 and 1977 does not allow for any conclusive remarks.

TABLE 10
Changes in Meat Consumption by Country (%)

Year	USA	Greece	Albania	Cyprus	Egypt	Israel	Italy	Spain	Turkey
1961:70	19.1	125.1	−4.5	100.7	−0.92	60.3	76.6	129.8	−2.59
1971:80	2.3	50	6.8	7	22.4	4.4	39.5	52.2	−3.46
1981:90	4.3	10.1	14.1	57.2	25.2	8.7	13.3	31.1	36.4
1991:97	4.6	10.06	35.1	16.9	25.2	15.9	−0.2	10.8	−1.2

It has been repeatedly said that the negative growth rate means that the quantity of meat consumed by the average person is less than when compared with the previous period studied. This may make the data of Table 7 appear contradictory. However, the rate of consumption refers to two consecutive time periods. Increase in total consumption is a reality, but in theory, this can reach a very low level at a given time period. For countries in the EU, the phenomenon of decrease in consumption is not unknown. It was foreseen as an eventuality — at least for Germany and France — decades ago.[55]

There are various reasons that explain consumption patterns. The most obvious is the standard of living enjoyed in the society analyzed. Historically, meat consumption reached very high levels after World War II, perhaps as a response to the rationing and scarcity during the war. Along with the dawn of the consumer age, increased spending ability turned meat from a special to an everyday food. In real terms, meat prices were also falling in comparison to prewar levels.

Despite the fact that we now recognize the need for quality protein for mental activity, meat consumption appears to be reaching a saturation point. Decrease in consumption growth has also been influenced by the "bad press" meat has received, blaming it for a number of problems associated with public health. Meat may contribute under certain conditions, but its consumption does not involve more risks than the consumption of any other foodstuff of animal or vegetable origin. One example is the case for nitric and nitrate salts. It is a well-established fact that meat contains only a low amount of nitrate (0.05 to 20 ppm), while meat products contain them in a ratio of no more than 150 ppm.[56] By comparison, the nitrate content in some vegetable foods, as well as water and beer, is notably higher.[57]

Lifestyle, age and income, and local customs, as well as marketing and retailing methods (for example the availability of ready-cut meat portions) can also influence meat consumption.

The question posed in view of meat's importance to a balanced diet is how far the trend in declining consumption will go. We speculate that the decline will continue for fresh bovine meat, while meat products' share of the market will increase. This is already evident in the U.S. and Germany. Ultimately, meat will recuperate when it becomes clear that, when consumed as it should be, meat has no negative effects on human health.

Such a diet is in remarkable accordance with the nutritional patterns seen in Mediterranean countries, and especially Greece. As has already been indicated, this model of nutrition has been in use since the time of Homer, changed little over the years to adapt to modern needs.

There is evidence that in Ancient Greece the diet of athletes — and especially that of Olympic Games winners — was very carefully balanced and high in meat proteins. This diet included meat, bread, vegetables, cereals, and fruits on an almost everyday basis.[66]

Hippocrates' fundamental principle, as described in his work *About Diet*, that "food is nutrition and pleasure" was absolutely respected by everybody. People used to eat grilled or boiled meat (pork, beef, goat, game, etc.) after religious sacrifices, and the aristocrats and rich people ate meat more often. Later, during the Roman Age, the Romans' diet included bread and cheese for breakfast, cold meat, vegetables, fruits, and wine for lunch, and appetizers (mussels, oysters etc), eggs, vegetables, and cooked meat for dinner. So, the roots of the Mediterranean Diet are in Ancient Greece.[67] Since then, through the centuries, it has passed to the rest of the Mediterranean populations.[65] Through the ages, it has gradually adapted to the circumstances and needs of human beings in every era.

Exemplary among Greek regions is the diet of Crete. Cretans are known for keeping an admirable balance between foods deriving from animal and vegetable origin. Milk, yogurt, cheese, meat — especially that of small animals, game, and fish — form the basis of the protein provision. These are complemented by bread and nuts, which offer carbohydrates, while virgin olive oil completes the body's needs in calorific foods. Abundant fruits and vegetables — with which all countries of the Mediterranean are blessed — provide vitamins and trace elements. Indeed, this is an exemplary diet that has developed over the millennia, wherein meat plays an important role.

The data presented indicate the trends apparent in the rest of the Mediterranean countries under examination. Countries where meat consumption is low have been making efforts toward long-term consumption by investing in production (Table 1) while, in the short term, they cover their needs by importing meat (Tables 2 and 5). On the contrary, countries such as Spain and Italy, where meat consumption is already high, are moving toward a decline in consumption. This is more clearly seen in the data presented in Table 10, where diachronic changes in the ratio of consumption of vegetable and animal protein are shown.

VII. QUALITY AND SAFETY ISSUES

Foodstuffs, especially those of animal origin, and meat in particular, are vulnerable to deterioration and have the potential to pose important health hazards to individuals and public health in general. Such problems may have a physical, chemical, or biological cause. In a classification based on the frequency and risk involved, physical problems will have a negligible position. These usually involve foreign bodies such as pieces of wood, wire, etc. Chemical problems represent 20–25% of cases, while biological hazards represent 75–80%. Biological problems are usually of the large-outbreak type involving large numbers of the population and might even grow to an epidemic dimension. The danger for public health can potentially be great. According to Bean et al.,[60] in the U.S.A., there were 909 outbreaks during 1983–1987 that involved 54,540 cases. The causative hazards were as follows:

- Physical hazard: none.
- Chemical hazard: 202 outbreaks (25.52%) involving 1244 (2.28%) cases. It should be noted that these include cases of poisonous mushrooms and cases of fish poisoning. Cases of purely chemical origin were only 1.5%.
- Biological hazard: 677 outbreaks (74.48%) involving 53,296 (97.72%) cases. Causative agents included bacteria, mainly *Salmonellae* and *Shigellae*, viruses, and parasites.

Data derived from DGE[61] show that, during the years 1986–1990, 410,941 food-poisoning cases were reported and investigated, while 421 related deaths were recorded. These were all due to biological hazards, involving mainly *Salmonellae, Shigellae, Yersinia* and *Clostridia*. In total, 69,749 cases of food poisoning were recorded in the U.K., Japan, Holland, Canada, and the U.S. during the period 1973–91, of which purely chemical factors covered only 372 cases (0.6%) , unidentifiable 10,696 (15.3%), while the remaining 58,408 (83.7%) were of biological causes.[64]

Obviously, these are data derived from countries with high standards of living and education. Similar situations apply to some Mediterranean countries with comparable standards of living. It is understandable that in other countries the cases of biologically caused health problems through consumption of food will reach a much higher number. Notably in the developing world, it has been estimated that more than 5 million newborns and children younger than 5 years of age die yearly as a result of food-related contamination.[62] Based on this indicative data, it becomes clear that biological hazards are the most common and the risk they pose can cause huge damage in both public health and national economies.

Figure 3 demonstrates how factors of food poisoning interrelate.

Bacterial hazards usually involve *Salmonella, Shigella, Clostridia, E. coli, Yersinia enterocolitica, Vibrio paraemolyticus, Cambylobacter jejuni* and others. Other biological hazards include biogenetic amines (histamine, tyramine, tryptamine, mycotoxines etc). Viruses and parasites are statistically less responsible.

Chemical hazards include residues (pesticides, veterinary drugs, radioactive substances, environmental pollutants) that are carried in the animal and its meat,

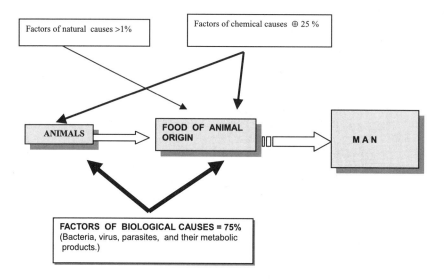

FIGURE 3   Relation and transmission pattern of food-derived health risks.

which is then consumed by humans. Natural causes usually refer to foreign bodies (wood, nails, etc.) that might be found accidentally or are used in the preparation of the foods.

Among the foods that were identified to cause food poisoning, meat and meat products participated at about 38%.[64] According to Pöhn,[68] 1,602 cases (34.6%) out of 4,127 food poisonings were due to consumption of meat and meat products and especially ground meat. It is obvious that food-poisoning cases due to meat and its products have the largest percentage (34.6 to 38%) when all the rest of foods together are considered to be responsible for food poisoning at about 60%.

Clearly, dangers in foods of both animal and vegetable origin exist, independent of the diet that an individual follows. Because meat, and meat products in particular, are susceptible to bacterial growth and represent 35–40% of food-poisoning cases,[64] every effort should be made to eliminate the risks as much as possible. Food ready for consumption should be hygienic, safe, and of a certain quality standard. The Mediterranean Diet is not only relevant to the kinds and quantities of foods consumed but also to hygiene, safety, and quality.

The modern science of hygiene and food technology safeguards these conditions by advocating preventive measures and thorough veterinary control through application of a multi-level Hazard Analysis Critical Control Points (HACCP) system. The first level is the reared animal, its health, nutrition, care, and conditions of exploitation. The next level is the production of the food, whether this is a dairy product or meat. Finally, the system involves slaughter, processing, transport, and retailing conditions, ending at the moment of sale to the consumer.

Proper veterinary control in all these levels along with the application of an HACCP system in all levels of production from "stable to table" can safegard the safety of meat foods.

REFERENCES

1. Judge, M., Aberle, E., Forrest, J., Hedrick, H. and Merkel, R., *Principles of Meat Science*. Kendall-Hunt, Iowa, 1989. Chapter 1.
2. Hofmann, K., Was ist Fleisch? *Fleischwirtschaft*, 53, 485, 1983.
3. Karaioannoglou, P., *Meat Hygiene* (in Greek). Kyriakidis Bross, Thessaloniki, 1994.
4. Oeker. P., Postmortale Veränderungen. in *Fleischtechnologie,* Sielaf, O. B., Verlag, Hamburg 1996. Chapter 5.
5. Schwägele, F., Honikel, K.O., von Lengerken, G. and Troeger, K., Kühl-Kühllagerung und Fleischreifung, *Fleischwirtschaft* 79 (6) 103, 1999.
6. Honikel, K.O. and Schwägele, F., Reifung von Fleisch, in *Qualität von Fleisch und Fleischwaren,* Branscheid, W., Honikel, K.O.,von Lengerken, G., and Troger, K., Deutsche Fachverlag, Frankfurt/Main 1998. Chapter 17.6.
7. Dransfield, E., Modeling postmortem tenderization. IV, *Meat Sci.* 34, 217, 1993.
8. Fehlhaber, K. and Janetschke, P. *Veterinärmedizinische Lebensmittelhygiene.* Verlag G. Fischer, Jena, Stuttgart, 1992, pp. 146–150.
9. Tarrant, P.V., The occurrence, changes, and consequences of dark cutting beef, in *Qualität von Fleisch und Fleischwaren,* Branscheid,W., Honikel, K.O., von Lengerken, G. and Troger, K., Deutscher Fachbuch Verlag, Frankfurt, 1998. Chapter 17.4.
10. Riever, H., Die Postmortale Veränderungen des Fleisches und Fettes, in *Lehrbuch der Tierärtzlichen Lebensmittel Überwachung.* Lerche, M., Goertler, V. and Rievel, H., Verlag M & H. Schaper, Hannover 1957, pp. 216–224.
11. Sinell, H. –J., Haltbarmachung und sonstige Behandlung von Lebensmitteln, in *Einführung in die Lebensmittelhygiene* 3. Aufl., Verlag P. Parey, Berlin, 1992. Chapter 4.1.
12. Lerche, M., *Die deutschen Wursterzeugnisse - eine Systematik der Wurstarten und Wurstsorten in Bundesreplublik und West – Berlin.* Arbeiten der DLG, Band 134, Frankfurt 1972.
13. Troeger, K., Fleischwaren-Systematik, in *Qualität von Fleisch und Fleischwaren,* Branscheid, W., Honikel, K.O., Lengerken, G., and Troeger, K., Deutsche Fachbuch Verlag, Frankfurt, 1998. Chapter 20.1.
11. Sinell, H – J., Systematik der Fleischerzeugnisse, in *Einführung in der Lebensmittelhygiene, 3. Auf.,* Sinell, Verlag P. Parey, Berlin, 1992. Chapter 4.3.
15. Bank of Greece. *Monthly Bulletin.* Athens, August, 1996.
16. Bank of Greece. *Monthly Bulletin.* Athens, February, 1999.
17. FAO Databank, Agriculture, Food, 1999.
18. FAO Databank, Agriculture , Livestock, 1999.
19. Sielaf. H., Fleischerzeugung und Ernährungsphisiologische Aspekte, in *Fleischtechnologie,* Sielaf, H., Verlag Behr's, Hamburg, 1996. Chapter 1.
20. Anon. Bio-Produktion wird internationaler. *Fleischwirtschaft* 79, 126, 1999.
21. FAO. Databank, Agriculture, Food Balance Sheet, Meat, 1999.
22. FAO. Databank, Agriculture, Food Balance Sheet, Meat Products, 1999.
23. FAO. Database, Agriculture, Food Balance Sheet, Import von Fleisch in U.S., 1999.
24. Niinivaara, F.P. and Antila, P., *Der Nährwert des Fleisches.* Verlag der Rheinhessische Druckwerkstätte, Alzey, 1972.
25. Georgakis, S.A., Chemical composition of meat, in *Food Technology of Animal Origin,* (in Greek) University Studio Press, Thessaloniki, 1988.
26. National Livestock and Meat Editorial Board, Chemical composition of meat, in *Lesson on Meat*, Chicago, 1994. Chapter 1.
27. Souci, S.W., Fachmann, W. and Kraut, H., *Die Zusammensetzung der Lebensmitteln. Nährtabellen.* 5. Aufl., Wisseschaftliche Verlagsgesellschaft mbH, Stuttgart, 1994.

28. FAO Databank, Agriculture. Food Balance Sheet. Meat consumption, 1999.
29. Gremer, H.D. and Hötzel, D. *Angewahndte Ernährungslehre.* Bd III, G. Thieme Verlag, Stuttgart, 1974. Chapter 4.
30. Deutsche Gesellschaft für Ernährung. *Jahrebericht.* Frankfurt, 1984.
31. National Research Council, Target levels and current dietary patterns, in *Designing Foods,* National Academy Press, Washington, 1988.
32. National Research Council. Diet, nutrition and cancer, in *Designing Foods,* National Academy Press, Washington, D.C.1982.
33. Sielaf, H., Fette, in *Fleischtechnologie,* Sielaf, H. Verlag Behr's, Hamburg, 1996, chapter 3.2.1.
34. Grau, R., *Handbuch der Lebensmittelchemie,* Bd III/2 Springer Verlag, Berlin, Heidelberg, New York, 1968, chapter B, II.
35. Glatzel, H., *Fett- ein Stück Natur,* Fischer Druck AG, Münsingen, 1977. Chapter 2.
36. Aspiotis, N., *Physiology.* (in Greek) Thessaloniki, 1984.
37. Trakatellis, A. *Biochemie* (in Greek), Kyriakidis Bros, Thessaloniki, 1994.
38. Michail, S., *Histology* (in Greek), Kyriakidis Bros, Thessaloniki, 1991.
39. AIDA, *Speisefette* Heft No. 1012, Bonn 1998.
40. Arneth, W., Über die Bestimmung des intramuskulären Fettes. *Fleischwirtschaft,* 76, 907, 1996.
41. Honikel, K.O. and Arneth, W., Cholisteringehalt in Fleisch und Eien. *Fleischwirtschaft* 76, 1244,1996.
42. Committee on Technological Options, *Designing Foods,* National Academy Press, Washington D.C, 1988,pages 72, 76.
43. Hofmann, E., Oxidation des Cholesterins und seine Beziehung zur Fleischqualitäs. *Fleischwirtschaft,* 77, 243, 1997.
44. Trichopoulou A., Food Composition Tables (in Greek), Athens, 1992.
45. Boskou D., *Food Chemistry* (in Greek), Gartaganis, D., ed.,Thessaloniki, 1983.
46. U.S. Department of Agriculture. Nationwide food consumption survey, 1985.
47. Arsenos, G., Effect of genotype and management factors on fatty acid composition of carcass fat, in Boutsko, Serres, and Karagouniko, Lambs. Doctoral Thesis. Faculty of Veterinary Medicine, Aristotle University of Thessaloniki, 1997.
48. Judgee, M., Aberle E., Forrest J., Hedrickk H. and Merkel R., *Principles of Meat Science.* Kendall-Hunt, Iowa 1989, Chapter 13.
49. Kennz, T.A., Development opportunities in animal by-products. *Meat Research Series No 8.* An Foras Toluntais, Ireland, 1981.
50. Scheller, E., Hochwertiges Eisweiß als Nervennahrung, in Schweisfurt, K.L. and Baumgartner, O., *Ökologische Qualität in Fleischerhandwerke.* Deutsche Fachbucheverlag, Frankfurt, 1996, chapter 1.
51. Sielaf, H., Zusammensetzung von Organen, in *Fleischtechnologie,* H. Behr's Verlag, Hamburg, 1996, Chapter 3.
52. National Livestock and Meat Board, Lessons on Meat, Chicago, 1994, Chapter 2.
53. Dahl, O., *Schlachtfette.* Verlag der Rheinhessischen Druck werhstatte Abzey, 1973, p. 26.
54. Bjorn Rasmussen, E. and Hallberg, L., Effect of animal protein on the absorption of food iron in man. *Nutr. Metab.* 23, 192, 1979, and Branscheid, W., Honikel, K.O., von Lengerken, G., and Troger, K., in *Fleisch und Fleischwaren,* Deutsche Fachbuchverlag, Stuttgart, 1988, Chapter 18.
55. Branscheid, W., Honikel, K.O., von Lengerkken, G., and Troeger, K., *Fleisch und Fleischwaren.* Vol. I Chapter 1.3. Deutsche Fachbuchverlag, Stuttgart, 1998.
56. European Union, Directive number 95/2.

57. Reuter, W. and Wolkerstrofer, W., Nitrate in vegetables. *Zeitschrif für Lebensmitteluntersuchung und Fosrschung,* 175, 123, 182.
58. Münch, S., Arneth, W., and Grosch, W., Formation of oxidation products of cholesterol. *Fleischwirtschaft,* 79, 84, 1999.
59. Nindhorst, H.W., Weißfleisch setz Erforgsstorz fort. *Fleischwirtschaft* 79, 49, 1999.
60. Bean, N., Griffin, P.M., Goulding, J.S., and Ivey, C.B., Foodborne disease outbreaks. 5-year summary 1983–1987. *J. Food Protection* 53, 711, 1990.
61. Deutsche Gesellschaft für Ermährung, *Ernahrungsberscht.* Frankfurt, 1992.
62. Sinell, H.J., *Einfuhrung in die Lebensmittelhygiene.* 3. Auf. Verlag P. Parey, Berlin, 1992, Chapter 2.3.
63. Baltes, J., *Gewinnung und Verarbeitung von Nahrungsfetten*, Verlag P. Parey, Berlin, 1975, pp. 20.
64. Genigeorgis, K., International statistics for foodborne dieseases from food of animal origin (in Greek). Lessons in the Veterinarian Medical Faculty of Aristotle University of Thessaloniki, 1998.
65. Tromaras, L.M., *Roman Cooking* (in Greek), University Studio Press, 1988, Thessaloniki, pp. 12–21.
66. Korobilas, K., What did the ancient Olympic champions eat? (in Greek), *Food and Beverages*, 220, Triaina, Athens, 1999, pp. 94–100.
67. Lambaki–Mixa, A., The diet of the Ancient Greeks. Doctoral Thesis. School of Philosophy, University of Athens, Athens, 1984.
68. Pöhn, H., Ph. Salmonellose–Überwachung beim Menschen in der Bunderepublik. Deutschland, Jahreberict 1978–80, in Sinell, *Einführung in die Lebensittelhygiene.* Verlag P. Parey, Berlin, 1992.

8 Alcoholic Beverages

Mary Yannakoulia and Tonia Vassilakou

CONTENTS

I. INTRODUCTION

The so-called Mediterranean Diet has gained enormous popularity during the last 40 years. Much research has been focused on the analysis of its components and their relation to health. Alcohol, mainly in the form of wine, has been consumed in moderate amounts as part of the meals of the day (noon, evening, and even mid-morning meals) by Christians for centuries, whereas for Moslems, wine consumption is forbidden.[1,2] Much of the attention on wine and its constituents was the result of the recent observation regarding the French paradox, that is, people with a relatively high proportion of saturated fatty acids in their habitual diets manage to keep the cardiovascular mortality and morbidity rates at low levels, partly due, it is believed, to the concurrent consumption of moderate amounts of red wine.[3]

In general, beverages are appreciated for their flavor and for the pharmacological action of some of their ingredients. The majority also contribute to total dietary energy intake. Discovery of the fermentation process resulted in the invention of several types of alcoholic drinks as dilute solutions of ethyl alcohol. Alcohol, apart from having mood-altering effects, also contributes to the energy intake (7.1 kcal/g in the bomb calorimeter), being utilized as efficiently as carbohydrates and fats by the body of healthy nonalcoholic individuals.[4] In addition, alcoholic beverages contain a variety of other substances whose role has not been fully identified.

The scope of this chapter is to discuss the role of alcohol in the Mediterranean Diet. The main interest will be first on issues concerning production and availability patterns of alcoholic beverages and second, on the composition of wine and some other types of drinks consumed in the Mediterranean basin.

II. TRENDS IN ALCOHOLIC BEVERAGE PRODUCTION AND AVAILABILITY

Profound socioeconomic and cultural changes in Mediterranean countries during the past decades have been closely related to changes in both life-style and nutrition patterns. Consumption and, consequently, production of alcoholic beverages have been greatly affected. The assessment of alcohol consumption remains a rather difficult task because people tend to underreport alcoholic beverage intake.[5] Furthermore, the methodology used for data collection in the context of studies on alcohol consumption is not uniform and, thus, the information obtained is not comparable. As a result, remarkably variable data from several sources can be observed. In this review, to evaluate trends in production and availability of alcoholic beverages over the period 1961–1997, the 5-year averages (for the period 1991–1997, the 7-year average) as appearing in the standardized Food Balance Sheets compiled by the Food and Agriculture Organization (FAO) have been mainly used,[6] as well as selected data from comparable sources.

The production of alcoholic beverages has been steadily increasing in Europe,[6,7] in the U.S., and in the rest of the world.[6] It is noteworthy that the increase in total alcoholic beverage production was not attributed to changes in wine production, but mainly to a sharp increase in the production of beer and distilled beverages. Wine production in France and Italy still accounts for more than 40% of the world's production,[6,8] but wine has been losing ground, and this is of particular interest for the Mediterranean countries, where it has been traditionally related to the habits and culture of the people.

According to the standardized Food Balance Sheets for the period 1961–1997,[6] alcohol-consumption patterns have been subjected to serious changes regarding both the total quality and its distribution among various products. Daily alcoholic beverage availability per capita is presented in Tables 1–4. Trends in availability vary significantly among the Mediterranean countries.[6] Total availability declined in France[9] and Italy, but it increased in Greece, Portugal, and Spain. Regarding the availability of specific alcoholic beverages, no uniform pattern can be identified, apart from a critical decrease in wine and a concomitant increase in beer consumption. Furthermore, considerable differences are observed in availability levels of specific alcoholic beverages in the Mediterranean area.

The decrease in the total availability of alcoholic beverages in France was mainly due to a constant decline in wine availability. France is the only Mediterranean country where beer availability did not increase over the last four decades; although an upward trend was observed until 1980, a substantial decline has occurred since then. Only distilled-beverage availability has been expanded. Similar conclusions have been drawn from producers' data and household budget surveys.[9,10]

TABLE 1
Secular Trends (1961–1997) in Alcoholic-Beverage Availability for Human Consumption in the Mediterranean Countries, Europe, the U.S., and the World[6]

Country	1961– 1965	1966– 1970	1971– 1975	1976– 1980	1981– 1985	1986– 1990	1991– 1997	Differences 1961–1997
			(grams per capita per day)					(%)
France	490	470	461	451	405	340	307	– 37.5
Greece	105	116	107	128	165	178	159	+ 51.4
Italy	321	343	342	306	281	244	224	– 30.2
Portugal	230	293	331	341	352	349	368	+ 60.0
Spain	218	250	280	313	299	319	299	+ 37.2
Europe	263	293	326	335	327	316	240	– 8.7
U.S.	190	219	256	294	312	303	286	+ 50.5
World	75	82	90	95	93	90	88	+ 17.3

Note: Values are given as averages.

TABLE 2
Secular Trends (1961–1997) in Wine Availability for Human Consumption in the Mediterranean Countries, Europe, the U.S., and the World[6]

Country	1961– 1965	1966– 1970	1971– 1975	1976– 1980	1981– 1985	1986– 1990	1991– 1997	Differences 1961–1997
			(grams per capita per day)					(%)
France	326	300	288	265	235	199	172	– 47.2
Greece	88	88	67	64	74	63	46	– 47.7
Italy	294	308	299	258	223	176	159	– 45.9
Portugal	182	234	229	214	212	164	159	– 12.6
Spain	164	155	164	164	140	123	107	– 34.8
Europe	106	110	112	108	101	88	62	– 41.5
U.S.	9	12	17	20	24	23	20	+ 122.2
World	19	19	19	18	17	13	11	– 42.1

Note: Values are given as averages.

In Italy, total consumption of alcoholic beverages decreased after 1975 due to a decline in wine and distilled-beverage availability. On the other hand, beer availability is constantly increasing. Similar trends have been identified in Greece and Spain. The main characteristics of the changes taking place in these countries are, first, the notable increase in overall availability of alcoholic beverages (+ 51% and + 37%, respectively) resulting from a significant increase in beer and distilled-beverage availability, and, second, the accompanying decrease in wine availability. These changes are much more pronounced in Greece than in Spain. Finally, in Portugal, although total availability

TABLE 3
Secular Trends (1961–1997) in Beer Availability for Human Consumption in the Mediterranean Countries, Europe, the U.S., and the World[6]

Country	1961–1965	1966–1970	1971–1975	1976–1980	1981–1985	1986–1990	1991–1997	Difference 1961–1997
			(grams per capita per day)					(%)
France	104	111	119	126	115	98	92	– 11.5
Greece	14	25	35	57	80	100	102	+ 628.6
Italy	23	30	38	43	55	65	62	+ 169.6
Portugal	13	26	66	95	105	155	180	+ 1284.6
Spain	46	85	107	138	150	187	183	+ 297.8
Europe	140	167	194	204	209	209	159	+ 13.6
U.S.	168	193	222	256	272	267	253	+ 50.6
World	40	45	51	55	55	56	58	+ 45.0

Note: Values are given as averages.

TABLE 4
Secular Trends (1961–1997) in Distilled-Beverage Availability for Human Consumption in the Mediterranean Countries, Europe, the U.S., and the World[6]

Country	1961–1965	1966–1970	1971–1975	1976–1980	1981–1985	1986–1990	1991–1997	Difference 1961–1997
			(grams per capita per day)					(%)
France	3	5	7	8	8	8	7	+ 133.3
Greece	3	3	5	8	11	16	12	+ 300.0
Italy	4	4	5	5	4	3	3	– 25.0
Portugal	34	33	36	32	35	29	30	– 11.8
Spain	6	7	7	8	8	8	7	+ 16.7
Europe	8	9	13	15	14	13	15	+ 87.5
U.S.	12	14	17	18	17	13	13	+ 8.3
World	6	7	8	9	10	10	10	+ 66.7

Note: Values are given as averages.

of alcoholic beverages fluctuates from year to year, an overall increase is noticed, mainly due to a dramatic increase in beer availability (+ 1295%) at the expense of wine and distilled-beverage availability, which declined slightly.[6]

Given the variable content of ethyl alcohol in alcoholic beverages, neither total nor specific distilled-beverage availability allows us to draw conclusions on the alcohol availability among the Mediterranean countries. Therefore, pure alcohol

TABLE 5
Secular Trends (1961–1997) in Ethyl Alcohol Availability for Human Consumption in the Mediterranean Countries, Europe, the U.S., and the World[6]

Countries	1961–1965	1966–1970	1971–1975	1976–1980	1981–1985	1986–1990	1991–1997	Differences 1961–1997
	(grams per capita per day)							(%)
France	43.8	42.0	41.7	39.8	35.8	30.8	27.0	– 38.3
Greece	12.0	12.5	11.4	13.3	16.7	18.3	15.0	+ 25.0
Italy	36.5	38.4	38.2	33.7	29.9	24.6	22.5	– 38.2
Portugal	34.5	40.8	43.3	41.5	42.9	37.6	38.7	+ 12.1
Spain	23.4	24.2	26.9	28.8	26.6	26.5	24.1	+ 2.9
Europe	22.2	24.4	27.5	28.3	27.4	25.5	20.8	– 6.5
U.S.	14.0	16.4	19.5	21.9	22.8	20.9	19.9	+ 42.1
World	6.5	7.1	7.8	8.2	8.5	8.1	8.0	+ 23.2

Note: Values are given as averages.

availability was estimated, using the following reference values for the ethyl alcohol content of wine, beer, and distilled beverages: 11.5%, 5% and 38% respectively. As shown in Table 5, ethyl-alcohol availability increased substantially worldwide and in the U.S., but it decreased slightly in Europe. Among Mediterranean countries, it increased significantly in Greece (+ 25%) and Portugal (+ 12%), as a result of the increase in distilled beverages and beer availability respectively, and slightly in Spain (+ 3%). On the other hand, it decreased meaningfully in France and Italy (- 38% in both countries), mainly due to the decline in wine availability.

As already mentioned, substantial shifts occurred in alcoholic-beverage consumption during the period from 1961–1965 to 1991–1997 among Mediterranean countries. The most significant change is the so-called modernization of preferences, where a traditional drink is replaced by other, more modern, and "westernized" drinks. Similar changes have been observed in most European countries.[9,11,12] The extent of this modernization in Mediterranean countries is presented in Table 6, which displays the distribution of total distilled-beverage availability into their main components.[6]

In the Mediterranean wine-producing countries, a major change was the decrease in the proportion of wine and the increase in the proportion of beer. In Italy and Greece, wine dominated alcoholic beverage availability early in the 1960s. From 1961–1997, the greatest decrease in the proportion of wine, as well as the greatest increase in the proportion of beer, took place in Greece. In Portugal, the contribution of distilled beverages in the total alcoholic beverage availability was high during early 1960s, but it declined significantly in the following decades. In particular, the increase in the proportion of beer totally outweighed the decrease in the proportion of both wine and distilled beverages. In France, a notable decrease in the proportion of wine availability and a considerable increase in the proportion of beer availability

TABLE 6
Secular Trends (1961–1997) of the Distribution (%) of Alcohol Availability into Wine, Beer, and Distilled Beverages* in the Mediterranean Countries[6]

	France			Greece			Italy		
Years	Wine	Beer	Distilled Beverages	Wine	Beer	Distilled Beverages	Wine	Beer	Distilled Beverages
1961–1965	67	21	0.6	84	13	3	92	7	1
1966–1970	64	24	1	76	22	3	90	9	1
1971–1975	62	26	2	63	33	5	87	11	2
1976–1980	59	28	2	50	45	6	84	14	2
1981–1985	58	28	2	45	48	7	79	20	1
1986–1990	59	29	2	35	56	9	72	27	1
1991–1997	56	30	2	29	64	8	71	28	1

	Portugal			Spain		
Years	Wine	Beer	Distilled Beverages	Wine	Beer	Distilled Beverages
1961–1965	79	6	15	75	21	3
1966–1970	80	9	11	62	34	3
1971–1975	69	20	11	59	38	3
1976–1980	63	28	9	52	44	3
1981–1985	60	30	10	47	50	3
1986–1990	47	44	8	39	59	3
1991–1997	43	49	8	36	61	2

* Alcoholic beverages also include fermented beverages and non-food alcohol, not shown here.
Note: Values are given as average %.

were observed. Similar patterns were also observed in Spain, but changes were much more profound.

Another important issue concerning these trends is the internationalization of beverage consumption, which refers to the consumption of imported beverages compared with locally produced (or native) drinks.[10] To examine this internationalization in the Mediterranean countries, data in Tables 7–10 present the proportion of imported alcoholic beverages in relation to total distilled-beverage availability.[6] The trends did not match in all Mediterranean countries and for all beverages. The main finding is the total or partial replacement of traditional drinks by imported or international drinks. In particular, early in the 1960s, alcoholic-beverage imports were insignificant in most Mediterranean countries, with the exception of France and Greece. They increased substantially in the following decades, and, according to recent FAO data, they account for 18% and 14% of the alcoholic beverages available for human consumption in France and Greece, respectively. In the other Mediterranean countries, consumption is rather low. In the 1991–1997 period, wine imports were found to be meaningful only in France (16%) and Portugal (9%), while

TABLE 7
Secular Trends (1961–1997) in the Proportion (%) of Alcoholic-Beverage Imports in Relation to Total Availability in the Mediterranean Countries[6]

Country	1961–1965	1966–1970	1971–1975	1976–1980	1981–1985	1986–1990	1991–1997
France	16	10	11	12	13	13	18
Greece	0.3	0.8	5	3	3	8	14
Italy	0.5	0.8	2	2	5	7	9
Portugal	0.2	0.3	2	2	0.8	6	8
Spain	0.1	0.3	1	1	1	4	10

Note: Values are given as average %.

TABLE 8
Secular Trends (1961–1997) in the Proportion (%) of Wine Imports in Relation to Total Availability in the Mediterranean Countries[6]

Country	1961–1965	1966–1970	1971–1975	1976–1980	1981–1985	1986–1990	1991–1997
France	22	13	14	14	14	12	16
Greece	0.02	0.2	6	0.2	0.2	1	4
Italy	0.1	0.2	0.8	0.4	0.6	1	1
Portugal	0.02	0.02	0.02	2	0.008	7	9
Spain	0.009	0.03	1	0.06	0.1	0.4	4

Note: Values are given as average %.

they were insignificant in the other Mediterranean countries, where locally produced wine is consumed. During the same period, beer imports were considerable in Italy (23%) and France (17%), but were very low in Portugal (2%). In Greece and Spain, beer imports account for 6% and 7% respectively. Portugal is the only Mediterranean country where a great part of available distilled beverages are produced locally (75%). In other countries, imports account for more than 92% of total distilled-beverage availability.

Another source of information on alcohol availability in Greece during the late 1980s and mid-1990s and in Spain during early 1990s is Data Food Networking (DAFNE) project. [13,14] The DAFNE databank summarizes several nutritional and sociodemographic data originating from Household Budget Surveys conducted by national statistical offices in 10 European countries. This databank tabulates, among other statistics, information on beverage availability within the household; beverages consumed outside household are not included. Comparison between FAO and

TABLE 9
Secular Trends (1961–1997) in the Proportion (%) of Beer Imports in Relation To Total Availability in the Mediterranean Countries[6]

Country	1961–1965	1966–1970	1971–1975	1976–1980	1981–1985	1986–1990	1991–1997
France	2	5	8	10	11	13	17
Greece	2	2	1	1	0.7	3	6
Italy	3	4	6	8	15	16	23
Portugal	1	0.4	0.1	0.03	0.1	1	2
Spain	0.2	0.3	0.5	0.5	1	3	7

Note: Values are given as average %.

TABLE 10
Secular Trends (1961–1997) in the Proportion (%) of Distilled-Beverage Imports in Relation to Total Availability in the Mediterranean Countries[6]

Country	1961–1965	1966–1970	1971–1975	1976–1980	1981–1985	1986–1990	1991–1997
France	44	28	40	47	49	74	92
Greece	3	10	23	29	29	57	97
Italy	6	11	27	34	53	83	99
Portugal	0.3	1	8	8	6	21	25
Spain	3	8	15	27	23	55	147

Note: Values are given as average %.

DAFNE data on distilled-beverage availability may help in identifying drinking habits in Mediterranean countries.

By reviewing DAFNE data, it becomes evident that absolute values of alcoholic beverage availability in Greece and Spain are substantially lower than those resulting from Food Balance Sheets.[6] This indicates that only a small amount of alcoholic beverages is consumed within the household; the greatest part is consumed outside during social events. In Greece, an important increase in wine availability within the household has been observed during the period 1987–1994, which is in disagreement with the trend of wine availability according to the FAO data. Furthermore, data from the DAFNE project show a higher proportion of wine than beer availability within the household, both in Greece and Spain. These observations suggest that, in Greece and Spain, wine is the most popular alcoholic beverage within households, while beer is mostly preferred in outside household social life.[13,14] The same pattern was also observed in France.[9] Distilled beverages are equally preferred within and outside the household in Greece, whereas in Spain they are consumed mostly outside the home.[13,14]

Biological as well as socioeconomic factors (gender, age, urbanization, and education) influence alcoholic beverage availability. Alcoholic beverages are consumed more often and in greater amounts among men than among women, in both the Mediterranean region and northern Europe.[15-17] This pattern is observed in all age groups; however, among young persons, it becomes weaker because they adapt more easily to modern life-styles.[18] The percentage of energy from alcohol varied considerably among elderly persons from the Mediterranean countries. According to the Euronut-Seneca study,[19] alcohol contributed 3.9–4.5% to the total energy intake of males in Greece, 6.3–6.4% in France, 6.9% in Portugal, 7.3% in Spain, and 10.7–11.1% in Italy. For comparison, the corresponding values are considerably lower in women, namely 0.1–0.5% in Greece, 0.5% in Portugal, 1.4–2.7% in France, 2.6% in Spain and 3.5–6.0% in Italy.

Exploring information from the Household Budget Surveys for Greece and Spain,[13,14] total alcoholic beverage availability is higher in rural areas of Greece. Beer and spirits availability is higher among persons living in urban areas of Spain, whereas wine is preferred by residents of rural and semi-urban areas. In Greece and Spain, wine is selected mostly by persons of lower education, while spirits are consumed in greater amounts among persons of higher education. In Greece, beer is preferred by persons of higher education, whereas in Spain education does not seem to be associated with beer availability.[13,14]

III. WINE

Wine is considered to be the traditional drink in the Mediterranean countries, at least in those of the European coast. Vineyards, olive trees, and wheat make up a great proportion of the Mediterranean flora, and their products — wine, olives, and wheat — are characteristic ingredients of the Mediterranean Diet. Most researchers believe that the domestication of the wine grape, as well as the art of winemaking, or at least its development, originated in southern Caucasia (an area that today includes parts of Turkey, northern Iraq, Azerbaijan, and Georgia).[20] From this area, wine production and winemaking spread southward to Palestine, Syria, Egypt, Mesopotamia, and then around the Mediterranean region. This colonization of the eastern Mediterranean is still viewed as the predominant reason for expanding the knowledge of winemaking in southern and central Europe. Wine, together with beer, constituted a safe source of fluid in people's diets before the relatively recent availability of clean, pure water.[21]

During antiquity, wine was widely consumed in Greece and Rome, mainly after dilution with at least an equal amount of water. In ancient Athens, wine production was sufficient to allow a part of the wine produce, along with olives, to be exported, thus generating funds to buy grain imported from the Black Sea.[22] The existence of specific gods for wine, such as Dionysius, or Bacchus, in Greek and Roman mythology, denotes its importance for ancient people in the Mediterranean.[23]

Moving to the 1960s, alcohol consumption in the Greek island of Crete, the region with the lowest cardiovascular disease rates, according to the findings of the

Seven-Countries Study, was 15 g per person per day.[24] Cretans consumed wine, but they did so in moderate amounts, mainly as part of a meal. Alcoholism was rare and wine drinking was not associated with alcohol abuse.[25] This is in accordance with similar observations in contemporary societies: wine is more often consumed at home with meals, whereas alcoholic problems, especially the serious ones, are mostly related to the preference for spirits and/or beer than to wine drinking.[26]

A. COMPOSITION OF WINE

Wine, as a composite mixture of organic and inorganic substances, is rich in a variety of non-alcoholic compounds. Its composition is more complex than that of grapes, since several metabolites are produced during winemaking, storage, and maturation. Research in the area is ongoing and new substances are being discovered. In this chapter, an overview of the most widely recognized and explored ones will be given.

1. Water

Water is the predominant constituent of grapes and wine. It plays a significant role in establishing the basic characteristics of the beverage, acting as vehicle for a variety of important compounds (compounds insoluble or slightly soluble in water rarely play a significant role in wine) and determining flow properties. It remains an essential component for many chemical reactions during winemaking and aging.[20,27]

2. Alcohol

Ethyl alcohol is the alcohol of foremost importance in wine. Its primary source, as the main organic by-product, is the yeast fermentation of the grape sugars. It is a strong activator of enzymes and other compounds responsible for several wine characteristics, and crucial for the stability, aging, and sensory characteristics of the wine, namely its color, body, and flavor. Ethyl alcohol also acts as a solvent in the extraction of tannins and pigments. It influences the amount of aromatic compounds, and contributes to the dilution of compounds produced during fermentation and maturation in wood cooperage. From a nutritional point of view, it is essential to know the alcohol content of wine to evaluate its contribution to the dietary energy intake. Alcohol concentration in ordinary wines ranges between 10 and 14% (v/v); higher levels are found in the so-called fortified wines.[27,28]

3. Sugars and Polysaccharides

The main grape sugars are glucose and fructose. Other sugars are also present but in insignificant amounts. Sucrose is rarely found in grapes of the *Vitis vinifera* cultivars. The sugar content of the grape is critical for the vinification process, the yeast growth, and metabolism, given the fact that *Saccaromyces cerevisiae* derives most of its energy from sugars. Unfermented sugars constitute the so-called residual sugars of the wine. In dry wines, the residual sugars are at low concentrations, undetectable on the palate. Their nutritive value is also negligible; they may, however, increase the microbial hazard, especially if the wine acid and alcohol content are low. When residual sugars rise to levels above 0.2%, exceptionally sensitive individuals may detect sweetness; however, the majority of people detect distinct sweetness at concentration over 1%. The detection of sweetness is also influenced by the presence of other constituents, namely alcohol, acids, and tannins. In very sweet wines, sugar content may be well above 10%.[20]

The polysaccharide content of the final product in the vinification process is at low levels, and its significance to the sensory characteristics of the wine has not been evaluated, though believed to be negligible.[20]

4. Acids

Wine contains two types of acids: the volatile (acetic acid) and the fixed acids (tartaric, lactic, oxalic, fumaric, mallic, succinic, and citric acids). The distillation process can readily remove the former, whereas the latter are responsible for controlling wine's pH.[27]

5. Nitrogen

Nitrogen-containing compounds in grapes and wines play an important role in the growth of yeast and bacteria, and, consequently, in the fermentation rate as well as the production of flavor compounds.[29]

6. Vitamins and Minerals

The same vitamins and minerals that are present in the grape are also present in wine at levels that are insignificant for human nutrition, but may be important for microbial growth. However, it is noteworthy that higher levels of some minerals may result from wine storage or contamination. For example, elevated calcium levels are found in wines stored in unlined cement tanks, whereas high levels of iron and copper can result from contact with corroded winery equipment and chemicals sprayed on vines. From an enological point of view, higher than normal levels of iron and copper are generally undesirable, causing cloud formation, oxidation-reduction reactions, and yeast and flavor impairment. Magnesium and manganese are also detected in very small quantities, but aluminum constitutes a normal constituent of this alcoholic beverage.[20,29,30]

7. Phenols

It is widely accepted among health professionals that wine is a unique beverage, mainly due to its content of a wide range of polyphenols. Phenolic compounds, flavonoids, and nonflavonoids are being investigated for their beneficial effects on health. Among the large group of flavonoids, the major classes found in wine and grape juice are the flavonols (quercetin, rutin, myricetin, kaempferol, isorhamnetin), flavanols (catechin, gallocatechin, procyanidins, condensed tannins) and, in red wine, anthocyanins. Nonflavonoids are mostly represented by phenolic acids (benzoic acids and hydroxycinnamic acids) and stilbenes (trans-resveratrol). Phenolic and related compounds can affect wine's organoleptic characteristics (appearance, taste, mouth-feel, fragrance) and they also exhibit anti-microbial properties.[27,31,32] During wine aging (i.e., the chemical reactions that occur during red wine conservation and maturation that result in positive organoleptic changes), the grape anthocyanins transform into new pigments much more stable in this fluid aqueous environment. Consequently, as wine ages, its polyphenolic content becomes different from what it was at the beginning of the winemaking process. Brouillard and his co-workers[33] speculate that the better antioxidant activities reported elsewhere for red wines arise from the presence of new phenolic compounds produced during maturation.

As a result of the vinification process, red wines are richer in phenolic compounds than white wines. White wines are made with free-run juices, without pomace, and consequently there is no contact with the grape skins, which are a rich source of phenols. In contrast, red wines are macerated with the skins, which results in levels of phenolics approximately ten times higher than those of white wines. However, the phenolic content of the latter can be increased by modifying the winemaking process. For example, cold maceration with skins to expand pomace contact can be used for increasing the extract of phenolic compounds associated with pomace as well as some flavoring substances.[34]

Anthocyanins constitute pigment compounds, that confer red wine its color and other organoleptic characteristics. The amount and type of anthocyanins present in the grape depend on the species, variety, degree of maturation, and seasonal conditions, whereas the concentration of anthocyanins in wine is affected by the conditions of fermentation and aging.[35]

Taste and mouth-feel of red wine are greatly influenced by the flavonoid tannins. From a chemical point of view, wine tannins consist essentially of polymers of flavanols, also called condensed tannins, or proanthocyanidins. In addition, wine tannins also include non-proanthocyanidin tannin-like structures, formed during wine aging. All these compounds are mostly responsible for the wine's taste of bitterness and astringency.[36]

Reviewing their relation to health, quercetin, catechin, and other flavonoids have been shown to modify eicosanoid synthesis with implications in both inflammatory and vascular disease. The inhibition of the oxidation of the low-density lipoprotein cholesterol and flavonoids' effects on the platelet aggregation and endothelial vasodilation further suggest that flavonoids may be involved in the primary and secondary prevention of cardiovascular disease.[37,38] Additionally, it has been shown that flavonoids have antiviral properties and exert anti-mutagenic activities.[37] Since little is known on the pharmacokinetics of flavonoids, further research is needed in the area of their absorption and their *in vivo* biological effects.[32]

Stilbenes are phenolics acting as natural antifungal compounds that enable plants to overcome pathogen attack. They occur in very few fruits and vegetables, and the grapevine is one of them.[39] Trans-resveratrol is a stilbene extensively studied for its concentration in grapes and wines, as well as for its potential health benefits. The concentration of resveratrol in wine depends on a number of factors, namely the species of the grape, environmental, and enological practices. Several *in vivo, in vitro*, and animal experiments have shown that resveratrol may protect against atherosclerosis, mainly through its antioxidant properties, inhibition of platelet aggregation, inhibition of the hepatic synthesis, and secretion of apolipoprotein B and AI, as well as through eicosanoid synthesis of human platelets.[40] Additionally, its structure, which is similar to the synthetic estrogenic agent diethylstilbestrol, suggests that resveratrol acts as a phytoestrogen. Alcoholic beverages were known to contain estrogenically active substances,[41] but, quite recently, wine resveratrol was also identified as such. By binding to estrogen receptors, it has been speculated that it exerts beneficial effects on the female reproductive system, menopause, osteoporosis, and cancer.[42]

8. Aroma Precursors

Apart from polyphenols, precursors of aromas constitute an important group of secondary metabolites occurring during wine fermentation and aging. They can be classified as terpene compounds, norisoprenoids, and benzenoids. Some of them turn into odorless or low-threshold, odor-producing structures that are more stable under thermodynamic conditions. The role of these compounds has not been fully investigated; they seem, however, to be important from an enological viewpoint and may have a positive impact on drinkers' health.[28]

9. Other Constituents

White and red wines have been found to contain relatively high concentrations of the lignans matairesinol and secoisolariciresinol (range for total lignans 152.7–1376 µg/L), which act as biologically active phyto-estrogens — precursors of hormone-like compounds in mammalian systems.[43] Wine, like many plants, also constitutes a source of salicylic acid. Its content depends on a number of factors, such as variety, vine health, and processing practices. Again, salicylic acid levels are higher in red than in white wines. Plants produce salicylic acid as a chemical for natural defense. It is effective against some viral and bacterial infections, may be protective against the common cold, and has been shown to exert antioxidant action.[44]

B. Wine Regions in the Mediterranean and Wine Cultivars: Quality Issues

Traditional production of wine by grape fermentation in the past resulted in beverages with a lower alcoholic content than the wines familiar to the present-day consumer. These early wines also contained a high percentage of acetic and other organic acids, produced during fermentation, that would bother the tastebuds of modern enophiles, as the wines would resemble vinegar, with some hints of cider.[21]

There is no universal system of wine classification. Wines may be categorized according to several characteristics, namely color, sweetness, alcohol content, carbon dioxide content, grape variety, fermentation, or maturation involved. They are often also classified by geographic origin, associated with the traditional use of particular grape cultivars, as well as grape growing and winemaking techniques. Grapes in the Mediterranean region belong to the species of *Vitis vinifera L.*, which grows best in this type of climate with long, relatively dry, summers and mild winters. Based on their alcoholic content, wines are classified into table wines and fortified wines. Table wines can be further subdivided into still and sparkling, depending on the carbon dioxide level retained in the bottle. In fortified wines, alcohol content reaches levels from 17 to 22% (v/v). Around the Mediterranean region, some very famous fortified wines are produced, namely sherry in Spain, port in Portugal, vermouth in Italy, and Marsala in Sicily.[20]

France has a worldwide reputation for the quality of its wines as well as for the significant role that this beverage plays in the French cuisine and culture. It is the leading wine-producing country in the world, and the third in grape hectarage. It is famous for its red wines as well as champagne, the preeminent sparkling wine. Bordeaux, Alsace, Champagne, Burgundy, Beaujolais, the Loire and Rhone valleys, and Languedoc-Roussillon are the most important French viticultural regions in terms of quantity, quality, and world trade; Merlot, Cabernet Sauvignon, Cabernet franc, Petit Verdot, Sauvignon, Semillon, Muscat, Pinot, Chardonnay, and Sirah are some of the predominant cultivars. Government regulation of regional wine types, known as *appellations contrôlées*, are of major importance to the French wine industry and the improvement of wine quality.[29,45,46]

Italy is the second country in worldwide wine production and consumption. One of the most famous Italian wines is the red Chianti, Tuscany's and Italy's largest appellation. There are no general taste descriptions that apply to all Chianti wines. Sangiovese blended with smaller quantities of the red cultivars Canaiolo and Colorino and the white cultivars Trebbiano and Malvasia are used to make Chianti. In addition, the sweet Italian vermouth, a type of flavored fortified wine that originated in the Turin region, is one of the world's classic wines, but it is now widely produced in most wine-producing countries. Original Italian vermouth consists of a muscat-based wine plus the infusion of herbs, sugar, caramel, and alcohol. The custom of adding herbs is an ancient practice, and probably the presence of so many native herbs in northern Italy facilitated its development. The quality of the final product largely depends on the quality of the base wine, the mixing and the quality of the herbs, the aging, and the finishing process. Interestingly, most Italian wine is produced in southern Italy, but the great proportion of it goes to inexpensive blends or for distillation into industrial alcohol. The application of modern enological practices has been gradually improving the quality and consequently the production of better wines, which are bottled and traded under their own names.[20,29]

Spain is the third wine-producing country but the first worldwide in grape hectarage. Table wines are produced from La Mancha to the Pyrenees, but the region of Rioja has a long tradition of producing the finest table wines in Spain. Several types of wine are produced, with dessert being the most important Spanish wines. One famous Spanish wine is sherry. The making of sherry has been evolved in southern Spain since the early 1800s. In this country, the designation sherry is used as geographical appellation, restricted to the wines produced in and around Jerez, Andalucia. Spanish sherry is divided into three major categories, namely *finos, amontillados,* and *olorosos*.[20,29,47]

Portugal is also an important viticultural area. Port, or porto, the red sweet wine, is produced from red grapes grown and fermented in the upper Douro

Valley in northern Portugal. Samples from several vintages and localities are blended for creating the formula of a brand name with consistent character.[20,47]

In Greece, an ancient winemaking technique, the addition of resin during fermentation, is still in use, giving to retsina a terpene-like character. Resin is usually derived from the pine (*Pino halepensis*) that grows south of Athens in central Greece, and retsina is mainly produced in Attiki (the greater Athens area) from Savatiano white grapes. In recent decades, the production of resinated wines has diminished greatly. When it is practiced, much less resin is added in the fermenting must (less than 0.5% resin, in comparison with up to 2% in the past) (unpublished data from wine producers). The Peloponnese covers a quarter of the Greek wine production, and Aghiorgitiko, Moshofilero, Muscat, and Roditis are among the traditional cultivars. Recently, an upward trend has been noted in the production and quality of Greek wines. Macedonia and Thrace seem to have made progress in the wine industry, with Xinomavro being the most traditional cultivar of the region. The Aegean and Ionian islands also have interesting enological profiles, which vary greatly from island to island (Rombola, Asyrtiko, Limnio). Sweet wines have been traditionally produced in Greece, such as the sweet muscat wine in the island of Samos, and *Mavrodaphne*, a sort of tawny port-type wine that has a caramel flavor.[48] It is important to mention that a great proportion of Greek wines is distributed in bulk — approximately 40–50% of the total wine production (unpublished data from wine producers). As a whole, the Greek wine industry is a dynamic sector of growing importance for the country's economy. Among the positive points are the great number of indigenous varieties that result in a variety of products with particular characteristics, the improvements observed in the quality of winemaking at all stages, and the efficient adaptation to the market's local and international needs.[49]

C. WINE AND HEALTH

Vineyards and grapes, widespread in the Mediterranean landscape, are a part of traditional medicine. In Greece, grapes were traditionally recommended for the cure of diabetes, atherosclerosis, hypertension, cancer, and for keeping the body in good health.[50]

In scientific research, wine has been proven to be beneficial to a number of systems and diseases.[50] The cardioprotective anticarcinogenic effects of red wine consumption are studied most closely. The protection wine offers against cardiovascular disease may be attributed partly to its ethanol content (alcohol intake increases serum concentration of high density lipoprotein cholesterol) and partly to the antioxidant and platelet-inhibitory properties of its flavonoids and other phenolic compounds (such as resveratrol).[27,52,53,54] At the same time, wine still emerges as the companion drink of everyday meals, and seems to be preferable to other alcoholic drinks. Its consumption is perceived as transmitting messages of communication and warmth.[55] Of course, the beneficial effects of wine refer to moderate drinking, corresponding to two or three glasses of wine per day, consumed at a leisurely pace throughout the meal.[56]

IV. OTHER ALCOHOLIC BEVERAGES

A. BEER

Beer-making has a long tradition in the Mediterranean region. The first yeast was obtained from the froth of beer made in Spain, introducing the leavening process in human nutrition very early.[22] However, there is evidence that the beer-making process was also known in other parts of the Mediterranean region. For example, it has been recently discovered that ancient Greeks used to consume an alcoholic beverage that was similar to beer or a mixture of beer and wine.[57] Despite the fact that it was not originally a constituent of the traditional Mediterranean Diet, its popularity is gaining ground and tends to be considered, nowadays, as the typical drink in the diet of Mediterranean people.

Beer is a complex mixture made from malted barley. More than 400 different constituents have been identified so far. Some of them derive from the starting material (barley) and remain unchanged during the brewing process, whereas others are the result of several chemical transformations during the beer-making. Concentrations of these substances vary greatly among various types of beer, and they contribute to the particular sensory characteristics. The major constituent of beer is water, the solvent medium for all other substances. As a natural product of fermentation, beers contain carbon dioxide at recommended levels of 3.5–4.5 g/l. Beer may also include minor amounts of carbohydrates, remaining unfermented sugars (values ranging from 0.89 to 5.98% w/v as glucose are found). Complete carbohydrate fermentation results in the production of beers with very low sugar concentration. Protein and nitrogenous compounds are detected at nonsignificant levels (on average 0.2–0.3 g/100ml).[58,59] The alcohol content of beer, regarded as a measure of its strength, varies greatly from 3–7.5 g alcohol/100 ml, though some special brews may contain a lot more. It also determines the caloric content of beer (together with minor amounts of the residual carbohydrates and protein). Beer also contains small quantities of nicotinic acid and riboflavin, and, to a lesser extent, thiamine, biotin, pantothenic acid, B_6, folic acid, and vitamin B_{12}. Potassium, sodium, magnesium, and calcium are also present in beers.[59] Interestingly, beer provides a significant dietary source of readily available silicon, most of which is rapidly absorbed and excreted. Since some evidence suggests that silicon may play a role in excluding aluminum from organisms and fish and in gastrointestinal absorption, beer drinking should be evaluated in disease states conjectured to be related to aluminum intake.[60]

B. TRADITIONAL DISTILLED ALCOHOLIC BEVERAGES IN THE MEDITERRANEAN REGION

Ouzo is a traditional distilled spirit made with anise and produced in Greece. The term ouzo is recognized exclusively as a Greek name, after the consolidation by the EU regulations.[61] It is the most popular distilled spirit consumed in Greece, with considerable economic importance both as a domestic and an export product. It is produced by the distillation of the seeds of *Illicium verum* (star anis), *Pimpinella anissum* (aniseed), *Foeniculum vulgare* (fennel), *Pistacia Chia lentiscus* (mastic), and other aromatic plants (coriander, cinnamon, nutmeg), with ethyl alcohol of agricultural origin.[62] Ouzo must have alcohol content above 37.5% (v/v) (most made for commercial purposes has 40–42%), and sugar concentration lower than 50 g/l (most commonly 20g/l, whereas some have none). The characteristic taste and aroma of ouzo are attributed to anethole, an essential flavoring component of the above-mentioned seeds. Anethole is almost insoluble in water; it forms an emulsion when water or ice is added, because of the insolubility of anethole when the alcohol concentration decreases. The characteristic "milky" hue of ouzo depends on its alcohol and anethole concentration, the amount of water added, and the temperature.[62] Differences in aroma and flavor between several ouzo products are attributed to differences in the concentration of other minor components, as a result of the use of different flavoring materials added by local manufacturers.[63,64]

Concurrent with, or following, the production of ouzo, several Mediterranean countries produce anis-flavored alcoholic beverages, i.e. beverages produced by the flavoring of pure alcohol with star anis, aniseed, or fennel. The most representative and popular are the *pastis* in France and the *anis* in Spain. Some analogous liqueurs, like *anesone* in Spain and *sambuca* in Italy, are also popular in the Mediterranean region.[30,62]

Brandy is a generic name used for the alcoholic drinks produced traditionally by wine distillation.[30] Famous brandies are Cognac and Armagnac in France (produced in the corresponding regions), but brandies of good quality are also produced all over the wine-making Mediterranean countries.[62]

Alcoholic drinks produced by the distillation of the pomace are widely known across the Mediterranean. *Grappa* in Italy, *tsipouro* and *tsikoudia* in Greece, *bagaceira* in Portugal, and *marc* in France, all constitute part of the tradition of this region. Depending on the regulations governing the distillation process, sucrose may be added in small amounts as well as aniseeds and other botanical aromatic ingredients. The alcoholic content of these commercial products must be higher than 37.7% (v/v).[30,62,65,66]

V. CONCLUSIONS

Alcoholic beverages constitute an important component of the Mediterranean Diet. In the past, alcohol was consumed daily in moderation and during meals, mainly in the form of wine, the traditional drink of this region since ancient times. Wine is closely associated with the culture and life-style of the Mediterranean people, excluding the Moslems. During recent decades, wine has been further appreciated for its beneficial effects on health; in particular, its protective role against cardiovascular disease is fairly well documented.

Due to the profound socioeconomic and cultural changes in the area, alcohol-consumption patterns have been considerably affected. Total alcohol-beverage availability decreased in France and Italy, whereas wine availability decreased in all Mediterranean countries. Recently introduced international beverages have replaced wine consumption in various degrees. Beer, in first place, followed by distilled beverages, is gaining ground in the preferences of people living in this basin. The decrease in wine consumption has come about in spite of improvement and standardization of wine-production quality and the increase in consumer information about wine quality issues and health benefits.

REFERENCES

1. Nestle, M., Mediterranean diets: historical and research overview, *Am. J. Clin. Nutr.* 61, 1313S, 1995.
2. Keys, A., Mediterranean diet and public health: personal reflections, *Am. J. Clin. Nutr.* 61, 1321S, 1995.
3. Renaud, S. and de Lorgeril, M., Wine, alcohol, platelets, and the French Paradox for coronary heart disease, *Lancet* 339, 1523, 1992.
4. Atwater, W. O. and Benedict, F. G., An experimental inquiry regarding the nutritive value of alcohol, *Mem. Natl. Acad. Sci.* 8, 235, 1902.
5. Pernanen, K., Validity of survey data on alcohol use, *Research Advances in Alcohol and Drug problems*, Vol 1, Gibbins, R .J. et al., Eds., John Wiley & Sons, New York, 1974, 355.
6. Food and Agriculture Organization (FAO) Databank, Standardized Food Balance Sheets, 1999.
7. Anderson, P., Management of drinking problems, WHO Regional Publication, European Series No 32, WHO Regional Office for Europe, Copenhagen, 1990.
8. Buora, N., Tendenze e consumi — il beverage in Italia, *Imballaggio*, 519, 74, 1999.
9. Sulkunen, P., Drinking in France 1965–1979: An analysis of household consumption data, *Addiction,* 84, 61, 1989.
10. Pyörälä, E., Trends in alcohol consumption in Spain, Portugal, France, and Italy from the 1950s until the 1980s, *Br. J. Addict.*, 85, 469, 1990.
11. Hupkens, C. L. H., Knibbe, R. A., and Drop, M. J., Alcohol consumption in the European Community: uniformity and diversity in drinking patterns, *Addiction*, 88, 1391, 1993.
12. Simpura, J., Paakkanen, P., and Mustonen, H., New beverages, new drinking contexts? Signs of modernization in Finnish drinking habits from 1984 to 1992, compared with trends in the European Community, *Addiction*, 90, 673, 1995.
13. Trichopoulou, A. and Lagiou, P., Eds., *DAFNE (Data Food Networking): Methodology for the exploitation of HBS data and results on food availability in five European countries*, Office for Official Publications of the European Community, Luxembourg, 1997, 89, 90, 98.
14. Trichopoulou, A. and Lagiou, P., Eds., *DAFNE (Data Food Networking), Methodology for the exploitation of HBS data and results on food availability in six European countries*, Office for Official Publications of the European Community, Luxembourg, 1998, 127, 128, 136.
15. Ritson, E. B., Community response to alcohol-related problems: review of an international study, *Public Health Paper No 81*, World Health Organization, Geneva, 1981.
16. Barnes, G., Welte, J., and Dintcheff, B., Alcohol misuse among college students and other young adults: findings from a general population study in New York State, *Int. J. Addict.* 27, 917, 1992.
17. Madianos, M. G., Gefou-Madianou, D., and Stefanis, C., Patterns of alcohol consumption and related problems in the general population of Greece, *Addiction*, 90, 73, 1995.

18. Choquet, M., Menke, H., and Ledoux, S., Self-reported alcohol consumption among adolescents and the significance of early onset, *Soc. Psychiatry Psychiatr Epidemiol.*, 24, 102, 1989.

19. Moreiras-Varela, O., van Stavaren, W. A., Cruz, J. A., Nes, M., and Lund-Larsen, K., EURONUT-SENECA: Intake of energy and nutrients, *Eur. J. Clin. Nutr.*, 45 (Suppl 3), 105, 1991.

20. Jackson, R. S., *Wine Science: Principles and Applications*, Academic Press, San Diego, 1994, Chaps. 1, 6, 10.

21. Vallee, B. L., Alcohol in the Western World, *Sci. Am.* 278, 80, 1998.

22. Waterlow, J. C., Diet of the classical period of Greece and Rome, *Eur. J. Clin. Nutr.* 43 (Suppl. 2), 3, 1989.

23. Haas, C., L'orge, l'olive et le vin, triade dietetique et therapeutique des anciens peuples de la Mediterranée, *Ann. Med. Interne* 149, 275, 1998.

24. Kromhout, D., Keys, A., Aravanis, C., Buzina, R., Fidanza, F., Giamaoli, S., Jansen, A., Menotti, A., Nedeljkovic, S., Pekkarinen, M., Simic, B. S., and Toshima, H., Food consumption patterns in the 1960s in seven countries, *Am. J. Clin. Nutr.* 49, 889, 1989.

25. Christakis, G., Severinghaus, E. L., Maldonado, Z., Kafatos, F. C., and Hashim, S. A., Crete: a study in the metabolic epidemiology of coronary artery disease, *Am. J. Cardiol.* 15, 320, 1965.

26. Smart, R. G., Behavioral and social consequences related to the consumption of different beverage types, *J. Stud. Alcohol* 57, 77, 1996.

27. Soleas, G. J., Diamandis, E. P., and Goldberg, D. M., Wine as a biological fluid: history, production, and role in disease prevention, *J. Clin. Lab. Anal.* 11, 287, 1997.

28. Di Stefano, R., Advances in the study of secondary metabolites occurring in grapes and wines, *Drugs Exp. Clin. Res.* 25, 53, 1999.

29. Amerine, M. A., Berg, H. W, Kunkee, R. E., Ough, C. S., Singleton, V. L., and Webb, A. D., *The Technology of Winemaking*, 4th ed., AVI Publishing Company, Westport, 1980, chaps. 1, 5.

30. Kourakou-Dragona, S., *Wine Choices*, Athens, Trohalia, 1997 (in Greek).

31. Simonetti, P., Pietta, P., and Testolin, G., Polyphenol content and total antioxidant potential of selected Italian wines, *J. Agric. Food Chem.* 45, 1152, 1997.

32. Lairon, D. and Amiot, M. J., Flavonoids in food and natural antioxidants in wine, *Curr. Opin. Lipidol.*, 10, 23, 1999.

33. Brouillard, R., George, F., and Fougerousse, A., Polyphenols produced during red wine ageing, *Biofactors* 6, 403, 1997.

34. Lamuela-Raventos, R. M. and De La Torre-Boronat, M. C., Beneficial effects of white wine, *Drugs Exp. Clin. Res.* 25, 121, 1999.

35. Mazza, G., Anthocyanins in grapes and grape products, *Crit. Rev. Food Sci. Nutr.* 35, 341, 1995.

36. Cheynier, V., Fulcrand, H., Brossaud, F., Asselin, C., and Moutounet, M., Phenolic composition as related to wine flavor, ACS Symp. Series 714, American Chemical Society, Washington, DC, 1998, p. 124.

37. Formica, J. V. and Regelson, W., Review of the biology of quercetin and related bioflavonoids, *Fd. Chem. Toxic.* 33, 1061, 1995.

38. Croft, K. D., The chemistry and biological effects of flavonoids and phenolic acids, *Ann. NY Acad. Sci.* 854, 435, 1998.

39. Bavaresco, L., Fregoni, C., Cantu, E., and Trevisan, M., Stilbene compounds: from grapevine to wine, *Drugs Exp. Clin. Res.* 25, 57, 1999.

40. Soleas, G. J., Diamandis, E. P., and Goldberg, D. M., Resveratrol: a molecule whose time has come? And gone?, *Clin. Biochem.* 30, 91, 1997.

41. Gavaler, J. S., Imhoff, A. F., Pohl, C. R., Roseblum, E. R., and van Thiel, D. H., Alcoholic beverages: a source of estrogenic substances, *Alcohol* Suppl. 1, 545, 1987.

42. Calabrese, G., Nonalcoholic compounds of wine: the phytoestrogen resveratrol and moderate wine consumption during menopause, *Drugs Exp. Clin. Res.* 15, 111, 1999.

43. Mazur, W., Phytoestrogen content in foods, *Baillieres Clin. Endocrinol. Metabol.* 12, 729, 1998.

44. Muller, C. J., Wine and health — it is more than alcohol, in *Wine Analysis and Production*, Zoecklein, B.W., et al., Eds., Chapman & Hall, New York, 1995, 14.

45. Bell, B. and Dorozynski, A., *Le Livre du Vin*, Editions des Deux Coqs d' Or, Paris, 1968.

46. Navarre, C., *L' Oenologie*, Lavoisier Tec. & Doc., Paris, 1998, chap. 9.

47. Johnson, H., *Wine*, Simon & Schuster Inc., New York, 1974.

48. Tsakiris, A., *Knowledge of the Greek Wines*, Iniohos, Athens, 1995 (in Greek).

49. Bamiatzis, Y., Wine and economy: upward trends in exports, *Oineas' News* 22, 24, 1999 (in Greek).

50. Wahlquist, M., Kouris-Blazos, A., and Polychronopoulos, E., The wisdom of the Greek cuisine and way of life, *Age Nutr.* 2, 163, 1991.

51. Finkel, H. E., Wine and health: a review and perspective, *J. Wine Res.* 7, 157, 1996.

52. Hulley, S. B. and Gordon, S., Alcohol and high density lipoprotein cholesterol: causal inference from diverse study designs, *Circulation* 64, 57, 1981.

53. Maalej, N., Demrow, H. S., Slane, P. R., and Folts, J. D., Antithrombotic effect of flavonoids in red wine, ACS Symp. Series 661, American Chemical Society, Washington, DC, 1997, pp. 247.

54. Goldberg, D. M., Hahn, S. E. and Parkes, J. G., Beyond alcohol: beverage consumption and cardiovascular mortality, *Clin. Chim. Acta* 237, 155, 1995.

55. Tzimitra-Kalogianni, I., Papadaki-Kavdianou, A., Alexaki, A., and Tsakiridou, E., Wine routes in Northern Greece: consumer perceptions, *Br. Food J.* 101, 884, 1999.

56. Trichopoulou, A., Kouris-Blazos, A., Vassilakou, T., Gnardellis, C., Polychronopoulos, E., Venizelos, M., Lagiou, P., Wahlqvist, M. L., and Trichopoulos, D., Diet and survival of elderly Greeks: a link to the past, *Am. J. Clin. Nutr.* 61(suppl.), 1346S, 1995.

57. Greek Ministry of Culture and National Archaeological Museum, Minoans' and Mycenaeans' Flavors, Ministry of Culture, Athens, 1999.

58. Holland, B., Welch, A. A., Unwin, I. D., Buss, D. H., Paul, A. A., and Southgate, D. A. T., *McCance & Widdowson's The Composition of Foods*, 5th ed., Royal Society of Chemistry, Cambridge, 1991.

59. Hough, J. S., Briggs, D. E., Stevens, R., and Young T. W., *Malting and Brewing Science*, Vol. II, Chapman & Hall, London, 1982, chap. 22.

60. Bellia, J. P., Birchall, J. D., and Roberts, N. B., Beer: a dietary source of silicon, *Lancet* 343, 235, 1994.

61. European Commission, Regulation 1576/89.

62. Tsakiris, A., *Potographia*, Psychalos, Athens, 1999 (in Greek).

63. Kontominas, M. G., Volatile constituents of Greek ouzo, *J. Agric. Food Chem.* 34, 847, 1986.

64. Geronti, A., Spiliotis, C., Liadakis, G. N., and Tzia, C., Effect of distillation factors on ouzo flavors examined by sensory evaluation, *Dev. Fd. Sci.* 40, 219, 1998.

65. Da Porto, C., Grappa and grape-spirit production, *Crit. Rev. Biotechol.* 18, 13, 1998.
66. Soufleros, E. and Bertrand, A., Etude sur le Tsipouro, eau-de-vie de marc traditionelle de Grèce, precurseur de l' ouzo, *Connaisance Vigne Vin* 21, 93, 1987.

Part III

Health Promotion and Disease Prevention

9 Mediterranean Diet and Longevity

George Mamalakis and Anthony Kafatos

CONTENTS

I. INTRODUCTION

The virtues of the Mediterranean Diet have been advocated since the Renaissance. Efforts at facilitating change in dietary patterns toward the Mediterranean prototype have been manifested in the works of American and European authors since 1614. The impetus came from a book on Italian herbs, fruits, and vegetables by Giacomo Castelvetro, an exile from Modena, Italy.[1] Since the 1950s and the work by Ancel Keys,[2] the Mediterranean Diet has served as a prototype for dietary recommendations in the U.S. and elsewhere. Growing evidence indicates that the Mediterranean Diet is protective against a number of diseases, particularly coronary heart disease and some forms of malignancy.[3] It is characterized by high consumption of fruit, vegetables, legumes, and whole grains; frequent consumption of fish; moderate intake of alcohol, mainly wine; moderate or low consumption of milk and dairy products, mostly cheese; and low intake of animal products and refined carbohydrates. The Mediterranean Diet is rich in monounsaturated fat, fiber, vitamins, and natural antioxidants, and poor in polyunsaturated, saturated, and hydrogenated fats.

Although there are several variants,[3] the common denominator, the typical Mediterranean Diet, is characterized by lower intakes of meat and animal fat and higher intakes of fish, fruit, vegetables, and olive oil. Perhaps the cardinal characteristic of the Mediterranean Diet is that olive oil serves as the principal source of dietary fat.[3,4] Olive oil, or "liquid gold," as ancient historian Homer used to call it, is extracted from the stone fruits, or drupes, of *Olea Europaea*.[5] Since antiquity, the olive tree has been widely grown in the areas of southern Europe, hence its name. The therapeutic virtues of olive oil were acknowledged by doctors of antiquity such as Galen, Hippocrates, and Dioscorides.[5,6]

II. THE MEDITERRANEAN DIET AND ALL-CAUSES MORTALITY DATA

There are numerous indications that adoption of a Mediterranean Diet is associated with longevity or decreased all-cause mortality. Mediterranean populations, Greeks and Italians in particular, have been reported to have among the highest life expectancies in the world, and among the lowest prevalence rates in certain forms of cancer and diet-related chronic diseases.[7] According to a recent report,[8] adult mortality in Albania, a Mediterranean country, is similar to that of other Mediterranean countries. An examination of the regional distribution of the 1978 mortality there indicated that mortality was lowest in the southwest part of the country, where there is greatest production and consumption of fruits, vegetables, and olive oil. Results of the Seven Countries Study,[9] after 25 years of follow-up, indicated that, among the 16 different cohorts studied, the Greeks and Italians had among the lowest all-cause mortality (Figure 1). The cumulative mortality from all causes for the Italian group was 48.3%, whereas that for the Greek group was 35.3%.[10]

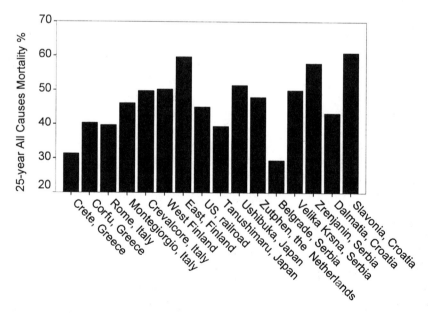

FIGURE 1   All-causes mortality for the Seven Countries Study cohorts.

Among the 16 cohorts of the surviving men of the Seven Countries Study, the Cretan cohort and that from Belgrade, Serbia, had the lowest all-cause mortality 25 years after the initiation of the study.[9] In another study, survival of elderly men and women was studied in relation to adherence to the Greek variant of the Mediterranean Diet. Degree of adherence to the traditional Greek diet was reflected by a composite dietary score, based on eight characteristics. It was found that each unit increase in the diet score was associated with a significant 17% reduction in overall mortality. The authors concluded that life expectancy in the elderly is positively affected by the degree of adherence to the Greek variant of the Mediterranean Diet.[11]

In a recent randomized prospective prevention trial (Lyon Diet Heart Study),[12] the effects of the Step 1 American Heart Association prudent diet and the Cretan Mediterranean Diet were tested on 605 patients recovering from myocardial infarction. It was found that, within a few months (27 months), recurrent myocardial infarction, cardiovascular events, and cardiac and all-cause mortality were reduced by more than 70% in the group consuming the Cretan diet. The authors concluded that the high life expectancy of the Cretans appears to stem largely from their dietary habits. Similar findings were indicated after 4 years of follow-up. Specifically, with reference to all-cause mortality, there was a significant 56% reduction in total deaths in the subjects consuming the Cretan diet as opposed to those on the prudent diet.[13] Finally, it was observed that the Cretan diet was associated with a 70% decrease of all-cause mortality after 5 years of follow-up.[14]

III. THE MEDITERRANEAN DIET AND MORTALITY FROM CANCER AND CHD

There are indications that, besides reducing deaths from all causes, consumption of a Mediterranean diet is associated with decreased mortality from diseases that are leading causes of death, such as coronary heart disease and cancer. Mortality data indicates that, compared with eastern, central, and northern European populations, Mediterranean populations have lower all-cause mortality rates and lower morbidity and mortality rates from coronary heart disease and cardiovascular disease, and from many neoplastic diseases, despite a high prevalence of smoking.[15-17] As indicated by the Lyon Diet Heart Study,[13] besides the significant reduction in total and cardiac deaths, there was a significant (61%) reduction in cancer deaths in the Cretan diet group as opposed to that on the AHA prudent diet, at 4 years of follow-up. In addition, results from the Seven Countries Study[18] indicated that, compared with northern European groups, Mediterranean groups had five times lower 25-year mortality from coronary heart disease (Figure 2). With reference to cancer, the Greek group had the lowest 25-year cancer mortality, compared with all other groups (Figure 3).[9]

The decreased coronary heart disease, cancer, and all-cause mortality associated with the Mediterranean Diet appears to be due to the increased consumption of fruit and vegetables and the associated elevated intake of fiber, vitamins, and antioxidant flavonoid and polyphenolic constituents that characterize this diet. It has been reported that high dietary intakes of fruit and vegetables are associated with elevated

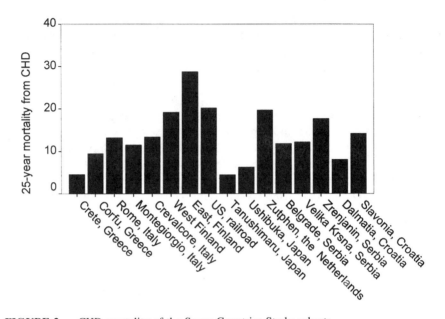

FIGURE 2   CHD mortality of the Seven Countries Study cohorts.

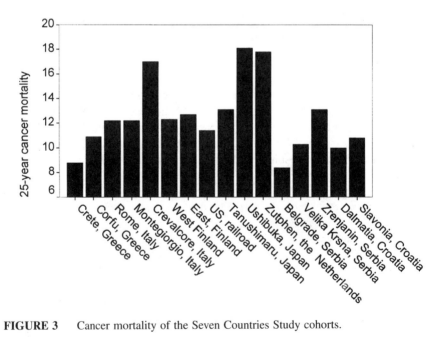

FIGURE 3   Cancer mortality of the Seven Countries Study cohorts.

plasma vitamin levels.[19] On the other hand, there is considerable evidence that, besides fruits and vegetables,[20-22] certain vitamins confer protection against neoplastic diseases. For example, high-plasma antioxidants such as vitamins C, A, and E, ceruloplasmin, and carotenoids (alpha- and beta carotene, cryptoxanthin, lycopene, lutein, zeaxanthin) were found in a randomly selected population subsample in an area with low frequency of cancer.[23] A prospective study on 2974 men (Basel Study),[24] indicated that overall mortality from cancer was associated with decreased plasma carotene and vitamin C levels at both 12 and 17 years of follow-up.[25] Along the same lines, a large-scale study in 65 counties in the People's Republic of China[26] indicated consistent negative correlation between cancer mortality rates and dietary antioxidants, particularly vitamin C.

A recent review study[27] indicated that the decrease in cancer risk associated with fruit and vegetable consumption may be due to the vitamin, carotenoid, and flavonoid content of this diet. The study presented experimental evidence indicating that these dietary constituents have the potential to quench the carcinogenecity of known carcinogens, such as N-nitrosocompounds and free radicals, and to reduce DNA damage and mutagenesis. The authors concluded that, although there is as yet insufficient direct evidence for a cancer protective effect by these micronutrients, recommendations should be made toward increasing fruit and vegetable intake, as there are clear indications that such a diet decreases the risk of cancer.

Much like cancer, the risk of coronary heart disease also appears to be reduced by micronutrient compounds such as vitamins, flavonoids, and polyphenols.[19,28-31]

It has been suggested that the lower incidence and mortality from cancer and coronary heart disease associated with the Mediterranean Diet may be, at least in part, due to its high content of vitamins, flavonoids, and polyphenols.[32] Moreover, there are indications that, in addition to decreasing cancer and coronary heart disease mortality risks, certain vitamins appear to be associated with longevity or decreased all-cause mortality. Specifically, the Established Populations for Epidemiologic Studies of the Elderly[29] examined the effects of vitamin supplementation on all-cause mortality risk in 11,178 elderly persons. There were 3490 deaths within a 9-year period. It was found that vitamin E supplementation reduced significantly the risk of all-cause mortality. Moreover, simultaneous supplementation with vitamins E and C was associated with an even further decrease in all-cause mortality risk. Similarly, in a study of 29,584 adults,[33] the effects of vitamin and mineral supplementation were tested with reference to all-cause mortality within a time period of 5 years. It was found that selenium, beta carotene, and vitamin E supplementation was associated with a significantly reduced all-cause mortality. In addition, a study of 5133 men and women aged 30–69 indicated an inverse relation between dietary flavonoid intake and total mortality after 15–20 years of follow-up.[30] Finally, the Seven Countries Study data[34] indicated a significant inverse relation between vitamin C intake and 25-year all-cause mortality. The higher life-span and decreased all-causes, cancer, and coronary heart disease mortality in the Mediterranean region, therefore, may be due, at least partly, to the elevated content of Mediterranean Diet in certain vitamins, flavonoids, and polyphenols.

IV. THE FREE RADICAL AND MITOCHONDRIAL THEORY OF AGING

The health and longevity associated with the adoption of a Mediterranean diet appears to stem from the effects of vitamins and antioxidants in this diet on free radical production and scavenging, and on the associated effects on cellular and DNA integrity, cellular respiration and energy production, and immunity. In an attempt to study aging and longevity, many theories have been formulated in the last decades. Among them, the free radical theory of aging[7] has received much attention and support from an increasing body of evidence. According to this theory, aging is very dependent on oxidative stress, free radical attack, and damage on cellular constituents such as membranes, proteins, lipids, RNA and DNA.[35-36] Free radicals are found as environmental pollutants (e.g. tobacco smoke, smog) or can be produced during irradiation exposure (e.g., U.V. irradiation), autooxidation of various chemicals and biomolecules (e.g., polyunsaturated fats), lipid peroxidation of polyunsaturated fatty acids, and mitochondrial respiration. The mitochondria is the power factory of the body. O_2 consumption and respiration in the mitochondria are the means of supplying the body with chemical energy or ATP. In healthy tissues, more than 90% of the O_2 is consumed by the mitochondria, and, for this reason the mitochondrion is the major intracellular O_2-radical producing unit. On the other hand, mitochondrial DNA (mtDNA), is very close to and eventually contacts the inner mitochondrial membrane, the chief free radical production site within the mitochondrion.[37]

Another reason for the vulnerability of mtDNA to oxidative damage is that human mtDNA replicates rapidly in the absence of efficient proofreading and repair systems.[38-39] Most cellular genes are at the nuclear, not the mitochondrial DNA. However, mtDNA is much more susceptible to oxidative damage than nuclear DNA.[37,40] An increasing body of literature suggests an association between mtDNA damage and aging (mito-chondrial theory of aging). Specifically, deletions, point mutations, tandem duplica-tions, and rearrangements of mtDNA have been identified in various tissues of elderly humans.[41-46] Moreover, the extent of various such mtDNA deformations/damage has been found to increase as a function of age and to correlate with oxidative damage to mtDNA.[45,47-49] Apart from predisposing toward developing a number of diseases, there are indications that oxidative damage to mtDNA might also impair mitochondrial respiration and ATP production,[50-54] leading to inadequate energy supply to cells and tissues and energy depletion and possibly fatigue in the elderly (bioenergetic disease). Nevertheless, in addition to mitochondrial respiration impairment,[53-54] aging has been reported to be associated with a deficiency in degrading and disposing the aberrant proteins that have resulted from oxidative modifications.[55-57]

One of the causes of free radical formation and oxidative stress and possibly mtDNA damage, is peroxidation of polyunsaturated fats (PUFA). Lipid peroxidation or, simply, peroxidation, refers to free radical attack on, or oxidative modification of lipids, PUFA in particular. Lipid peroxidation results in reversible or irreversible cell and tissue damage, and is thus implicated in the aging process. The peroxidative breakdown of PUFA by free radicals in the cellular membranes leads to degradation of the cellular membranes and the generation of new free radicals. Peroxidation of polyunsaturates leads to the formation of toxic lipid peroxides such as lipid hydro-peroxide (LOOH), lipid peroxyl radical (LOO·), lipid alkoxyl radical (LO·), and lipofuscins. Lipofuscins are believed to result from the cross-linking of proteins that have undergone free radical attack (aberrant proteins) and lipid peroxides.[58-59] Lipo-fuscins are definitely implicated in the aging process, therefore the name "age pigments." [58-61] In addition to lipofuscins, there are indications that other deleterious products of PUFA oxidation such as malondialdehyde (MDA) and thiobarbituric acid-reacting substances (TBARS) also may be elevated in the elderly.[36,62-64] In addition, there are indications that glutathione peroxidase, the main enzyme for the biodegradation of lipid hydroperoxides, is reduced in the elderly.[65-67] Most of the studies we have found show an increase in PUFA peroxidation and peroxidation products in the elderly, as opposed to younger age groups.[36,66,68-69] It has been reported that lipid peroxides may damage biomembranes, thereby facilitating cellular aging.[70-71] In addition, there are indications that peroxidation of PUFA may be implicated in the aging of human erythrocytes both *in vivo* and *in vitro*. [72-74] Moreover, there are indications that there is a simultaneous increase in PUFA peroxidation and mtDNA damage during aging in both animals and humans.[36,58-59,75-76] For example, Miquel and associates [74-76]demonstrated that in animals there was a simultaneous increase in mtDNA damage and lipofuscin content during aging.

Along the same lines, a human study showed a simultaneous and age-dependent increase in PUFA peroxidation, and oxidatively damaged and deleted mtDNA in the human lung.[74] Also, similar findings were indicated by another human study[36] that showed that the 4977-bp and 7436 mtDNA deletions, the most abundant and prev-alent mtDNA deletions, show an age-dependent increase. Second, it was found that there is also an age-dependent increase in the mitochondrial lipid peroxide content in several different human tissues. Finally, there was a positive relation between the proportion of 4977-bp mtDNA deletions and mitochondrial lipid peroxides in various human tissues. On the other hand, the possibility of a causal link between PUFA peroxidation and aging via mtDNA damage was further strengthened by another, albeit animal, study. This study showed that administration of coenzyme Q_{10}, a free radical scavenger, decreased lipid peroxide content and prevented mtDNA deletion in mouse heart mitochondria.[76]

V. THE MEDITERRANEAN DIET AND OXIDATIVE STRESS

There are indications that certain dietary constituents of the Mediterranean Diet such as olive oil, vitamins, flavonoids, polyphenols, and herbal antioxidant ingredients may inhibit free radical formation and PUFA peroxidation, and protect against DNA dam-age. Furthermore, there are indications that some of these ingredients may enhance immunity and facilitate mitochondrial respiration and ATP production. Specifically, it has been reported that, unlike PUFA-containing oils such as sunflower and soy, olive oil is particularly resistant to high-temperature heating (180°C). High-temperature heating resulted in loss of antioxidant defense potential and increase in toxic lipid peroxidation products in PUFA oils, but not in olive oil.[77] There are indications that certain polyphenolic olive oil constituents, such as hydroxytyrosol, oleuropein, caffeic acid, rutin, protocatecuic acid, 3,4-dihydroxyphenylethanol-elenolic acid (3,4-DHPEA-EA), and 3,4-dihydroxyphenylethanol (3,4-DHPEA) are endowed with strong antioxidant properties.[78-80] For example, an *in-vitro* human study showed that 3,4-DHPEA conferred complete protection against oxidative damage to intestinal epithelium cells at a concentration as small as 100 micromol/L.[81]

In a cross-cultural study,[82] the effects of the Mediterranean Diet vs. those of a northern European diet were compared with reference to lipid peroxidation. The two groups consisted of young healthy people from Naples (southern Italy) and Bristol (U.K.). Compared with the Bristol group, the Italian group had significantly reduced serum lipid peroxidation indices, such as lipid peroxides, conjugated dienes, and diene conjugation index. In another study,[83] 80 men were supplemented with either menhaden oil (fish oil) or olive oil, over a period of 6 weeks. Fish oil supplementation resulted in a significant elevation in plasma malondialdehyde and other products of lipid peroxidation, while no such elevations were evidenced for olive oil.

Another human study reported that oleic acid, the main fatty acid in olive oil, inhibited lipid peroxidation and protected gastrointestinal mucosal membranes and liver microsomes from oxidative damage *in vitro*.[84] Similarly, there was an increase in reactive oxygen species (ROS) and lipid peroxidation products following incubation of cultured human fibroblasts with either n-3 or n-6 polyunsaturates. However, no increases in ROS or lipid peroxides were evidenced after incubation with oleic acid.[85]

Finally, in another study,[86] 59 healthy adults were supplemented with either sunflower oil (rich in PUFA) or low-erucic-acid rapeseed oil (rich in monounsaturated fatty acids). Compared with the monounsaturated fat-containing oil, the PUFA oil resulted in higher levels of malondialdehyde, the major product of lipid peroxidation, and DNA adducts in white blood cells. In fact, compared with the monounsaturated fat-containing oil, the PUFA oil resulted in 3.6-fold higher levels of DNA adducts of malondialdehyde. In addition to olive oil and its constituents, other Mediterranean Diet components, such as vitamins, flavonoids, and herbal micronutrients, also inhibit ROS and lipid peroxidation. For example, all, vitamins C, E, and beta-carotene have been reported to inhibit free radical formation and lipid peroxidation, and protect biological membranes from oxidative damage.[87-92] There are indications that there is antioxidant synergism between vitamins C and E.[90-92] Also, there are indications that, among these vitamins, vitamin E has the most effective antioxidant action.[87-88] In addition to vitamins, flavonoids also have been reported to inhibit free radical formation and lipid peroxidation, and to confer cytoprotection, and, specifically, protect biomembranes from oxidative damage.[80,93-97] Although, as yet, there are no complete accounts, the use of herbs such as sage, thyme, oregano, and rosemary, to mention only a few, is believed to be a common practice in Crete. Much like olive oil constituents, vitamins and flavonoids, herbal ingredients, also have been reported to inhibit free radical formation. Several ingredients present in rosemary, sage, oregano, and thyme are reported to have antioxidant effects.[98-104]

In addition to protecting from free radical-induced membrane damage, certain Mediterranean Diet constituents appear also to protect against oxidative damage to the mitochondria. As shown by a study, dietary polyunsaturated fat was associated with a decrease in mitochondrial coenzyme Q, an antioxidant agent, whereas monounsaturated fat was associated with elevated mitochondrial coenzyme Q levels.[105] As indicated by an animal study, there was a higher degree of protection of the mitochondrial membranes of rats fed virgin olive oil than those fed sunflower oil, a polyunsaturated fat-containing oil.[106] In another study,[107] the effects of olive oil, coenzyme Q_{10} (an antioxidant), and sunflower oil (rich in n-6 PUFA) on the rat heart mitochondria were tested. It was found that olive oil and coenzyme Q_{10}, but not sunflower oil, effectively reduced lipid peroxidation and protected rat mitochondrial membranes against oxidative damage. Moreover, a series of experiments on rats[108] showed that dietary olive oil was associated with successful protection of mitochondrial and microsomal membranes from peroxidation, a fact not evidenced for dietary polyunsaturated fat.

VI. THE MEDITERRANEAN DIET AND MITOCHONDRIAL RESPIRATION

As has already been stated,[53-54] sufficient energy production and supply to the body is contingent on mitochondrial respiration, a function that has been reported to decline with aging. As shown by animal studies, there are indications that certain Mediterranean Diet constituents, such as vitamins C and E, may stimulate mitochondrial respiration and ATP production.[109-112]

VII. THE MEDITERRANEAN DIET AND DNA DAMAGE

As indicated in a recent review study,[27] micronutrient components of the Mediterranean Diet, such as some vitamins, carotenoids, and flavonoids, have the potential to reduce DNA damage. Both animal and human studies indicate that vitamins E and C, and maybe to a lesser extent vitamin A and beta carotene, protect against oxidative DNA damage in various types of cells.[113-122] It has been suggested that, because they protect against oxidative DNA damage, vitamins may also protect from diseases that are leading causes of death, such as cancer for example, thereby contributing to longevity. In addition to vitamins, a number of studies indicate that naturally occurring polyphenols and flavonoids also protect against oxidative DNA modifications.[115,123-126] Some studies indicated that flavonoids were more effective than vitamins in protecting against oxidative DNA modifications,[115,123] while other studies suggested that, in the presence of metal ions (e.g., Fe^{+3}, copper), some flavonoids act as pro-oxidants rather than antioxidants, and inducers of oxidative DNA damage.[127-130] Still another study[131] indicated that some flavonoids act as anticarcinogens via stimulating tumor suppressor protein p53 accumulation, cancer cell growth arrest, and apoptosis or destruction of cancer cells.

A recent intervention study evaluated the effects of a high-fat diet and a Mediterranean diet, and their supplementation with red wine on, among other things, oxidative DNA damage in human leukocytes. Two groups of male participants, 21 subjects in each group, received either a high-fat diet or a Mediterranean diet over a period of 3 months. Both diets were supplemented with wine during the second month of intervention. Total serum antioxidant capacity increased for the Mediterranean but not for the high-fat group. Wine supplementation resulted in an increase in total antioxidant capacity in both groups, 56% and 23%, respectively. Oxidative damage to leukocyte DNA was markedly elevated in the high-fat group. Wine supplementation resulted in marked reductions in oxidative damage to leukocyte DNA (to about 50% baseline levels) in both groups.[132] These findings are probably due to the elevated flavonoid content of wine[97] and the increased vitamin and flavonoid content of the Mediterranean Diet. There are indications that because they protect against oxidative DNA damage, Mediterranean Diet constituents such as vitamins and naturally occurring flavonoids and polyphenols may protect from diseases that are leading causes of death, such as cancer for example,[113,118,129,131] thereby contributing to longevity.

VIII. THE MEDITERRANEAN DIET AND IMMUNITY

It has been suggested that aging is coupled with a decline in immunological vigor and an associated increase in infectious and neoplastic diseases.[133,134] This decline in immune response is believed to be contributing to the elevated morbidity and mortality in the elderly.[134] On the other hand, Mediterranean Diet ingredients such as vitamins E, C, A, and beta-carotene have been reported to have immunoenhancing effects.[133-140]

IX. THE MEDITERRANEAN DIET AND DETOXIFICATION

It has been suggested that one of the mechanisms contributing to maintenance and longevity in mammals is detoxification. Detoxification refers to the process of degrading and disposing deleterious or toxic chemicals endogenously produced or arising in the environment or diet. A wide array of enzymes responsible for detoxification, localized in the liver, are known as the P_{450} cytochromes.[141] There are indications that certain micronutrient ingredients of herbs and spices in the Mediterranean Diet are implicated in the detoxification process. A human study indicated that, in addition to inhibiting oxidative stress and DNA adduct formation, carnosol and carnosic acid, active components of rosemary (*Rosmarinus officialis*), exhibited anticarcinogenic action. The two mechanisms proposed to underlie this action were: (1) inhibition of procarcinogen activation via mobilization of detoxification phase I cytochrome P_{450} enzymes, and (2) via mobilization of phase II detoxification enzymes, such as glutathione S-transferase.[102] Animal studies have shown that ingredients present in rosemary inhibit tumor initiation and promotion.[104] An *in vitro* human study indicated that both whole rosemary extract and its antioxidant constituents, carnosol or carnosic acid, inhibited DNA adduct formation by 80% after 6 hours' co-incubation with a procarcinogen. Although inhibiting cytochrome P_{450} enzyme activity (70–90%), carnosol brought a 3- to 4-fold increase in expression of phase II detoxification enzyme glutathione-S-transferase, and a parallel increase in NAD(P)H:quinone reductase, another phase II detoxification enzyme. The authors concluded that the ability of rosemary ingredients to reduce mobilization and detoxify an important human carcinogen renders them promising potential chemopreventive candidates.[104]

X. ANTIMICROBIAL EFFECTS OF THE MEDITERRANEAN DIET

In addition to possibly impacting on detoxification pathways, certain micronutrients in herbs and spices in the Mediterranean Diet are credited with potent antiviral and antimicrobial actions. For example, a study[101] showed that both Herbor 025, a rosemary extract, and Spice Cocktail, a Provençal extract of herbs, inhibited human immunodeficiency virus (HIV) infection at very low concentrations. However, cytotoxicity was also evidenced. In addition, carnosol, an antioxidant in rosemary, showed definite anti-HIV activity at a concentration as low as 8 μM, while being devoid of any cytotoxic effects.[101] An *in vitro* study[142] tested the effects of extracts of several plants for possible inhibitory action against *Helicobacter pylori*. Among the different extracts tested, the most effective were thyme (aqueous extract) and cinnamon (alcoholic extract). Unlike several antibacterials, thyme extract had significant inhibitory action against *Helicobacter pylori* growth and activity. These observations led the authors to suggest that the apparent therapeutic potential of thyme aqueous extract is worth validating by clinical studies. Not only thyme, but also oregano, may be endowed with antimicrobial properties. Specifically, another *in vitro* study tested the effects of 52 plant oils and extracts against *Acinetobacter baumanii, Aaromonas veronii* biogroup *sobria, Candida albicans, Enterococcus faecalis, Escherichia coli, Klebsiella pneumoniae, Pseudomonas aeruginosa, Salmonella enterica* subsp. *enterica* serotype *typhimurium, Serratia marcescens,* and *Staphylococcus aureus*. Oregano, bay, and lemongrass inhibited all organisms, while, among the 52 different plant oils and extracts tested, thyme oil exhibited the minimum inhibitory concentrations against *Escherichia coli* and *Candida albicans*.[143] In addition to thyme and oregano, basil[144-146] and, perhaps, sage,[147] are credited with antimicrobial actions.

XI. THE MEDITERRANEAN DIET AND CELLULAR SENESCENCE

There are indications that cells lose their proliferative or replicative capacity with aging or reach the stage of so-called proliferative senescence. It has been suggested that cellular senescence results from, or is concomitant to, telomere shortening, and that telomere shortening is caused by damage to the telomeric DNA by free radicals (telomeric theory of aging).[148] A human study[149] indicated that intracellular enrichment of vascular endothelial cells with vitamin C resulted in a 52–62% reduction in telomere shortening and an extension of cellular life span and prevention of cellular senescence.

XII. CONCLUSIONS

In summary, there are indications that the reported longevity and reduced mortality rates of Mediterranean populations are attributed, at least in part, to their dietary habits. Evidence indicates that certain Mediterranean Diet constituents, such as oleic acid, vitamins, flavonoids, and polyphenols, may protect health and foster longevity via inhibiting free radical formation and PUFA peroxidation, protecting against biomembrane and DNA damage, facilitating mitochondrial respiration and ATP production, stimulating detoxification processes, exerting antiviral and antimicrobial effects, enhancing immunity, and possibly protecting against cellular senescence.

REFERENCES

1. Buzina R., Suboticanec K., and Saric M., Diet patterns and health problems: diet in southern Europe, *Ann. Nutr. Metab.*, 35 (Suppl 1), 32, 1991.
2. Richter C., Gogvadze V., Laffranchi R., Schlapbach R., Schnizer M., Suter M., Walter P., and Yaffee M., Oxidants in mitochondria: From physiology to disease, *Biochim. Biophys. Acta*, 1271: 67, 1995.
3. Willett W.C., Sacks F., Trichopoulou A., Drescher G., Ferro-Luzzi A., Helsing E., and Trichopoulos D., Mediterranean Diet pyramid: a cultural model for healthy eating, *Am. J. Clin. Nutr.*, 61 (Suppl 6), 1402, 1995.
4. Nestle M., Mediterranean diets: historical and research overview, *Am. J. Clin. Nutr.*, 61 (Suppl 6), 1313, 1995.
5. Haber B., The Mediterranean diet: a view from history, *Am. J. Clin. Nutr.*, 66 (Suppl 4), 1053., 1997.
6. Trichopoulou A. and Lagiou P., Healthy traditional Mediterranean diet: an expression of culture, history and lifestyle, *Nutr. Rev.*, 55, 383, 1997.
7. Harman D., Ageing: Theory based on free radical and radiation chemistry, *J. Gerontol.*, 11, 298, 1956.
8. Gjonca A. and Bobak M., Albanian paradox, another example of protective effect of Mediterranean lifestyle?, Lancet, 350, 1815, 1997.
9. Hertog M.G.L., Kromhout D., Aravanis C., Blackburn H., Buzina R., Fidanza F., Giampaoli S., Jansen A., Menotti A., Nedejikovic S., Pekkarinen M., Simic B.S., Toshima H., Feskens E.J.M., Hollman P.C.H., and Katan M.B., Flavonoid intake and long-term risk of coronary heart disease and cancer in the Seven Countries Study, *Arch. Intern. Med.*, 155, 381, 1995.
10. Dontas A.S., Menotti A., Aravanis C., Ioannidis P., and Seccareccia F., Comparative total mortality in 25 years in Italian and Greek middle-aged rural men, *J. Epidemiol. Comm. Health.*, 52, 638, 1998.
11. de Groot L.C., van Staveren W.A., and Burema J., Survival beyond age 70 in relation to diet, *Nutr. Rev.*, 54, 211, 1996.
12. Renaud S., de Lorgeril M., Delaye J., Guidollet J., Jacquard F., Mamelle N., Martin JL., Monjaud I, Salen P., and Toubol P., Cretan Mediterranean diet for the prevention of coronary heart disease, *Am. J. Clin. Nutr.*, 61 (Suppl 6), 1360, 1995.
13. de Lorgeril M., Salen P., Martin J.L., Monjaud I., Boucher P., and Mamelle N., Mediterranean dietary pattern in a randomized trial: prolonged survival and possible reduced cancer rate, *Arch. Intern. Med.*, 158, 1181, 1998.
14. de Lorgeril M., Renaud S., Mamelle N., Salen P., Martin J.L., Monjaud I., Guidollet J., Touboul P., and Delaye J., Mediterranean alpha-linolenic acid-enriched diet in secondary prevention of coronary heart disease, *Lancet*, 343, 1454, 1994
15. Menotti A., Food patterns and health problems: health in southern Europe, *Ann. Nutr. Metab.*, 35, 69, 1991.
16. World Health Organization, World Health Statistics Annual. Geneva, Switzerland: WHO, 1992.
17. Keys A., Menotti A., Aravanis C., et al., The Seven Countries Study: 2289 deaths in 15 years, *J. Prev. Med.*, 13, 141, 1984.

18. Kromhout D., Serum cholesterol in cross-cultural perspective. The Seven Countries Study, *Acta. Cardiol.*, 54, 155, 1999.

19. Ghiselli A., D'Amicis A., and Giacosa A., The antioxidant potential of the Mediterranean diet, *Eur. J. Cancer. Prev.*, 6 (Suppl 1), 15, 1997.

20. Hirayama T., A large scale cohort study of dietary habits and cancer mortality, *Gan. No. Rinsho.*, 32, 610, 1986.

21. Tavani A. and La Vecchia C., Fruit and vegetable consumption and cancer risk in a Mediterranean population, *Am. J. Clin. Nutr.*, 61 (Suppl 6), 1374, 1995.

22. Mobarhan S., Micronutrient supplementation trials and the reduction of cancer and cerebrovascular incidence and mortality, *Nutr. Rev.* 52, 102, 1994.

23. Caperle M., Maiani G., Azzini E., Conti E.M., Raguzzini A., Ramazzotti V., and Crespi M., Dietary profiles and antioxidants in a rural population of central Italy with a low frequency of cancer, *Eur. J. Canc. Prev.*, 5, 197, 1996.

24. Stahelin H.B., Gey K.F., Eichholzer M., Ludin E., Bernasconi F., Thurneysen J., and Brubacher G., Plasma antioxidant vitamins and subsequent cancer mortality in the 12-year follow-up of the prospective Basel Study, *Am. J. Epidemiol.*, 133, 766, 1991.

25. Eichholzer M., Stahelin H.B., Gey KF., Ludin E., and Bernasconi F., Prediction of male cancer mortality by plasma levels of interacting vitamins: a 17-year follow-up of the prospective Basel Study, *Int. J. Cancer.*, 66, 145, 1996.

26. Chen J., Geissler C., Parpia B., Li J., and Campbell T.C., Antioxidant status and cancer mortality in China, *Int. J. Epidemiol.*, 21, 625, 1992.

27. Schorah C.J., Micronutrients, vitamins, and cancer risk, *Vitam. Horm.*, 57, 1, 1999.

28. Jossa F. and Mancini M., The Mediterranean diet in the prevention of arteriosclerosis, *Recenti. Prog. Med.*, 87, 175, 1996.

29. Losonczy K.G., Harris T.B., and Havlik R.J., Vitamin E and vitamin C supplement use and risk of all-cause and coronary heart disease mortality in older persons: the established populations for epidemiologic studies of the elderly, *Am. J. Clin. Nutr.*, 64, 190, 1996.

30. Knekt P., Jarvinen R., Reunanen A., and Maatela J., Flavonoid intake and coronary mortality in Finland: a cohort study, *Brit. Med. J.*, 312, 478, 1996.

31. Lugasi A., Blazovics A., Dworschk E., and Feher J., Cardio-protective effect of red wine as reflected in the literature, *Orv. Hetil.*, 138: 673, 1997.

32. Visioli F., Bellosta S., and Galli C., Oleuropein, the bitter principle of olives, enhances nitric oxide production by mouse macrophages, *Life. Sci.*, 62, 541, 1998.

33. Blot W.J., Li JY., Taylor P.R., Guo W., Dawsey S., Wang G.Q., Yang C.S., Zheng S.F., Gail M., and Li G.Y., Nutrition intervention trials in Linxian, China: supplementation with specific vitamin/mineral combinations, cancer incidence, and disease-specific mortality in the general population, *J. Natl. Cancer.* Inst., 85, 1483, 1993.

34. Kromhout D., Bloemberg B., Feskens E., Menotti A., and Nissinen A., Saturated fat, vitamin C and smoking predict long-term population all cause mortality rates in the Seven Countries Study, *Int. J. Epidemiol.*, (in press).

35. Richter C., Gogvadze V., Laffranchi R., Schlapbach R., Schnizer M., Suter M., Walter P., and Yaffee M., Oxidants in mitochondria: from physiology to disease, *Biochim. Biophys. Acta.*, 1271: 67, 1995.

36. Wei Y.H., Kao S.H., and Lee H.C., Simultaneous increase of mitochondrial DNA deletions and lipid peroxidation in human aging, *Ann. N. Y. Acad. Sci.*, 786: 24, 1996.

37. Richter C., Park J.W., and Ames B.N., Normal oxidative damage to mitochondrial and nuclear DNA is extensive, *Proc. Natl. Acad. Sci. U.S.A.*, 85: 6465, 1988.

38. Clayton D.A., Doda J.N., and Friedberg E.C., The absence of a pyrimidine dimer repair mechanism in mammalian mitochondria, *Proc. Natl. Acad. Sci. U.S.A.*, 71, 2777, 1974.
39. Tomkinson A.E., Bonk R.T., Kim J., Bartfel N., and Linn S., Mammalian mitochondrial endonuclease activities specific for ultraviolet-irradiated DNA, *Nucl. Acids.*, 18, 929, 1990.
40. Fraga C.G., Shigenaga M.K., Park J.W., Degan P., and Ames B.N., Oxidative damage to DNA during aging: 8-Hydroxy-2-deoxyguanosine in rat organ DNA and urine. *Proc. Natl .Acad. Sci. U.S.A.*, 87, 4533, 1990.
41. Cortopassi G.A. and Arnheim N., Detection of a specific mitochondrial DNA deletion in tissues of older humans, *Nucl. Acids.*, 18, 6927, 1990.
42. Wei Y.H., Mitochondrial DNA alterations as aging-associated molecular events, *Mutat. Res.*, 275, 145, 1992.
43. Zhang C., Linnane A.W., and Nagley P., Occurrence of a particular base substitution (3243 A to G) in mitochondrial DNA of tissues of aging humans, *Biochem. Biophys. Res. Comm.*, 195, 1104, 1993.
44. Manscher C., Rieger T., Muller-Hocker J., and Kadenbach B., The point mutation of mitochondrial DNA characteristic for MERRF disease is found also in healthy people of different ages, *FEBS. Lett.* , 317, 27, 1993.
45. Lee HC., Pang CY., Hsu HS, and Wei YH., Aging-associated tandem duplications in the D-loop of mitochondrial DNA of human muscle, *FEBS. Lett.*, 354, 79, 1994.
46. Lee HC., Pang CY., Hsu HS and Wei YH., Differential accumulations of 4,977 bp deletion in mitochondrial DNA of various tissues in human aging, *Biochim. Biophys. Acta.*, 1226, 37, 1994.
47. Agarwal S. and Sohal R.S., Differential oxidative damage to mitochondrial proteins during aging, *Mech. Ageing. Dev.*, 85, 55, 1995.
48. Wei Y.H., Pang C.Y., You B.J., and Lee H.C., Tandem duplications and large-scale deletions of mitochondrial DNA are early molecular events of human aging process, *Ann. N. Y. Acad. Sci.*, 786, 82, 1996.
49. Hayakawa M., Katsumata K., Yoneda M., Tanaka M., Sugiyama S., and Ozawa T., Age-related extensive fragmentation of mitochondrial DNA into minicircles, *Biochem. Biophys. Res. Comm.*, 226, 369, 1996.
50. Mecocci P., MacGarvey U., Kaufman A.E., Koontz D., Shoffner J.M., Wallace D.C., and Beal M.F., Oxidative damage to mitochondrial DNA shows marked age-dependent increases in human brain, *Ann. Neurol.*, 34, 609, 1993.
51. Hsieh R.H., Hou J.H., Hsu H.S., and Wei Y.H., Age-dependent respiratory function decline and DNA deletions in human muscle mitochondria, *Biochem. Mol. Biol. Int.*, 32, 1009, 1994.
52. Lezza AMS., Boffoli D., Scacco S., Cantatore P., and Gadaleta MN., Correlation between mitochondrial DNA 4977-bp deletion and respiratory chain enzyme activities in aging human skeletal muscles, *Biochem. Biophys. Res. Comm.*, 205, 772, 1994.
53. Yoneda M., Katsumata K., Hayakawa M., Tanaka M., and Ozawa T., Oxygen stress induces an apoptotic cell death associated with fragmentation of mitochondrial genome, *Biochem. Biophys. Res. Comm.*, 209, 723, 1995.
54. Ames B.N., Shigenaga M.K, and Hagen T.M., Oxidants, antioxidants, and the degenerative diseases of aging, *Proc. Natl. Acad. Sci. U.S.A.*, 90, 7915, 1993.
55. Stadtman ER., Protein oxidation and aging, *Science*, 257, 1220, 1992.
56. Sohal R.S., Agarwal S., Dubey A., and Orr W.C., Protein oxidative damage is associated with life expectancy of houseflies, *Proc. Natl. Acad. Sci. U.S.A.*, 90, 7255, 1993.

57. Lavie L., Reznick A.Z., and Gershon D., Decreased protein and puromycinyl-peptide degradation in livers of senescent mice, *Mutat. Res.*, 275, 217, 1992.

58. Miquel J, Economos J.E., and Johnson J.E. Jr., Mitochondrial role in cell aging, *Exp. Gerontol.*, 15: 575., 1980.

59. Miquel J. An integrated theory of aging as the result of mitochondrial DNA mutation in differentiated cells, *Arch. Gerontol. Geriatr.*, 12: 99, 1991.

60. Ivy G.O., Schottler F., Wenzel J., Baudry M., and Lynch G., Inhibitors of lysosomal enzymes: Accumulation of lipofuscin-like dense bodies in the brain., *Science*, 226, 985, 1984.

61. Durand G. and Desnoyers F., Polyunsaturated fatty acids and aging. Lipofuscins: structure, origin and development, *Ann. Nutr. Aliment.*, 34, 317, 1980.

62. Rondanelli M., Melzi d'Eril G.V., Anesi A., and Ferrari E., Altered oxidative stress in healthy old subjects, *Aging.*, 9, 221, 1997.

63. Rodriguez-Martinez M.A. and Ruiz-Torres A., Homeostasis between lipid peroxidation and antioxidant enzyme activities in healthy human aging, *Mech. Ageing Dev.*, 66, 213, 1992.

64. Coudray C., Roussel A.M., Arnaud J., and Favier A., Selenium and antioxidant vitamin and lipidoperoxidation levels in preaging French population, *Biol. Trace. Elem. Res.*, 57, 183, 1997.

65. Lagarde M., Lemaitre D., Calzada C., and Vericel E., Involvement of lipid peroxidation in platelet signaling, *Prostagl. Leukot. Essent. Fatt. Acids*, 57, 489, 1997.

66. Tokunaga K., Kanno K., Ochi M., Nishimiya T., Shishino K., Murase M., Makino H. and Tokui S., Lipid peroxide and antioxidants in the elderly, *Rinsho. Byori.*, 46, 783, 1998.

67. Lagarde M., Vericel E., Chabannes B., and Prigent AF., Blood cell redox status and fatty acids, *Prostagl. Leukot. Essent. Fatt. Acids*, 52, 159, 1995.

68. Meydani M., Vitamin E requirements in relation to dietary fish oil and oxidative stress in elderly, *EXS.*, 62, 411, 1992.

69. Vericel E., Rey C., Calzada C., Haond P., Chapuy P.H., and Lagarde M., Age-related changes in arachidonic acid peroxidation and glutathione-peroxidase activity in human platelets, *Prostagland.*, 43, 75, 1992.

70. Matsumoto M., Tatsumi H., and Murai A., Lipid metabolism and aging, *Rinsho. Byori.*, 38, 530, 1990.

71. Leibovitz B.E. and Siegel B.V., Aspects of free radical reactions in biological systems: aging, *J. Gerontol.*, 35, 45, 1980.

72. Jain S.K., Evidence for membrane lipid peroxidation during the *in vivo* aging of human erythrocytes, *Biochim. Biophys. Acta.*, 937, 205, 1988.

73. Einsele H., Clemens M.R., and Remmer H., *In vitro* aging of red blood cells and lipid peroxidation, *Arch. Toxicol.*, 60, 163, 1987.

74. Mills D.E., Murthy M., and Galey W.R., Dietary fatty acids, membrane transport, and oxidative sensitivity in human erythrocytes, *Lipids*, 30, 657, 1995.

75. Lee H.C., Lim M.L., Lu C.Y., Liu V.W., Fahn H.J., Zhang C., Nagley P., and Wei Y.H., Concurrent increase of oxidative DNA damage and lipid peroxidation together with mitochondrial DNA mutation in human lung tissues during aging: smoking enhances oxidative stress on the aged tissues, *Arch. Biochem. Biophys.*, 362, 309, 1999.

76. Adachi K., Fujiura Y., Mayumi F., Nozuhara A., Sugiu Y., Sakanashi T., Hidaka T., and Toshima H., A deletion of mitochondrial DNA in murine doxarubicin-induced cariotoxicity, *Biochem. Biophys. Res. Comm.*, 195, 945, 1993.

77. Durak I., Yalcin S., Kacmaz M., Cimen M.Y., Buyukkocak S., Avci A., and Ozturk H.S., High-temperature effects on antioxidant systems and toxic product formation in nutritional oils, *J. Toxicol. Environ. Health*, 57, 585, 1999.

78. Masella R., Cantafora A., Modesti D., Cardilli A., Gennaro L., Bocca A., and Coni E., Antioxidant activity of 3,4-DHPEA and protocatechuic acid: a comparative assessment with other olive oil biophenols, *Redox. Rep.*, 4, 113, 1999.

79. Visioli F., Bellomo G., and Galli C., Free radical-scavenging properties of olive oil polyphenols, *Biochem. Biophys. Res. Comm.*, 247, 60-64, 1998.

80. Saija A., Scalese M., Lanza M., Marzullo D., Bonina F., and Castelli F., Flavonoids as antioxidant agents: importance of their interaction with biomembranes, *Free. Radic. Biol. Med.*, 19, 481, 1995.

81. Manna C., Galletti P., Cucciolla V., Moltedo O., Leone A., and Zappia V., The protective effect of the olive oil polyphenol (3,4-dihydroxyphenyl)-ethanol counteracts reactive oxygen metabolite-induced cytotoxicity in Caca-2 cells, *J. Nutr.*, 127, 286, 1997.

82. Mancini M., Parfitt V.J., and Rubba P., Antioxidants in the Mediterranean diet, *Can. J. Cardiol.*, 11 (Suppl G), 105, 1995.

83. Allard J.P., Kurian R., Aghdassi E., Muggli R., and Royall D., Lipid peroxidation during n-3 fatty acid and vitamin E supplementation in humans, *Lipids*, 32, 535, 1997.

84. Balasubramanian K.A., Nalini S., and Manohar M., Nonesterified fatty acids and lipid peroxidation, *Mol. Cell. Biochem.*, 111, 131, 1992.

85. Maziere C., Conte M.A., Degonville J., and Maziere J.C., Cellular enrichment with polyunsaturated fatty acids induces an oxidative stress and activates the transcription factors AP1 and NF Kappa B, *Biochem. Biophys. Res. Comm.*, 265, 116, 1999.

86. Fang J.L., Vaca C.E., Valsat L.M., and Mutanen M., Determination of DNA adducts of malondialdehyde in humans: effects of dietary fatty acid composition, *Carcinogen.*, 17, 1035, 1996.

87. McCall M.R. and Frei B., Can antioxidant vitamins maternally reduce oxidative damage in humans? *Free. Radic. Biol. Med.*, 26, 1034, 1999.

88. Evstigneeva R.P., Volkov I.M., and Chudinova V.V., Vitamin E as a universal antioxidant and stabilizer of biological membranes, *Membr. Cell. Biol.*, 12, 151, 1998.

89. Beyer R.E., The role of ascorbate in antioxidant protection of biomembranes: interaction with vitamin E and coenzyme Q, *J. Bioenerg. Biomembr.*, 26, 349, 1994.

90. Liebler D.C., The role of metabolism in the antioxidant function of vitamin E, *Crit. Rev. Toxicol.*, 23, 147, 1993.

91. Steinberg F.M. and Chait A., Antioxidant vitamin supplementation and lipid peroxidation in smokers, *Am. J. Clin. Nutr.*, 68, 319, 1998.

92. Courtiere A., Cotte J.M., Pignol F., and Jadot G., Lipid peroxidation in aged patients. Influence of an antioxidant combination (vitamin C-vitamin E-rutin), *Therapie*, 44, 13, 1989.

93. van Acker S.A., van Balen G.P., van den Berg D.J., Bast A., and van der Vijgh W.J., Influence of iron chelation on the antioxidant activity of flavonoids, *Biochem. Pharmacol.*, 56, 935, 1998.

94. Chen Z.Y., Chan P.T., Ho K.Y., Fung K.P., and Wang J., Antioxidant activity of natural flavonoids is governed by number and location of their aromatic hydroxyl groups, *Chem. Phys. Lipids.*, 79, 157, 1996.

95. Rice-Evans C.A., Miller N.J., Bolwell P.G., Bramley P.M., and Pridham J.B., The relative antioxidant activities of plant-derived polyphenolic flavonoids, *Free. Radic. Res.*, 22, 375.

96. Morel I., Lescoat G., Cogrel P., Sergent O., Pasdeloup N., Brissot P., Cillard P., and Cillard J., Antioxidant and iron-chelating activities of the flavonoids: catechin, quercetin and diosmetin on iron-loaded hepatocyte cultures, *Biochem. Pharmacol.*, 45, 13, 1993.

97. Paganga G., Miller N., and Rice-Evans C.A., The polyphenolic content of fruit and vegetables and their antioxidant activities. What does a good serving constitute? *Free Radic. Res.*, 30, 153, 1999.

98. Lamaison J.L., Petitjean-Freyet C., and Carnat A., Medicinal Lamiaceae with antioxidant properties, a potential source of rosmarinic acid, *Pharm. Acta. Helv.*, 66, 185, 1991.

99. Aeschbach R., Loliger J., Scott B.C., Murcia A., Butler J., Halliwell B., and Arnoma OI., Antioxidant actions of thymol, carvacrol, 6-gingerol, zingerone and hydrohytyrosol, *Food. Chem. Toxicol.*, 32, 31, 1994.

100. Alam K., Nagi M.N., Badary O.A., Al-Shabanah O.A., Al-Rikabi A.C., and Al-Bekairi A.M., The protective action of thymol against carbon tetrachloride hepatotoxicity in mice, *Pharmacol. Res.*, 40, 159, 1999.

101. Aruoma O.I., Spencer J.P., Rossi R., Aeschbach R., Khan A., Mahmood N., Munoz A., Murcia A., Butler J., and Halliwell B., An evaluation of the antioxidant and antiviral action of extracts of rosemary and Provençal herbs., *Food. Chem. Toxicol.*, 34, 449.

102. Offord E.A., Mace K., Avanti O., and Pfeifer A.M., Mechanisms involved in the chemoprotective effects of rosemary extract studied in human liver and bronchial cells, *Cancer. Lett.*, 114, 275, 1997.

103. Wang M., Shao Y., Zhu N., Rangarajan M., La Voie E.J., and Ho C.T., Antioxidative phenolic glycosides from sage (Salvia officinalis), *J. Nat. Prod.*, 62, 454, 1999.

104. Offord E.A., Mace K., Ruffieux C., Malnoe A., and Pfeifer A.M., Rosemary components inhibit benzo[a]pyrene-induced genotoxicity in human bronchial cells, *Carcinogen*, 16, 2057.

105. Mataix J., Manas M., Quiles J., Battino M., Cassinello M., Lopez-Frias M., and Huertas J.R., Coenzyme Q content depends upon oxidative stress and dietary fat unsaturation, *Mol. Aspects. Med.*, 18 (Suppl), 129, 1997.

106. Mataix J., Quiles J.L., Huertas J.R., Battino M., and Manas M., Tissue specific interactions of exercise, dietary fatty acids, and vitamin E in lipid peroxidation, *Free. Radic. Biol. Med.*, 24, 511, 1998.

107. Huertas J.R., Martinez-Velasco E., Ibanez S., Lopez-Frias M., Ochoa J.J., Parenti Castelli G., Mataix J., and Lenaz G., Virgin olive oil and coenzyme Q_{10} protect heart mitochondria from proxidative damage during aging, *Biofactors*, 9, 337, 1999.

108. Quiles J.L., Huertas J.R., Manas M., Battino M., Cassinello M., Littarrn G.P., Lenaz G., and Mataix F.J, Peroxidative extent and coenzyme Q levels in the rat: influence of physical training and dietary fats, *Mol. Aspects. Med.*, (Suppl 15), 89, 1994.

109. Donchenko G.V., Malen'Kykh L.B., Palyvoda O.M., and Zhalylo L.I., The role of a protein factor in the effect of alpha-tocopherol on mitochondrial respiration, *Ukr. Biokhim. Zh.*, 62, 115, 1990.

110. Ryuji H., The role of alpha-tocopherol and allopurinol in lipid peroxidation and mitochondrial respiration in the ischemic rat liver, Nippon. *Geka. Gakkai. Zasshi.*, 91, 95, 1990.

111. Donchenko G.V., Kuz'menko I.V., Kovalenko V.N., and Kunitsa N.I., Comparative study of the effects of alpha-tocopherol and a synthetic antioxidant on respiration and oxidative phosphorylation in rat liver mitochondria, *Biokhimia*, 48, 998, 1983.

112. Chen L.H. and Chang M.L., Effect of dietary vitamin E and vitamin C on respiration and swelling of guinea pig liver mitochondria, *J. Nutr.*, 108, 1616, 1978.

113. Lee B.M., Lee S.K., and Kim H.S., Inhibition of oxidative DNA damage, 8-OHdG, and carbonyl contents in smokers treated with antioxidants (vitamin E, vitamin C, beta-carotene and red ginseng), *Canc. Lett.*, 132, 219, 1998.

114. Cooke M.S., Evans M.D., Podmore I.D, Herbert K.E., Mistry N., Hickenbotham P.T., Hussieni A., Griffiths H.R., and Lunec J., Novel repair action of vitamin C upon oxidative DNA damage, *FEBS. Lett.*, 439, 363, 1998.

115. Noroozi M., Angerson W.J., and Lean M.E., Effects of flavonoids and vitamin C on oxidative DNA damage to human lymphocytes, *Am. J. Clin. Nutr.*, 67, 1210.

116. Sweetman S.F., Strain J.J., and McKelvey-Martin V.J., Effect of antioxidant vitamin supplementation on DNA damage and repair in human lymphoblastoid cells, *Nutr. Cancer.*, 27, 122, 1997.

117. Hartmann A., Niess A.M., Grunert-Fuchs M., Poch B., and Speit G., Vitamin E prevents exercise-induced DNA damage, *Mutat. Res.*, 346, 195, 1995.

118. Dyke G.W., Craven J.L., Hall R., and Garner R.C., Effect of vitamin C supplementation on gastric mucosal DNA damage, *Carcinogen*, 15, 291, 1994.

119. van Staden A.M., van Rensburg C.E., and Anderson R., Vitamin E protects mononuclear leucocyte DNA against damage mediated by phagocyte-derived oxidants, *Mutat. Res.*, 288, 257, 1993.

120. Sai K., Umemura T., Takagi A., Hasegawa R., and Kurokawa Y., The protective role of glutathione, cysteine and vitamin C against oxidative DNA damage induced in the rat kidney by potassium bromate, *Jpn. J. Cancer. Res.*, 83, 45, 1992.

121. Summerfield F.W. and Tappel A.L., Vitamin E protects against methyl ethyl Ketone peroxide-induced peroxidative damage to rat brain DNA, *Mutat. Res.*, 126, 113, 1984.

122. Webster R.P., Gawde M.D., and Bhattacharya R.K., Effect of different vitamin A status on carcinogen-induced DNA damage and repair enzymes in rats, *In Vivo*, 10, 113, 1996.

123. Duthie S.J., Collins A.R., Duthie G.G., and Dobson V.L., Quercetin and myricetin protect against hydrogen peroxide-induced DNA damage (strand breaks and oxidized pyrimidines) in human lymphocytes, *Mutat. Res.*, 393, 223, 1997.

124. Lean M.E., Noroozi M., Kelly I., Burns J., Talwar D., Sattar N., and Crozier A., Dietary flavonoids protect diabetic human lymphocytes against oxidative damage to DNA, *Diabetes*, 48, 176, 1999.

125. Sestili P., Guidarelli A., Dacha M., and Cantoni O., Quercetin prevents DNA single strand breakage and cytotoxicity caused by tert-butylhydroperoxide: free radical scavenging versus iron chelating mechanism, *Free. Radic. Biol. Med.*, 25, 196, 1998.

126. Deiana M., Aruoma OI., Bianchi ML., Spencer JP., Kaur H., Halliwel B., Aeschbach R., Banni S., Dessi MA., and Corongin FP., Inhibition of peroxynitrite dependent DNA base modification and tyrosine nitration by extra virgin olive oil-derived antioxidant hydroxytyrosol, *Free. Radic. Biol. Med.*, 26, 762, 1999.

127. Laughton M.J., Halliwell B., Evans PJ., and Hoult J.R., Antioxidant and pro-oxidant actions of plant phenolics quercetin, gossypol and myricetin. Effects on lipid peroxidation, hydroxyl radical generation and bleomycin-dependent damage to DNA, *Biochem. Pharmacol.*, 38, 2859, 1989.

128. Nakayama T., Suppression of hydroperoxide-induced cytotoxicity by polyphenols, *Canc. Res.*, 54 (Suppl 7), 1991, 1994.

129. Sahu S.C., Washington MC., Effect of ascorbic acid and curcumin on quercetin-induced nuclear DNA damage, lipid peroxidation and protein degradation, *Canc. Lett.*, 63, 237, 1992.

130. Duthie S.J., Johnson W., and Dobson V.L., Effects of dietary flavonoids on DNA damage (strand breaks and oxidisedpyrimidines) and growth in human cells, *Mutat. Res.*, 390, 141, 1997.

131. Plaumann B., Fritsche M., Rimpler H., Brandner G., and Hess R.D., Flavonoids activate wild-type p53, *Oncogene.*, 13, 1605, 1996.

132. Leighton F., Cuevas A., Guasch V., Perez D.D., Strobel P., San Martin A., Urzua U., Diez M.S., Foncea R., Castillo O., Mizon C., Espinoza M.A., Urquiaga I., Rozowski J., Maiz A., and Germain A., Plasma polyphenols and antioxidants, oxidative DNA damage and endothelial function in a diet and wine intervention study in humans, *Drugs. Exp. Clin. Res.*, 25, 133, 1999.

133. Meydani S.N. and Hayek M.G., Vitamin E and aging immune response, *Clin. Geriatr. Med.*, 11, 567, 1995.

134. Meydani S.N., Vitamin/mineral supplementation, the aging immune response, and the risk of infection, *Nutr. Rev.*, 51, 106, 1993.

135. Wang Y. and Watson RR., Ethanol, immune responses, and murine AIDS: the role of vitamin E as an immunostimulant and antioxidant, *Alcohol*, 11, 75, 1994.

136. Kolb E., The significance of vitamin A for the immune system, *Ber. Munch. Tierarztl. Wochenschr.*, 108, 385, 1995.

137. Beharka A., Redican S., Leka L., and Meydani S.N., Vitamin E status and immune function, Methods. *Enzymol.*, 282, 247, 1997.

138. Tengerdy R.P., The role of vitamin E in immune response and disease resistance, *Ann. N. Y. Acad. Sci.*, 587, 24, 1990.

139. Bendich A., Vitamin E and the immune functions, *Basic. Life. Sci.*, 49, 615, 1988.

140. Chew B.P., Immune function: relationship of nutrition and disease control. Vitamin A and beta-carotene on host defense, *J. Dairy. Sci.*, 70, 2732, 1987.

141. Holliday R., Causes of aging, *Ann. N. Y. Acad. Sci.*, 854, 61, 1998.

142. Tabak M., Armon R., Potasman I., and Neeman I., *In vitro* inhibition of Helicobacter pylori by extracts of thyme, *J. Appl. Bacteriol.*, 80, 667, 1996.

143. Hammer K.A., Carson C.F.,and Riley TV., Antimicrobial activity of essential oils and other plant extracts, *J. Appl. Microbiol.*, 86, 985, 1999.

144. Wan J., Wilcock A., and Coventry M.J., The effect of essential oils of basil on the growth of Aeromonas hydrophila and pseudomonas fluorescens, *J. Appl. Microbiol.*, 84, 152, 1998.

145. Lachowicz K.J., Jones G.P., Briggs D.R., Bienvenu F.E., Wan J., Wilcock A., and Coventry M.J., The synergistic preservative effects of the essential oils of sweet basil (*Ocimum basilicum L.*) against acid-tolerant food microflora, *Lett. Appl. Microbiol.*, 26, 209, 1998.

146. Fyfe L., Armstrong F., and Stewart J., Inhibition of Listeria monocytogenes and Salmonella enteriditis by combinations of plant oils and derivatives of benzoic acid: the development of synergistic antimicrobial combinations, *Int. J. Antimicrob. Agents*, 9, 195, 1997.

147. Masterova I, Misikova E., Sirotkova L., Vavarkova S., and Ubik K., Royleanones in the roots of *Salvia officinalis L.* of domestic provenance and their antimicrobial activity, *Ceska. Slov. Farm.*, 45, 242, 1996.

148. Von Zglinicki T., Telomeres: influencing the rate of aging, *Ann. N. Y. Acad. Sci.*, 854, 318, 1998.

149. Furumoto K., Inoue E., Nagao N., Hiyama E., and Miwa N., Age-dependent telomere shortening is slowed down by enrichment of intracellular vitamin C via suppression of oxidative stress, *Life. Sci.*, 63, 935, 1998.

10 Diabetes Mellitus, Obesity, and the Mediterranean Diet

Nicholas L. Katsilambros and Antonis Zampelas

CONTENTS

I. EPIDEMIOLOGY

Diabetes mellitus is a serious disease that is characterized by metabolic abnormalities of carbohydrate, fat, and protein. The most common abnormality is the presence of glucose intolerance or hyperglycemia, which is the result of reduced insulin synthesis by the pancreatic β-cells (Type I diabetes mellitus) or reduced tissue sensitivity and response to insulin (Type II diabetes mellitus).

Diabetes mellitus affects approximately 13 million Americans, about 5.2% of the total population and 6.6% of the population between 20 and 74 years of age. In the U.S., it has been estimated that there are 6.5 million undiagnosed cases of diabetes.[1] Type I diabetes mellitus is the least common type and accounts for 5 to 10% of all known cases of diabetes in the U.S., with most cases being diagnosed in people younger than 30. On the other hand, 85–90% of all known cases belong to Type II diabetes. Eighty percent of these patients are obese or have a history of obesity. Usually Type II diabetes occurs after the age of 30.

In Europe, prevalence rates of Type I diabetes mellitus differ between countries and also regionally within countries. In particular, with the exception of the Baltic region, incidence rates are higher in northern European countries (Finland, Norway, Sweden, Denmark, and the British Isles), than in Mediterranean, central- and eastern-European countries.[2] It is also noteworthy that, in Greece, where incidence rates are low, there is a difference between incidence rates in the region of Athens (10.9 for boys and 7.7 for girls per 100,000 per year, age between 0–14 years), and the northern region of Thessaloniki (5.3 for boys and 3.8 for girls). It seems that environmental factors, including dietary habits, contribute substantially to the variation in the incidence rates between the regions, since genetically similar populations exhibit similar incidence rates of Type I diabetes mellitus (Finland vs. Estonia and Hungary; Norway vs. Iceland).

It is also noteworthy that the incidence of diabetes mellitus has been constantly increasing through recent years. Thus, in a study[3] that was carried out in Greece, it was reported that the incidence of diabetes had increased in the Athens region. In particular, after including 21,410 persons in 1974 and 12,836 in 1990, it was observed that prevalence rates of diabetes had increased from 2.4% in 1974 to 3.1% in 1990. This study also reported that the changes in the prevalence rates that reached statistical significance were in the 50–59, 60–69 and 70–79 age groups. The observation that the increase in the prevalence rates of diabetes mellitus in the Athens region occurred in ages > 30 years suggests that it could be due to an increase in Type II diabetes mellitus, which is substantially influenced by changes in lifestyle, including dietary habits.

II. FAT INTAKE

A. TOTAL FAT INTAKE, INSULIN RESISTANCE, AND DIABETES MELLITUS

As mentioned above, Type II diabetes mellitus is very often associated with insulin resistance, and Type II diabetic patients are frequently overweight or obese. Insulin resistance could be acquired due to excessive calorie intake or to the inheritance of a gene or a set of genes that confer insulin resistance. Insulin resistance primarily affects muscle and involves both the oxidative and non-oxidative pathways of glucose disposal. In normal subjects, the β-cell recognizes the presence of insulin resistance and increases insulin secretion, and, in obese non-diabetics, this compensatory mechanism ensures the absence of glucose tolerance. On the other hand, in Type II diabetic patients, the response of β-cells is not adequate, and results in the development of glucose intolerance. It is also now known that persistently elevated plasma insulin levels can contribute to the development of hypertension, plasma lipid abnormalities, and atherosclerosis.[4]

It has been shown repeatedly that high-fat diets are associated with increased insulin resistance in animal models.[5] However, this association has yet to be established in humans, since the body of evidence is controversial.[6] Recent research suggests that high-fat, — particularly high-saturated-fat — diets may lead to insulin resistance as well as obesity. In contrast, polyunsaturated fatty acids are considered neutral or even protective, but data on the effects of monounsaturated fat on insulin resistance and obesity are still conflicting.[7] However, although no data on the prevalence of diabetes in the Seven Countries Study exist,[8] it is noteworthy that, in Crete, total dietary fat, as well as monounsaturated fat intakes, were high (approximately 40 and 20–25% of the total energy, respectively), but obesity was rare. This could be an indication that it is the saturated fat that is the main contributor to the onset of insulin resistance and, subsequently, to Type II diabetes, along with high energy intakes and a sedentary life-style.

B. MONOUNSATURATED FATTY ACIDS (MUFA)

As mentioned before, monounsaturated fatty acids, mainly present in olive oil, are the principal dietary fat and energy contributors in the populations of the Mediterranean basin. This major difference in the composition of the habitual diets between Mediterraneans and northern Europeans could affect metabolic responses to meals and consequently differentiate the risk for development of several degenerative diseases, including diabetes mellitus. According to a recently published study,[9] glucose-dependent insulinotrophic polypeptide, insulin, and hepatic lipase responses to test meals, rich either in saturated or monounsaturated fat, are higher in Greeks than in northern Europeans (British and Irish). The observed higher hepatic lipase levels are somewhat unexpected, since such activity is correlated with the presence of atherogenic small and dense low density lipoprotein (LDL) particles.[10] However, the researchers argue that involvement of hepatic lipase with remnant removal suggests that, under conditions where neutral lipid exchange is not enhanced and triglyceride enrichment of high density lipoprotein (HDL) and LDL is low, a raised hepatic lipase activity would be advantageous by promoting rapid uptake and clearance of remnant particles.

Regarding diabetes mellitus, according to some studies, high-MUFA diets decrease plasma glucose and insulin levels in Type II diabetic patients, compared with high-carbohydrate diets, which provide the same amount of energy.[7,11,12] In another study,[13] an improvement in insulin sensitivity was observed in Type II diabetic subjects when the diet changed from a high-carbohydrate to an isocaloric high monounsaturated fatty acid diet. Other research conducted on Type II diabetic patients reported that high-MUFA diets result in similar effects with isocaloric, high polyunsaturated fatty acid (PUFA) diets, in terms of glycemia and lipidemia.[14] Moreover, diets rich in MUFA consistently lower plasma total cholesterol and LDL-cholesterol levels in normolipidemic subjects compared with isoenergetic control diets (which are high in saturated fat, or high in carbohydrates), as well as decrease oxidative capacity.[15,16] It has also been observed that in Type II diabetic patients, a diet rich in MUFA resulted in formation of LDL, with a composition that rendered it less atherogenic.[17]

A meta-analysis of several studies comparing high-MUFA and low-saturated-fat, high-carbohydrate diets in patients with Type II diabetes, reported that high-MUFA diets, on the one hand, reduce plasma triglycerides and very low density lipoprotein-cholesterol (VLDL-cholesterol) levels, and on the other hand, moderately increase HDL-cholesterol without adversely affecting LDL-cholesterol concentrations.[18] In addition, high-MUFA diets do not lead to an increase in body weight, provided that dietary energy intake is not increased. It has also been observed that high-MUFA diets may reduce LDL susceptibility to oxidation and, consequently, reduce their atherogenicity.[19]

In a recent study,[20] it was reported that a change from a PUFA to a MUFA diet, in Type II diabetic subjects, reduced insulin resistance and restored endothelium-dependent vasodilation. In particular, the high-MUFA diet resulted in a decrease in fasting glucose/insulin, which is an index of insulin resistance, an improvement in insulin-stimulated glucose transport and on endothelium-dependent flow-mediated vasodilation. In addition, a significant correlation was observed between adipocyte membrane oleic/linoleic acid and insulin-mediated glucose transport, and a significant positive correlation between adipocyte membrane oleic/linoleic acid and endothelium-dependent flow-mediated vasodilation. These data suggest that high MUFA diets, such as the traditional Mediterranean Diet, are beneficial not only to plasma lipid levels but also to the function of endothelial cells.

C. Fish Oils

It has been extensively reported in the literature that dietary intake of fish decreases morbidity and mortality rates of cardiovascular diseases through their effect on known and newly established risk factors.[21] This beneficial effect of dietary fish has been attributed to the high content of fish in ω-3 PUFA, mainly eicosapentaenoic acid (EPA, C20:5 ω-3) and docosahexaenoic acid (DHA, C20:6 ω-3), since these fatty acids may have several anti-atherogenic and antithrombotic properties.

In the Zutphen study,[22] it was observed that a habitual fish consumption of about 30 g per day for more than 25 years resulted in a pronounced decrease in triglyceride levels. The lowering effect of EPA and DHA on plasma triglyceride levels has been widely reported in epidemiological and metabolic studies, and, since one of the adverse effects of Type II diabetes is the presence of increased triglyceride levels, high-fish diets may contribute to their improvement. However, fish oil supplementation has been reported to increase LDL-cholesterol concentrations. The mechanism that has been proposed for this action is the decrease in VLDL size through the decrease in triglyceride levels. Small VLDL tend to form LDL via hepatic lipase action, and not to be taken up by the liver. In addition, lipid peroxidation in Type II diabetes may be exacerbated by the consumption of fish oil.[23]

As far as fish oil supplementation is concerned, although the various studies showed a pronounced hypotriglyceridaemic effect, an adverse effect on HbA$_1$ was not reported in diabetics,[24,25] hyperlipidaemics, nor in patients with abnormal glucose tolerance.[26] However, an increase in fasting blood glucose was observed after fish oil supplementation in Type II diabetics, which probably was a result of increased energy intake and not of the increased consumption of ω-3 fatty acids per se.[27] Moreover, the suggestion that increased fish oil intake could worsen glucose metabolism could also be argued by the results of epidemiological studies that reported that Greenland natives, whose habitual diet contains large amounts of fish,[28] have low prevalence rates of CHD and Type II diabetes, despite their relative obesity.[29,30]

D. Postprandial Lipemia and the Diabetic Subject

Any physiological challenge of the equilibrated fasting state of the lipid transport system, such as the consumption of a fat-containing meal, constitutes postprandial lipemia. In healthy subjects, triglycerides can remain elevated in the circulation up to 8 hours after a meal containing a considerable amount of fat and, therefore, a person who normally ingests three meals in a day could be in a postprandial state most of the day. Abnormal triglyceride response to a meal constitutes a dysfunction of the lipid transport system that involves an exaggerated increase in postprandial triglyceride levels or an extension of their residence time in the circulation. An exaggerated postprandial triglyceride response could result in changes in blood levels and composition of all lipoprotein particles through the greater potential for exchange of triglycerides from chylomicrons and VLDL, and cholesterol esters from LDL and HDL.[31] The resulted lipoprotein profile is more atherogenic (increased cholesterol ester-enriched chylomicron- and VLDL-remnants, decreased HDL_2, and increased HDL_3 levels, as well as increased small and dense LDL particles). Consequently, increased postprandial triglyceride levels could be considered as an independent risk factor for CHD,[32] and it has been reported that extended postprandial lipemia is an inherent feature of diabetic dyslipidemia and highly prevalent in diabetic patients, even in those with normal triglyceride concentrations.[33]

Fatty acid composition of the diet plays an important role in postprandial lipemic response. Especially MUFA, which are the major source of fat in the traditional Cretan Mediterranean Diet, after being incorporated in mixed meals, are reported to lower postprandial triglyceride levels compared to isocaloric meals enriched in saturated fat, both in non-diabetic[34] and in diabetic persons.[35] Therefore, a diet consisting of 40% fat as energy (20-25% MUFA) could be of an overall benefit since it could improve postprandial lipaemic response.

III. CARBOHYDRATE INTAKE

A. Carbohydrate and Dietary Fiber

Traditionally, in many affluent societies, low-carbohydrate diets (i.e., diets providing carbohydrate at a level of 40% or less of total energy) were recommended for diabetic patients.[36] However, the consumption of high-carbohydrate diets has been associated with a deterioration of the glycemic control and an increase in serum triglycerides, if the intake of dietary fiber is low.[37] It is noted that, in some diabetic patients, there appears to be an increased response of plasma glucose after a high-carbohydrate meal, and the average glucose level throughout the day is often higher than on a high-fat diet.[38] Therefore, in contrast to non-diabetic subjects, the compensatory response to a high-carbohydrate diet in some Type II diabetic subjects may not be adequate. As a result, the response of β-cells to dietary carbohydrates may be low and the high resistance to the peripheral insulin action may not be overcome by a limited increase in insulin secretion induced by a high-carbohydrate diet.[38]

It has also been suggested that, if adequate amounts of dietary fiber are included in the daily diet, glycemic control can be improved.[39-42] Moreover, the EURODIAB

IDDM Complications Study Group[43] recently reported that high dietary fiber intake is independently related to beneficial modifications in serum cholesterol levels in men and to a lower risk for development of coronary heart disease (CHD) in European women with Type I diabetes.

There are two types of dietary fiber: (1) soluble, which includes gums, gels, mucilages, and pectic substances, and (2) insoluble, including cellulose, some of the hemicelluloses, and lignin.[36] Soluble fiber has the major effect on plasma glucose and lipid levels, and insoluble fiber decreases constipation. Foods with a high content of soluble fiber are legumes, lentils, some fruits, oats, and barley — foods that are commonly consumed in the Mediterranean region. The inclusion of these foods in the diet could result in an improvement of the glycemic control and a decrease in plasma LDL-cholesterol levels without a change in triglyceride levels or a deterioration of the LDL:HDL ratio.[36]

Early studies[44] suggested that approximately 15 g of soluble fiber daily intake may produce a decrease in fasting blood glucose, glycosylated hemoglobin, and serum total, as well as LDL-cholesterol concentrations in the average Type II diabetic patient. However, the inclusion of 15 g of soluble fiber in the diet would possibly increase the total fiber intake in levels that could exceed the total fiber intake of 20 g. More-recent studies suggest that diets relatively high in monounsaturated fatty acids could be equally or even more beneficial than high-carbohydrate, high-fiber diets,[45] and, as a consequence, the previous enthusiasm for very high-carbohydrate, high-fiber diets now seems to be questioned. Therefore, the traditional Mediterranean Diet, characterized by the daily consumption of olive oil (which provides adequate amounts of oleic acid) and fruits, vegetables, lentils, and legumes — good sources of soluble fiber — could be of benefit to the diabetic patient.

B. The Importance of the Glycemic Index (GI)

The GI has been defined as the ratio of the incremental blood glucose area following food ingestion to the corresponding area following ingestion of an isocarbohydrate portion of white bread. Therefore, it provides an estimate of the effect on blood glucose levels of equivalent amounts of carbohydrate contained in different foods. It has been observed that foods with similar macronutrient composition could influence blood glucose and insulin levels differently due to differences in digestion rates. The GI of several foods is given in Table 1. The GI is influenced by the form in which a food is consumed, its content of fat, protein, and fiber, as well as the way it is processed and prepared, and its rate of intake, digestion, and absorption. In particular, fat may decrease postprandial plasma glucose levels by delaying gastric emptying, and, as a result, the addition of butter to toast reduces the postprandial hyperglycemia in Type II diabetic subjects.[46] Moreover, the physical form of food also has important effects on postprandial hyperglycemia and insulin responses.[47,48] In general, the less processed an ingested food is, the lower the observed hyperglycemic response. Thus, apple juice results in a higher postprandial blood glucose response than raw apple.[49]

Currently, there is some evidence that consumption of foods with a low GI could be beneficial for diabetics to improve the control of plasma glucose levels.[36,50,51] It

TABLE 1
Glycemic Index of Various Foods

Food	Glycemic Index
Breakfast cereals	
Cornflakes	119
Weetabix	109
Oatmeal	97
Shredded wheat	85
All-Bran	73
Grains and cereal products	
Millet	103
White bread	100
Whole wheat bread	99
Rye bread	96
Spaghetti	38–61
Barley	31
Fruit	
Banana	79
Orange	66
Orange juice	67
Apple	53
Grapes	62
Grapefruit	36
Potatoes	
Baked	135
Mashed	100
Boiled	80
Legumes	
Canned baked beans	60
Beans, kidney	54
Butter beans	46
Soya beans	20
Lentils	43
Chick peas	49
Dairy products	
Yogurt	52
Ice cream	52
Whole milk	49
Skim milk	46
Sweeteners	
Maltose	152
Glucose	138
Honey	126
Sucrose	86
Fructose	30

is noteworthy that, in Type II diabetic patients, legume ingestion resulted, not only in a lower blood glucose response than after bread ingestion, but also in lower insulin levels, in both absolute and relative terms.[52] On the other hand, there are also data that suggest that foods with high GIs do not affect the glycemic response when given in mixed meals.[53-56]

The role of the GI has been questioned recently and some researchers[57] believe that the GI of meals is a better tool to assess glycemic responses than the GI of individual foods. However, it has been suggested that the GI can predict the ranking of the glycemic potential of different meals and low-GI diets could result in modest improvements in overall blood glucose control in Type I and Type II diabetic patients.[58,59] Therefore, the inclusion of legumes, pasta, and barley, foods that are part of traditional meals in the Mediterranean basin, could result in the lowering of glucose, insulin, and lipid levels.[60] Recently, in the Nurses' Study[61] it was observed that it was the diets with high GIs that could increase the risk for the development of CHD. A probable mechanism for the pronounced effect of a diet with high GI could be the decrease in insulin sensitivity, which has been shown to occur during short-term clinical studies.[62]

Furthermore, it was shown in six overweight Type II diabetic patients that a diet low in GI compared with one with high GI (57 and 86, respectively), resulted in lower fructosamine and cholesterol levels.[63] A small reduction in body weight was also observed on both diets. On average, low-GI diets are reported to moderately reduce glycosylated hemoglobin, fructosamine, C-peptide, glucose, cholesterol, and triglyceride levels, and consequently reduce the risk for complications observed in diabetes.[64]

C. SIMPLE SUGARS

Although milk, milk products, and fruits are good dietary sources of simple sugars, their intake need not be restricted so long as the appropriate total energy intake and the recommended carbohydrate intake are respected. It is noteworthy that, under certain circumstances, monosaccharides and disaccharides do not result in deterioration of glycemic control or elevated lipid levels.[65] Therefore, the American Diabetes Association[66] considers that a modest consumption of sucrose could be acceptable as long as glucose metabolic control is maintained. Furthermore, it was reported that the consumption of sesame-derived candies, commonly consumed in Greece, decreased blood glucose levels compared with bread, which provided equal amounts of glucose.[67] Since these candies are also a good source of PUFA, the authors concluded that — if desired — they could be consumed in moderate amounts by diabetic persons. In addition, in another study from the same group[68] it was observed that honey and bread produce similar degrees of hyperglycemia in Type II diabetic patients, even though honey contains significant amounts of simple sugars.

IV. PROTEIN

It has been suggested that the rate of protein degradation and conversion of protein to glucose in Type I diabetic subjects may partly depend on the degree of glycemic control, and, in Type II diabetic patients, the rate of gluconeogenesis could be rapid in the post-absorptive state. However, when glycemic control is optimal, the effect of dietary protein on plasma glucose levels is not significant.[69,70]

Although nephropathy is responsible for only 10% of all deaths, it accounts for 50–60% of the deaths of Type I diabetic patients.[71] It is widely recognized that nephropathy progresses without symptoms until renal failure is extensive. However, the effect of dietary manipulation on long-term renal function is still unknown, even though some research[72,73] suggest that an early intervention could be of benefit. Low-protein diets could modify the underlying glomerular injury as well as control hyperglycemia and hypertension. It is noteworthy that protein restriction in patients with incipient nephropathy resulted in a significant fall of the albumin excretion rate[74] and a decrease in the deterioration rate of renal function in individuals with diabetic nephropathy.[75] On the other hand, there is a risk for protein malnutrition when dietary protein intake is less than 0.6 g/kg/day.

In the traditional Mediterranean Diet, as it is described elsewhere in this volume, the daily intake of animal protein was low, since red meat was consumed only once per week and in small amounts. In studies with non-diabetics,[76] it was also observed that much of any observed benefit was due to a reduction in animal protein. Therefore, further investigation is necessary for the clarification of the role of vegetable protein on diabetic nephropathy. Currently, a dietary protein intake of 0.8 g/kg/day, which constitutes approximately 10% of total energy intake, could be recommended. This is not different from the U.S. Recommended Dietary Allowances (RDA) for non-diabetic adults.[77]

V. OBESITY

Obesity is related to diabetes mellitus and CHD in both men and women. From studies carried out in Finland, the U.S., and the Netherlands, it has been observed that, had there been no increase in body weight to levels of Body Mass Index (BMI) higher than 25 kg/m², 15–30% of all deaths from CHD[78-80] and 64% of male[81] and 77% of female[82] cases of Type II diabetes mellitus could theoretically have been prevented. It is noteworthy that, in the Netherlands, a 12% increase in the incidence of Type II diabetes mellitus has been observed, which may be partly the consequence of the increased prevalence of obesity during the same period.

In the Seven Countries Study,[83] hazard ratios for death from all causes, all cardiovascular diseases, and other causes were significantly higher in men who lost weight than in men whose weight remained constant. In addition, fluctuation in body weight was associated with an increased risk of all-cause mortality, CHD, and myocardial infarction. The data relating obesity and cardiovascular morbidity or overall mortality are not unanimous. In a more-recent paper[84] published by the same group, it was reported that a BMI of 25–30 kg/m² was not related to increased mortality. In addition, a BMI of > 30 kg/m² was not related to increased mortality among current smokers. In those who had never smoked, a BMI of > 30 kg/m² was related to increased mortality, but the hazard ratios were lower than those for BMI < 18.5 kg/m².

In a study[85] carried out in the Cretan low-risk population of Spili, it was reported that hypertension, diabetes, obesity, and hypercholesterolemia were at least as prevalent as in Sweden. In addition, the end points of the so-called Metabolic Syndrome X, including insulin resistance and hyperinsulinemia, also existed in the Spili population. These observations are in contrast to the low prevalence of myocardial infarction observed in Cretan men from Spili. The authors suggested that protective factors such as high intake of olive oil, cereals, and fruit existed in the village, as well as the social network that included low divorce rates and no male unemployment, which could — at least partly — justify these unexpected results.

There is also controversy over the role of dietary fat in the development of obesity. There are several epidemiological studies that reported a positive correlation between high-fat diets and an increased prevalence of obesity.[86-88] However, the Seven Countries Study[89] did not show the existence of such a relationship. It is noteworthy that the prevalence of obesity was lower in the Greek cohort than in the American, Finnish, or Dutch groups, even though the dietary fat intake was similarly high. In addition, in the Risk Factor and Life Expectancy (RIFLE) pooling project,[90] when the relation of BMI to short-term mortality in a large Italian cohort (32,471 men and 30,305 women) was evaluated, a U- or inverse J-shaped relation was not demonstrated. The minimum of the curve was located at 27.0 kg/m^2 and 31.8 kg/m^2 for young and mature women, respectively. No relation was found for young men, whereas for mature adult men, only the model for all subjects retained significant curvilinear relation. As the authors reported, the uncommon high values of BMI carrying the minimum risk of death observed in this study is in contrast to weight guidelines. The fact that dietary fatty acid composition, and consequently adipose tissue fatty acid composition, is different, and probably MUFA enriched, in Italians compared with Americans and northern Europeans, could possibly partly explain these interesting observations. This difference could also suggest that, for similar BMI values, the risk of death differs according to adipose tissue fatty acid composition.

In contrast to epidemiological studies, some metabolic studies in humans showed that high-fat diets do not result in weight gain when compared isocalorically with very low-fat diets.[91] It has been suggested that if there is an effect of high-fat diets on obesity rates, it could be due to the increase in active and passive hyperphagias that have been observed in subjects on high-fat diets.[92,93] The whole issue of the increased susceptibility for developing obesity when on high-fat diets is arguable, since, even recently in the U.S., it has been observed that the prevalence of obesity has increased, while the proportion of fat in the diet has decreased.[94]

The issue of low-fat diets vs. high-fat diets has also always to be addressed in conjunction with the carbohydrate intake. It is now widely known that a high percentage intake of carbohydrate will result in high postprandial insulin response which, hypothetically, would mean a long-term effect of an age-related decline in insulin secretion, and possibly lead to an earlier onset of Type II diabetes mellitus.[95] Interestingly, it has been reported that high-carbohydrate, compared with high-MUFA diets results in an increased resistance to the peripheral action of insulin,[93] and, therefore, the concept of dietary fat composition and the prevalence of diabetes and obesity requires further investigation.

VI. RECOMMENDATIONS

The American Diabetes Association[96] and the Nutrition Study Group of the European Association for the Study of Diabetes[97], have reached basic recommendations, and the Nutrition Study Group has renewed its recommendations, which have been recently published.[98] A summary of these recommendations follows.

- BMI should be between 18.5–25.0 kg/m². For patients with BMI > 25 kg/m² a lower dietary energy intake should be recommended (500 kcal less than the usual daily energy intake) through a reduction of energy-dense foods.
- Regular physical activity may improve glucose tolerance and the lipid profile, and, therefore, combination of a healthy and balanced diet and increased physical activity should be recommended.
- Regarding the dietary changes:
  - Saturated and trans fatty acids should be < 10% of daily energy intake, or even lower (< 8% of total energy) in the case of increased LDL cholesterol levels. The above suggested fatty acid intake is similar to the one recommended by the American Heart Association (AHA) in Step I and Step II diets for the treatment of hypercholesterolemia.
  - PUFA intake should be < 10% of total energy intake.
  - MUFA should provide between 10 and 20% of total energy intake. 20% of MUFA intake is similar to the traditional Cretan diet MUFA composition.
  - Cholesterol intake should be less than 300 mg per day.
  - Protein intake should be between 10 and 20% of total energy.
  - Combined carbohydrate and MUFA of cis-configuration should provide a total 60–70% of the daily dietary energy intake.
- An increase in consumption of rich-in-fiber, carbohydrate-containing, and low-glycemic-index foods should be encouraged.

It is noteworthy that the daily carbohydrate intake should be between 45 and 60%, whereas fat intake is recommended to be between 25 and 35% of total energy. MUFA intake, mainly from vegetable sources, should provide 10 to 20% of total energy. These recommendations are similar to the traditional Cretan diet, considering that carbohydrate intake was 40–45% of energy, fat intake was around 40%, and MUFA intake was half of the total fat intake. It is noteworthy that, in an 1800 kcal diet that could be recommended to some obese Type II diabetic patients in order to reduce their weight, a Mediterranean 40%-fat diet would provide 80 g of fat per day, whereas a 25%-fat diet that would be carbohydrate-rich would provide 50 g of fat per day. The 30-g difference of fat between these two diets is equal to 2 tablespoons of olive oil (approximately 30 ml), which is probably similar to the amount of olive oil that Cretans put in their salads on a daily basis.

Emphasis is also placed on the dietary antioxidant intake. This is of increasing importance, since diabetic patients have reduced antioxidant defenses and there is growing awareness that free radical processes may be of particular importance in the complications of diabetes.[99] A study indicated that flavonol-rich foods resulted in beneficial effects against oxidative stress in Type II diabetic patients.[100] In contrast, experimental data support the hypothesis that there is an increase in lipid peroxidation when on high-PUFA diets, and, therefore, increased dietary antioxidant intake could counteract this adverse effect.[101] However, research on recommended daily antioxidant intake is inconclusive. For example, the RDA for vitamin E is currently 10 mg, and this intake may be inadequate for the prevention or treatment of microvascular complications present in diabetics.[102] Certainly, further research is needed.

REFERENCES

1. American Diabetes Association: Diabetes 1993 Vital Statistics. Alexandria VA, American Diabetes Association, 1993.
2. Pickup, J. C. and Williams, G., The epidemiology of diabetes mellitus, in *Textbook of Diabetes*, Blackwell Science, 2nd ed., 1997.
3. Katsilambros, N., Aliferis, K., Darviri, Ch., Tsapogas, P., Alexiou, Z., Tritos, N., and Arvanitis, M., Evidence for an increase in the prevalence of known diabetes in a sample of an urban population in Greece, *Diab. Med.*, 10, 87, 1993.
4. DeFronzo, R. and Ferrannini E., Insulin resistance. A multifaceted syndrome responsible for NIDDM, obesity, hypertension, dyslipidemia, and atherosclerotic cardiovascular disease, *Diabetes Care*, 14, 173, 1991.
5. Pan, D. A., Hulbert, A. J., and Storljen, L. H., Dietary fats, membrane phospholipids, and obesity, *J. Nutr.*, 124,1555,1994.
6. Howard, B. V., Dietary fatty acids, insulin resistance, and diabetes, *Ann. N. Y. Acad. Sci.*, 827, 215, 1997.
7. Storlien, L. H., Kriketos, A. D., Jenkins, A. B., Baur, L. A., Pan, D. A., Tapsell, L. C., and Calvert, G. D., Does dietary fat influence insulin action? *Ann. N. Y. Acad. Sci.*, 827, 287, 1997.
8. Kromhout, D., Menotti, A., Bloemberg, B., Aravanis, C., Blackburn, H., Buzina, R., Dontas, A. S., Fidanza, F., Giampaoli, S., and Jansen, A., Dietary saturated and trans fatty acids and cholesterol and 25-year mortality from coronary heart disease: the Seven Countries Study, *Prev. Med.*, 24, 308, 1995.
9. Jackson, K. G., Zampelas, A., Knapper, J. M., Roche, H. M., Gibney, M. J., Kafatos, A., Gould, B. J., Wright, J. W., and Williams, C. M., Differences in glucose-dependent insulinotrophic polypeptide hormone and hepatic lipase in subjects of southern and northern Europe: implications for postprandial lipemia, *Am. J. Clin. Nutr.* 71, 13, 2000.
10. Karpe, F., Steiner, G., Olivecrona, T., Carlson, L. A., and Hamsten, A., Metabolism of triglyceride-rich lipoproteins during alimentary lipaemia, *J. Clin. Invest.* 91, 748, 1993.
11. Garg, A., Bantle, J. P., Henry, R. R., Coulston, A. M., Griver, K. A., Raatz, S. K., Brinkley, L., Chen, Y., Grundy, S. M., Huet, B. A., and Reaven, G. M., Effects of varying carbohydrate content of diet in patients with non-insulin-dependent diabetes mellitus, *J. Am. Med. Assoc.*, 271, 1421, 1994.
12. Rivellese, A. A., Monounsaturated and marine ω-3 fatty acids in NIDDM patients., *Ann. N. Y. Acad. Sci.*, 827,302, 1997.

13. Low, C. C., Grossman, E. B., and Gumbiner, B., Potentiation of effects of weight loss by monounsaturated fatty acids in obese NIDDM patients, *Diabetes*, 45, 569, 1996.

14. Katsilambros, N., Kostalas, G., Michalakis, N., Kapantais, E., Manglara, E., Kouzeli, Ch., Marangos, M., Alevizou, V., Sakellariou, Ch., and Richardson, S. C., Metabolic effects of long-term diets enriched in olive oil or sunflower oil in non-insulin-dependent diabetes, *Nutr. Metab. Cardiovasc. Dis.*, 6, 164, 1996.

15. Berry, E. M., Eisenberg, S., Friedlander, Y., Harats, D., Kaufmann, N. A., Norman, Y., and Stein, Y., Effects of diets rich in monounsaturated fatty acids on plasma lipoproteins. The Jerusalem Nutrition Study: Monounsaturated vs. saturated fatty acids, *Nutr. Metab. Cardiovasc. Dis.*, 5, 55, 1995.

16. Williams, C. M., Francis-Knapper, J. A., Webb, D., Brookes, C. A., Zampelas, A., Tredger, J. A., Wright, J., Meijer, G., Calder, P. C., Yaqoob, P., Roche, H., and Gibney, M. J., Cholesterol reduction using manufactured foods high in monounsaturated fatty acids: a randomized crossover study, *Br. J. Nutr.* 81, 439, 1999.

17. Dimitriadis, E., Griffin, M., Collins, P., Johnson, A., Owens, D., and Tomkin, G. H., Lipoprotein composition in NIDDM: effects of dietary oleic acid on the composition, oxidizability and function of low and high density lipoproteins, *Diabetologia*, 39, 667, 1996.

18. Garg, A., High-monounsaturated-fat diets for patients with diabetes mellitus: a meta-analysis, *Am. J. Clin. Nutr.*, 67(suppl), 577S, 1998.

19. Berry, E. M., Eisenberg, S., Friedlander, Y., Harats, D., Kaufmann, N. A., Norman, Y., and Stein, Y., Effects of diets rich in monounsaturated fatty acids on plasma lipoproteins – the Jerusalem Nutrition Study II: Monounsaturated fatty acids vs. carbohydrates, *Am. J. Clin. Nutr.*, 56, 394, 1992.

20. Ryan, M., McInerney, D., Owens, D., Collins, P., Johnson, A., and Tomkin, G, H., Diabetes and the Mediterranean Diet: a beneficial effect of oleic acid on insulin sensitivity, adipocyte glucose transport and endothelium-dependent vasoreactivity, *Q. J. M.*, 93, 85, 2000.

21. Nordøy, A., Fish consumption and cardiovascular disease: A reappraisal, *Nutr. Metab. Cardiovasc. Dis.*, 6, 103, 1996.

22. Kromhout, D., Katan, M. B., Havekes, L., Groener, A., Hornstra, G., De Lezenne, and Coulander, C., The effect of 26 years of habitual fish consumption on serum lipid and lipoprotein levels (The Zutphen Study), *Nutr. Metab. Cardiovasc. Dis.*, 6, 65, 1996.

23. McGrath, L. T., Brennan, G. M., Donnelly, J. P., Johnston, G. D., Hayes, J. R., and McVeigh, G. E., Effect of dietary fish oil supplementation on peroxidation of serum lipids in patients with non-insulin-dependent diabetes mellitus, *Atherosclerosis*, 121, 275, 1996.

24. Vessby, B., n-3 fatty acids and blood glucose control in diabetes mellitus, *J. Intern. Med.*, 225, 207, 1989.

25. Luo, J., Rizkalla, S. W., Vidal, H., Oppert, J-M., Colas, C., Boussairi, A., Guerre-Millo, M., Chapuis, A-S., Chevalier, A., Durand, G., and Slama, G., Moderate intake of n-3 fatty acids for 2 months has no detrimental effect on glucose metabolism and could ameliorate the lipid profile in type 2 diabetic men, *Diabetes Care*, 21, 717, 1998.

26. Sirtori, C. R,, Paoletti, R., Mancini, M., Crepaldi, G., Manzato, E., Rivellese, A., Pamparana, F., and Stragliotto, E., N-3 fatty acids do not lead to an increased diabetic risk in patients with hyperlipidemia and abnormal glucose tolerance. Italian Fish Oil Multicenter Study, *Am. J. Clin. Nutr.*, 65, 1874, 1997.

27. Borkman, M., Chisholm, D. J., Furler, S. M., Storlien, L. H., Kraegen, E. W., Simons, L. A., and Chesterman, C. N., Effects of fish oil supplementation on glucose and lipid metabolism in NIDDM, *Diabetes*, 38, 1314, 1989.

28. Bang, H. O., Dyerberg, J., and Sinclair, H. M., The composition of Eskimo food in northwestern Greenland, *Am. J. Clin. Nutr.*, 33, 2657, 1980.

29. Kromann, N., and Green, A., Epidemiological studies in the Upernavik district of Greenland, incidence of some chronic diseases 1950–1974, *Acta Med. Scand.*, 208, 401, 1980.

30. Mouratoff, G. J., Caroll, N. V., and Scott, E. M., Diabetes mellitus in Eskimos, *J. Am. Med. Assoc.*, 199, 107, 1967.

31. Zampelas, A., Postprandial lipaemia, coronary heart disease and dietary fatty acid compsition, *BNF Nutr. Bull.*, 19(Suppl), 25, 1994.

32. Ebenbichler, C. F., Kirchmair, R., Egger, C., and Patsch, J. R., Postprandial state and atherosclerosis, *Curr. Opin. Lipidol.*, 6, 286, 1995.

33. Coppack, S. W., Postprandial lipoproteins in non-insulin-dependent diabetes mellitus, *Diabet. Med.*, 14(suppl 3), S67, 1997.

34. Nicolaïew, N., Lemort, N., Martin, C., Linné, I., and Jacotot, B., Postprandial lipemia is differently affected by monounsaturated and saturated dietary fats in humans, *Nutr. Metab. Cardiovasc. Dis.*, 8, 315, 1998.

35. Michailidou, G., Perea, D., and Katsilambros, N., Monounsaturated fat and postprandial triglyceride levels in non-insulin-dependent diabetic persons, *Diabet. Med.*, 14, 406, 1997.

36. Mann, J. I., and Lewis-Barned, N. J. Dietary management of diabetes mellitus in Europe and North America, in *International Textbook of Diabetes Mellitus*, Alberti, K.G.M.M., De Fronzo, R.A., Keen, H., and Zimmet. P., Eds, Volume 1., John Wiley and Sons, Chichester, 1992, 685.

37. Aro, A., Uusitupa, M., Voutilainen, E., Hersio, K., Korhonen, T., and Siitonen, O., Improved diabetic control and hypocholesterolaemic effect induced by long-term dietary supplementation with guar gum in type 2 (insulin-independent) diabetes, *Diabetologia*, 21, 29, 1981.

38. Grundy, S. M., Dietary therapy in diabetes mellitus. Is there a single best diet? *Diabetes Care*, 14, 796, 1991.

39. Kiehm, T. G., Anderson, J. W., and Ward, K., Beneficial effects of a high carbohydrate, high fibre diet on hyperglycaemic men, *Am. J. Clin. Nutr.*, 29, 895, 1976.

40. Jenkins, D. J. A., Goff, D. V., Leads, A. R., Alberti, K. G., Wolever, T. M., Gassull, M. A., and Hockaday, T. D., Unabsorbable carbohydrates and diabetes: decreased postprandial hyperglycaemia, *Lancet*, 2, 172, 1976.

41. Simpson, H. C. R., Carter, R. D., Lousley, S., and Mann, J. I., Digestible carbohydrate – an independent effect on diabetic control in type 2 (non-insulin dependent) diabetic patients? *Diabetologia*, 23, 235, 1982.

42. Riccardi, G., Rivellese, A., Pacioni, D., Genovese, D., Mastranzo, P., and Mancini, M., Separate influence of dietary carbohydrate and fiber on the metabolic control in diabetes, *Diabetologia*, 26, 116, 1984.

43. Toeller, M., Buyken, A. E., Heitkamp, G., de Pergola, G., Giorgino, F., and Fuller, J. H., Fiber intake, serum cholesterol levels, and cardiovascular disease in European individuals with type 1 diabetes. EURODIAB TYPE I DIABETES Complications Study Group, *Diabetes Care*, 22(suppl 2), B21, 1999.

44. Fuessl, H. S., Williams, G., Adrian, T. E., and Bloom, S. R., Guar sprinkled on food: effect on glycaemic control, plasma lipids, and gut hormones in non-insulin-dependent diabetic patients, *Diabetic. Med.*, 463, 1987.

45. Nutrition Subcommittee of the British Diabetic Association's Professional Advisory Committee: Dietary recommendations for people with diabetes: an update for the 1990s, *Diabetic Medicine*, 9, 189, 1992.
46. Katsilambros, N., Philippides, Ph., Metaxatos, G., Frangaki, D., Marangos, M., and Daikos, G. K., Effect of butter and salami ingestion on the postprandial hyperglycemia in NIDDs, *Diabetes Res. Clin. Pract.*, 2(suppl 1), S291, 1985.
47. O'Dea, K., Nestel, P. J., and Antonoff, L., Physical factors influencing postprandial glucose and insulin responses to starch, *Am. J. Clin. Nutr.*, 33, 760, 1980.
48. Katsilambros, N., Saviolakis, A., Philippides, Ph., Tsakiri, I., Siskoudis, P., Manglara, E., and Kardari, A., Metabolic effects of chestnuts in non-insulin-dependent diabetics: role of the method of cooking, *Nutr. Metab. Cardiovasc. Dis.*, 4, 101, 1994.
49. Haber, C. B., Keaton, K. W., and Murphy, D., Depletion and disruption of dietary fiber. Effects of satiety, plasma glucose, and serum insulin, *Lancet*, I, 679, 1977.
50. Jenkins, D. J. A., Wolever, T. M. S., and Jenkins, A. L., Starchy foods and GI, *Diabetes Care*, 11, 149, 1988.
51. Bornet, F. R. J., Costagliola, D., Rizkalla, S. W., Blayo, A., Fontvieille, A. M., Haardt, M. J., Letanoux, M., Tchobroutsky, G., and Slama, G., Insulinemic and GIes of six starch-rich foods taken alone and in a mixed meal by type 2 diabetics, *Am. J. Clin. Nutr.*, 45, 588, 1987.
52. Voyatzoglou, D., Loupa, Ch., Philippides, Ph., Siskoudis, P., Kitsou, E., Alevizou, V., Manglara, E., and Katsilambros, N, Insulin response to legumes in type 2 diabetic persons, *Eur. J. Intern. Med.*, 6, 201, 1995.
53. Coulston, A. M., Hollenbeck, C. B., Swislocki, A. L. M., and Reaven, G. M., Effect of source of dietary carbohydrate on plasma glucose and insulin responses to mixed meals in subjects with type I diabetes, *Diabetes Care*, 10, 395, 1987.
54. Bantle, J. P., Laine, D. C., Castle, G. W., Thomas, J. W., Hoogwerf, B. J., and Goetz, F. C., Postprandial glucose and insulin responses to meals containing different carbohydrates in normal and diabetic subjects, *New Engl. J. Med.*, 309, 7, 1983.
55. Coulston, A. M., Hollenbeck, C. B., Liu, G. C., Williams, R. A., Starich, G. H., Massaferri, E. L., and Reaven, G. M., Effect of source of dietary carbohydrate on plasma glucose, insulin and gastric inhibitory polypeptide responses to meals in subjects with non-insulin-dependent diabetes mellitus, *Am. J. Clin. Nutr.*, 40, 965, 1984.
56. Nuttall, F. Q., Mooradian, A. D., DeMarais, R., and Parker, S., The glycemic effect of different meals approximately isocaloric and similar in protein, carbohydrate, and fat content as calculated using the A.D.A. exchange lists, *Diabetes Care*, 6, 432, 1983.
57. Wolever, T. M., The GI: flogging a dead horse? *Diabetes Care*, 20, 452, 1997.
58. Wolever, T. M., Jenkins, D. J., Jenkins, A. L., and Josse, R. G., The GI: methodology and clinical implications, *Am. J. Clin. Nutr.*, 54, 846, 1991.
59. Wolever, T. M., and Jenkins, D. J., The use of the GI in predicting the blood glucose response to test meals, *Am. J .Clin. Nutr.*, 43, 167, 1986.
60. Wolever, T. M., The GI, *World Rev. Nutr. Diet.*, 62, 120, 1990.
61. Liu, S., Stampfer, M. J., Manson, J. E., Hu, F. B., Franz, M., and Willett, W. C., A prospective study of glycemic load and risk of myocardial infarction in women, *FASEB J.*, 12, A260, 1998.
62. Frost, G., Keogh, B., Smith, D., Akinsanya, K., and Leeds, A., The effect of low glycemic carbohydrate on insulin and glucose response *in vitro* and *in vivo* in patients with coronary heart disease, *Metabolism*, 45, 669, 1996.
63. Wolever, T. M., Jenkins, D. J., Vuskan, V., Jenkins, A. L., Wong, G. S., and Josse, R. G., Beneficial effect of low-GI diet in overweight type I diabetes subjects, *Diabetes Care*, 15, 562, 1992.

64. Miller, J. C., Importance of GI in diabetes, *Am. J. Clin. Nutr.*, 59, 747S, 1994.
65. Bantle, J. P., Laine, D. C., and Thomas, J. W., Metabolic effects of dietary fructose and sucrose in types I and II diabetic subjects, *J. Am. Med. Assoc.*, 256, 3241, 1986.
66. American Diabetes Association: Glycemic effects of carbohydrates, *Diabetes Care*, 7, 607, 1984.
67. Katsilambros, N., Philippides, Ph., Davoulos, G., Gialouros, K., Kofotzouli, L., Manglara, E., Ioannidis, P. I., Siskoudis, P., and Sfikakis, P., Sesame-derived candies and glycemic response in Type II diabetic subjects, *Diab. Nutr. Metab.*, 4, 325, 1991.
68. Katsilambros, N. L., Philippides, Ph., Touliatou, A., Georgakopoulos, K., Kofotzouli, L., Frangaki, D., Siskoudis, P., Marangos, M., and Sfikakis, P., Metabolic effects of honey (alone or combined with other foods) in Type II diabetics, *Acta Diabetol. Lat.*, 25, 197, 1988.
69. Peters, A. L. and Davidson, M. B., Protein and fat effects on glucose response and insulin requirements in subjects with insulin-dependent diabetes mellitus, *Am. J. Clin. Nutr.*, 58, 555, 1993.
70. Nuttall, F. Q., Mooradian, A. D., Gannon, M. C., Billington, C., and Krezowski, P., Effect of protein ingestion on the glucose and insulin response to a standardized oral glucose load, *Diabetes Care*, 7, 465, 1984.
71. Zeman, F. J., *Clinical Nutrition and Dietetics,* MacMillan Publishing Co, New York, 2nd. ed., 1991, 398.
72. Mogensen, C. E. and Christensen, C. K., Predicting diabetic nephropathy in insulin-dependent patients, *New Engl. J. Med.*, 311, 89, 1984.
73. Viberti, G. C. and Keen, H., The patterns of proteinuria in diabetes mellitus: relevance to pathogenesis and prevention of diabetic nephropathy, *Diabetes* 33, 686, 1984.
74. Cohen, D., Dodds, R., and Viberti, G. C., Effect of protein restriction in insulin dependent diabetics at risk of nephropathy, *Br. Med. J.*, 294, 795, 1987.
75. Zeller, K., Whittaker, E., Sullivan, L., Raskin, P., and Jacobson, H. R., Effect of restricting dietary protein on the progression of renal failure in patients with insulin-dependent diabetes mellitus, *New Engl. J. Med.*, 324, 78, 1991.
76. Jibani, M. M., Bloodworth, L. L., Foden, E., Griffiths, K. D., and Galpin, O. P., Predominantly vegetarian diet in patients with incipient and early clinical diabetic nephropathy: effects on albumin excretion rate and nutritional status, *Diabet. Med.*, 8, 949, 1991.
77. National Research Council, *Recommended Dietary Allowances*, National Academy Press, 10th ed., Washington D.C., 1989.
78. Jousilathi, P., Tuomiletho, J., Vartainen, E., Pekkanen, J., and Puska, P., Body weight, cardiovascular risk factors, and coronary mortality: 15 year follow-up of middle-aged men and women in eastern Finland, *Circulation*, 93, 1372, 1996.
79. Willett, W. C., Manson, J. E., and Stampfer, M. J., Weight, weight change, and coronary heart disease in women. Risk within the "normal" range, *J. Am. Med. Assoc.*, 273, 461, 1995.
80. Seidell, J. C., Verschuren, W. M. M., vanLeer, E. M., and Kromhout, D., Overweight, underweight and mortality: a prospective study of 48,287 men and women, *Arch. Intern. Med.*, 156, 958, 1996.
81. Chain, J. M., Rimm, E. B., Colditz, G. A., Stampfer, M. J., and Willett, W. C., Obesity, fat distribution, and weight gain as risk factors for clinical diabetes in men, *Diabetes Care*, 17, 961, 1994.
82. Colditz, G. A., Willett, W. C., Rotnitzky, A., and Manson, J. E., Weight gain as a risk factor for clinical diabetes mellitus in women, *Ann. Intern. Med.*, 122, 481, 1995.

83. Peters, E. T., Seidell, J. C., Menotti, A., Aravanis, C., Dontas, A., Fidanza, F., Karvonen, M., Nedeljkovic, S., Nissinen, A., Buzina, R., et al., Changes in body weight in relation to mortality in 6441 European middle-aged men: the Seven Countries Study, *Int. J. Obes. Relat. Metab. Disord.*, 19, 862, 1995.

84. Visscher, T. L., Seidell, J. C., Menotti, A., Blackburn, H., Nissinen, A., Feskens, E. J., and Kromhout, D., Underweight and overweight in relation to mortality among men aged 40–59 and 50–69 years: the Seven Countries Study, *Am. J. Epidemiol.*, 1, 660, 2000.

85. Koutis, A. D., Lionis, C. D., Isacsson, A., Jacobsson, A., Fioretos M., and Lindholm, L. H., Characteristics of the "Metabolic Syndrome X" in a cardiovascular low risk population in Crete, *Eur. Heart J.*, 13, 865, 1992.

86. West, K., and Kalbfleisch, J., Influence of nutritional factors on prevalence of diabetes, *Diabetes*, 20, 99, 1971.

87. Pudel, V., and Westenhoefer, J., Dietary and behavioral principles in the treatment of obesity, *International monitor on eating patterns and weight control (Medicom/Servier)*, 1, 2, 1992.

88. Curb, J., and Marcus, E., Body fat and obesity in Japanese Americans, *Am. J. Clin. Nutr.*, 53, 1552S, 1991.

89. Keys, A., Coronary heart disease in seven countries, *Circulation*, XLI(Suppl 1), 1, 1970.

90. Seccareccia, F., Lanti, M., Menotti, A., and Scanga, M., Role of body mass index in the prediction of all-cause mortality in over 62,000 men and women. The Italian RIFLE Pooling Project. Risk Factor and Life Expectancy, *J. Epidemiol. Community Health*, 52, 20, 1998.

91. Hirsch, J., Hudgins, L. C., Leibel, R. L., and Rosenbaum, M., Diet composition and energy balance in humans, *Am. J. Clin. Nutr.*, 67(Suppl), 551S, 1998.

92. Colay, A., and Bobbioni, E., The role of dietary fat in obesity, *Intern. J. Obes.*, 21(Suppl 3), S2, 1997.

93. Grundy, S. M., The optimal ratio of fat-to-carbohydrate in the diet, *Ann. Rev. Nutr.*, 19, 325, 1999.

94. Cent. Dis. Control. Prev., Daily dietary fat and total food energy intakes, Third National Health and Nutrition Examination Survey. Phase 1, *Morbid.Mortal.Wkly. Rep.*, 43, 116, 1994.

95. Parillo, M., Rivellese, A. A., Ciardullo, A. V., Capaldo, B., and Giacco, A., A high-monounsaturated fat/low carbohydrate diet improves peripheral insulin sensitivity in non-insulin-dependent diabetic patients, *Metabolism*, 41, 1278, 1992.

96. American Diabetes Association: Nutrition recommendations and principles for people with diabetes mellitus, *Diabetes Care*, 22(suppl 1), S42, 1999.

97. Diabetes and Nutrition Study Group of the European Association for the Study of Diabetes: Recommendations for the nutritional management of patients with diabetes mellitus, *Diab. Nutr. Metab.*, 8, 186, 1995.

98. The Diabetes and Nutrition Study Group (D.N.S.G.) of the European Association for the Study of Diabetes (E.A.S.D.), 1999, Recommendations for the nutritional management of patients with diabetes mellitus, *Eur. J. Clin. Nutr.*, 54, 353, 2000.

99. Gazis, A., Page, S., and Cockcroft, J., Vitamin E and cardiovascular protection in diabetes, *Br. Med. J.*, 314, 1845, 1997.

100. Lean, M. E. J., Noroozi, M., Kelly, I., Burns, J., Talwar, D., Sattar, N., and Crozier, A., Dietary flavonols protect diabetic human lymphocytes against oxidative damage to DNA, *Diabetes*, 48, 176, 1999.

101. Eritsland, J., Safety considerations of polyunsaturated fatty acids, *Am. J. Clin. Nutr.*, 71, 197, 2000.
102. Jain, S. K., Should high-dose Vitamin E supplementation be recommended to diabetic patients? *Diabetes Care*, 22, 1245, 1999.

11 The Mediterranean Diet and Coronary Heart Disease

Antonis Zampelas, Michael Hourdakis, and Nikos Yiannakouris

CONTENTS

I. EPIDEMIOLOGICAL STUDIES

The Mediterranean Diet became widely known for the first time in the 1970s from the Seven Countries Study.[1] This study began in 1960 and compared the incidence of coronary heart disease (CHD) and the life-styles of populations from seven countries, namely the U.S., the Netherlands, Finland, Japan, Yugoslavia, Italy, and Greece. The main finding of the Seven Countries Study was that the Greek population from Crete had very low morbidity and mortality rates from CHD compared with the populations of the other countries. It was also observed that Cretans had lower plasma cholesterol levels than Americans, which led to the suggestion that this difference in plasma cholesterol levels might have influenced the difference in the prevalence of CHD in these two countries.[1,2] However, even though the Cretan cohort had relatively higher plasma cholesterol levels than the Italian and Yugoslavian in the Seven Countries Study, the mortality rates from CHD on this island remained lower even 25 years after the beginning of the study.[3] In addition, it was reported that the risk for the development of CHD varied from country to country even for people with similar plasma cholesterol levels.[4] The last two observations indicate that environmental factors, such as diet and its components, could influence the risk for developing CHD, irrespective of plasma cholesterol levels.

The Seven Countries Study revealed that the traditional Cretan Mediterranean Diet was rich in total fat, rich in monounsaturated fat, and poor in saturated fat. These findings were supported by another study by Christakis et al. in 1965[2] that observed differences in the adipose tissue fatty acid composition between an American and a Cretan cohort. In particular, the Cretans' adipose tissue had a higher proportion of monounsaturated fatty acids than the adipose tissue of the American cohort. Since adipose tissue fatty acid composition is a marker for the long-term background diet, the results of this study were an indication that the traditional Cretan diet was high in monounsaturated fatty acids, originating mainly from olive oil.

Apart from olive oil consumption, there were also other differences in the diets of the seven cohorts. In particular, large differences in food group consumption were observed, with high consumption of dairy products in northern Europe; meat in the U.S.; vegetables, legumes, fish, and wine in southern Europe; and cereals, soya products, and fish in Japan. Animal food groups were directly correlated, while vegetable food groups (except potatoes), as well as fish and alcohol were inversely correlated with CHD mortality. Univariate analysis showed significant positive correlation coefficients for butter (r = 0.887), meat (r = 0.645), pastries (r = 0.752), and milk (r = 0.600) consumption, and significant negative correlation coefficients for legumes (r = −0.822), oils — mainly olive oil (r = −0.571) — and alcohol (r = −0.609).[5]

Apart from monounsaturated fatty acids, the Mediterranean Diet is rich in antioxidants from olive oil, fruits, and vegetables. Several studies have indicated that vitamin E and, especially, α-tocopherol, plays an important role in the resistance against LDL oxidation. However, with respect to the Seven Countries Study, it was observed that dietary intake of flavonoids and saturated fatty acids, as well as smoking habits, were more important factors that could influence the development of CHD than dietary intakes of vitamins E, C, and carotenoids.[6]

Following the findings of the Seven Countries Study, several studies have been carried out to compare the Mediterranean Diet, characterized by high olive oil intake, to other diets in different populations. Even in secondary prevention, the Cretan Mediterranean Diet, slightly modified with increased intake of α-linolenic acid, was found to be beneficial.[7] In particular, in the Lyon Diet Heart Study[7] it was observed that deaths in patients with acute myocardial infarction were dramatically decreased when patients were on a Cretan Mediterranean Diet, compared with controls who followed a diet recommended by the American Heart Association for the decrease in plasma lipids levels.[8-11] In particular, 605 French volunteers who had survived a first myocardial infarction were randomized into either a control or a Cretan Mediterranean group. After 27 months of follow-up, there were 16 cardiac deaths in the control and only 3 in the Cretan Mediterranean group. In addition, the risk of new major cardiac events was reduced by 73%. In the Mediterranean Diet that French volunteers followed, dietary intake of oleic and α-linolenic acids were increased, whereas dietary saturated fatty acid intake was decreased. In addition, an increase in the consumption of dietary fiber and in the intake of vitamins E and C was also observed.[10]

Although the Mediterranean Diet is characterized by the high consumption of olive oil, fruit, vegetables, and legumes; the moderate consumption of dairy products; and the low consumption of red meat; there is no single widely accepted Mediterranean Diet. Each country of this region has its own adaptations, according to its culture. Therefore, the emphasis in this chapter will be on the Cretan Mediterranean Diet, which was the one mainly discussed in the Seven Countries Study.[1] It will address the effects of the diet's components on morbidity and mortality rates from CHD, as well as on the classical and newly emerging risk factors for this disease.

II. MOLECULAR AND METABOLIC ASPECTS OF CORONARY HEART DISEASE

A. INTRODUCTION

Atherosclerosis is a disease of the tunica intima of large and medium-sized arteries, characterized by the development of fat deposits called plaques or atheromas. It begins in early childhood and, over the years, often leads to a heart attack, stroke, or peripheral vascular disease. These diseases are currently responsible for more than half of all deaths in the U.S., and are the principal causes of death in Europe and Japan. In particular, cardiovascular disease accounts for 44% of mortality in the U.S. and a great proportion of its morbidity.[12] CHD is the most common atherosclerotic disease. In the U.S., CHD is responsible for two thirds of all deaths resulting from heart disease, and 70% of all deaths in people who are older than 75.[12] It is multifactorial in its nature, and the only possibility for its successful prevention and treatment is to take into account all the risk factors responsible for its development.

The pathogenesis of atherosclerosis involves inflammatory infiltration of the vessel wall, cellular proliferation, fibrous plaque formation, and, ultimately, plaque rupture and occlusive thrombosis.[13] The atherosclerotic plaque consists of an outer fibrous cap containing smooth muscle cells, collagen and lipid-rich macrophages, and a necrotic core of cellular debris, cholesterol, and calcium. Arterial fat deposition, and especially cholesterol, which is partly affected by diet, influences the progress of the formation of atherosclerotic plaque. When fat deposition is increased, the artery becomes occluded and normal blood flow is inhibited, which results in decreased oxygen supply to the heart. This inadequate oxygen supply leads to cardiac dystrophy and, possibly, subsequent CHD and myocardial infarction. The formation of the atherosclerotic plaque depends on three processes: endothelial injury, lipid accumulation, and platelet/endothelial interaction.[14]

B. ENDOTHELIAL INJURY

The process of atherogenesis involves the interaction of cells and molecules in an artery and their responses to "assaults" over the years. The cells include smooth muscle cells, platelets, endothelial cells, and monocyte/macrophages; the molecules are the lipoproteins. Current models of atherosclerosis are based on the "endothelial injury" hypothesis. According to this hypothesis, atherosclerosis begins with an injury to the lining of an artery. This injury of the endothelium changes its regulatory functions, leading to an imbalance between relaxing and contracting factors, between procoagulant and anticoagulant mediators, or between growth-inhibiting and growth-promoting factors.[15] Endothelial dysfunction results in attraction of platelets and monocytes, release of growth factors, penetration of sub-endothelium by lipoproteins carrying cholesterol, and smooth muscle cell migration and proliferation. Therefore, a core interest of atherosclerosis research is what causes this initial injury and how it initiates a chain of cellular and molecular reactions that lead (after decades) to the development of CHD.

Initially, it was believed that the initial injury was the loss of endothelium. However, current understanding is that one of the earliest events of atherogenesis is the adhesion of circulating monocytes to the intact surface of endothelium, due to the presence of adhesion molecules. These molecules are expressed on the endothelial surface during an inflammatory response. It has also been shown that high-cholesterol diets lead to the binding of monocytes to the endothelium. The vascular cell adhesion molecule (VCAM) expression preceded the binding of monocytes, and lipids were ultimately responsible for activating the gene for VCAM.

Lesion-prone sites are the branch points of an artery because they are susceptible to alterations in the direction and force of the local blood flow (shear stress) that result in a change of the adhesion molecules expression. Moreover, in areas of low hemodynamic shear stress-sites, the residence time of molecules, including low density lipoproteins (LDL) and cells such as monocytes and platelets, is prolonged. Other factors that can cause injury to the endothelium are smoking and hypertension. However, every day, endothelial injuries occur, but they do not lead to atherosclerosis without lipid deposition in the arterial wall in the presence of elevated LDL levels, and the infiltration of LDL particles in the intima. Therefore, even though the initiating event of endothelial dysfunction is unknown, it is believed that it is related to LDL or their oxidized derivatives.[16]

C. LIPID INFILTRATION AND ACCUMULATION

The arterial intimal monocyte-macrophage recruitment plays an important role in the progress of atherosclerosis and reflects, partly, the inflammatory nature of this disease. Modified LDL, monocytes, macrophages, and smooth muscle cells are involved in the formation of the atherosclerotic plaque through their role in cholesterol deposition on the arterial wall. LDL enters the arterial wall by passing between adjacent endothelial cells. In the intima, the presence of macrophages is crucial in the accumulation of cholesterol and in the production of foam cells.

A possible mechanism that has been proposed as being responsible for the initiation of atherogenesis is as follows:[17]

- Increased circulating LDL leads to an increase in the entry of these lipoprotein particles into the arterial wall, passing through adjacent endothelial cells (cell injury is not necessary).
- Oxidation of LDL occurs in the intima, resulting in recruitment of circulating monocytes through a chemotactic factor present in oxidized LDL.
- Reactive oxygen species or free radicals, which are generated primarily by activated macrophages and secondarily by smooth muscle cells and endothelial cells, oxidatively modify LDL particles. Oxidative modification of LDL includes not only oxidation of fatty acid and phospholipid moiety of this lipoprotein, but also oxidation of its apolipoprotein B-100. As a consequence, oxidized LDL is not recognized by the LDL receptor, but only by the scavenger receptor, which is not down-regulated as the LDL receptor.
- The oxidized LDL pathway leads to uncontrolled entry of cholesterol into macrophages and secondarily to the migrated smooth muscle cells.
- Modification of monocytes to macrophages, uptake of LDL into smooth muscle cells and macrophages (via the LDL receptor) and of oxidized LDL into macrophages via the "scavenger" receptor results in the formation of foam cells (lipid-laden macrophages and smooth muscle cells).
- Break-up of macrophages occurs due to their overloading with cholesteryl esters, with resulting uptake of the released cholesteryl esters by adjacent smooth muscle cells.

- A further loss of endothelial cells also occurs due to cytotoxicity of oxidized LDL.
- Thickening of the atheroma occurs through aggregation of platelets, release of growth factors, and proliferation of smooth muscle cells (Figure 1).

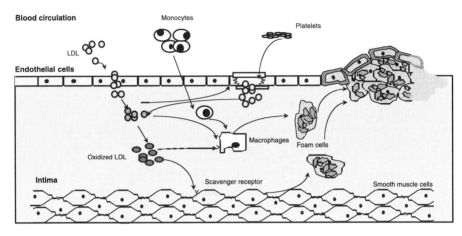

FIGURE 1   The process of atherogenesis.

It has also been suggested[18] that high concentrations of not only LDL, but also very low density lipoprotein (VLDL) particles, and especially their remnants, promote plaque growth and thrombosis through the following mechanisms:

- High concentrations of native LDL have been reported to promote the adhesion of monocytes to the endothelial cell. Oxidized LDL is more potent in this respect, and persistent exposure of the endothelium to such particles can eventually lead to cell injury.
- Activated endothelial cells promote thrombin generation and fibrin production.
- Oxidized LDL activate circulating monocytes when they also acquire procoagulant properties that favor thrombin production.
- Platelets show an increased tendency to aggregate when exposed to hypercholesterolemic plasma. These platelets adhere to activated endothelial cells. Platelets exposed to raised LDL levels also show reduced sensitivity to prostacyclin, an antiaggregatory agent. Oxidized LDL has been reported to stimulate platelet aggregation.
- Platelet aggregation and fibrin deposition at sites of endothelial injury will create microthrombi.
- Lipolysis of triglyceride-rich lipoproteins VLDL and chylomicrons at the endothelial cell surface leads to activation of coagulation mechanism with activation of factor VII, which is a potent procoagulant. In addition, hypertriglyceridemia is associated with an increased plasma concentration

of platelet activator inhibitor 1 (PAI-1) and a reduction in plasma fibrin-olytic activity.

D. ENDOTHELIAL RUPTURE AND THROMBOSIS

Thrombosis could cause sudden occlusion of the coronary artery, and myocardial infarction or sudden death could be the result of thrombus formation. Thrombus formation usually begins at a place where atheromatic plaque has been developed and the majority of acute coronary syndromes result from events such as rupture or disrupture of the atherosclerotic plaque, with intracoronary thrombosis and ischemia of the distal myocardium as a result.[19]

Thrombosis over atherosclerotic plaques is either due to superficial or to deep injury. In superficial injury, there is endothelial denudation with thrombi adherent to the surface of the plaque. In deep injury, major plaque disruption exposes the lipid core to the lumen. Blood enters the core of the plaque, where it is exposed to thrombogenic substances, and thrombus forms within the plaque, expanding its volume rapidly.[20,21]

Certain characteristics of plaques, such as the size and composition of the lipid core, the structure and composition of the fibrous cap and the presence of a local inflammatory process predispose plaque to disruption.[22] However, the risk for plaque rupture depends more on the composition of the plaque than its size. In particular, most of the ruptures occur in plaques containing a soft, lipid-rich core that is covered by a thin, inflamed cap of fibrous tissue.[23] Therefore, major determinants of plaque vulnerability and rupture are progressive lipid accumulation and cap weakening due to ongoing inflammation, with collagen degradation and impaired healing and repair.

E. DIETARY DETERMINANTS OF ATHEROSCLEROSIS AND NEWLY EMERGING RISK FACTORS

Diet plays an important role in the progress of atherogenesis, not only through its effects on lipoprotein levels and LDL oxidation, but also through its influence on the physiological function of the endothelium. Because of its constant exposure to blood components, including pro-oxidants, fats, and their derivatives, the endothe-lium is susceptible to oxidative stress and to injury. It has been suggested that unsaturated fatty acids enhance the formation of reactive oxygen intermediates, which can activate oxidative stress-responsive transcription factors. These factors, in turn, may promote cytokine production, adhesion molecule expression, and, ultimately, endothelial barrier dysfunction.[24] The resulting disturbances of endothe-lial integrity may allow increased penetration of cholesterol-rich lipoprotein rem-nants into the arterial wall.

Recently, emphasis has been put on dietary constituents that could lead to arginine deficiency or hyperhomocysteinemia.[25] Arginine is a key element for the activity of nitric oxide synthase, an enzyme responsible for the synthesis of nitric oxide (NO). NO is a potent vasodilator and an inhibitor of endothelial interactions, and a reduction of NO synthesis or activity may contribute to the progress of atherosclerosis. On the other hand, hyperhomocysteinemia leads to endothelial dysfunction with a loss of endothelium dependent vasodilation and antithrombotic properties, and proliferation of vascular smooth muscle cells, through a mechanism that possibly involves oxidative damage.[26] The observed relationship between poor vitamins B_6, B_{12} and folic acid nutritional status and high plasma homocysteine levels [27,28] probably renders diet a key determinant of the onset of hyperhomocysteinemia.

III. GENETIC PREDISPOSITION OF CORONARY HEART DISEASE AND THE ROLE OF GENE–DIET INTERACTIONS.

A. INTRODUCTION

The incidence and prevalence of CHD vary among individuals, families, and nations. Genetic predisposition, diet, and other environmental factors contribute to variations in both the incidence and prevalence of the disease.[29,30] Over the past two decades, evidence has accumulated to demonstrate that susceptibility to CHD is, to a great extent, genetically determined. It is now well established that several risk factors or protective factors with respect to cardiovascular diseases are strongly influenced by genes.[31-33] Hyperlipidemia and hypertension, for example, which are powerful and independent predictors of CHD, have strong genetic determinants. Scientists estimate that genetics explains roughly 50% of the variance in serum cholesterol concentrations[34] and 30–60% of variance in blood pressure levels.[35] In addition to the above, diabetes and obesity, which themselves are important risk factors for CHD, have also a genetic component.[36,37] Several major gene defects causing hyperlipidemia in humans, such as familial hypercholesterolemia with defective LDL receptors, have long been well characterized.[38] Most of these defects, however, are not common enough and account for a small percentage of CHD in the population. In recent years, advances in molecular genetics have enabled researchers to identify many genes and their variants or polymorphisms contributing to cardiovascular risk (particularly genes involved in lipid metabolism, as well as genes involved in hemostasis, coagulation, and hypertension). These findings have added support to the concept of CHD as a polygenic disease, and that environmental factors— diet being a factor of major importance — act on this genetic background.

B. APOLIPOPROTEIN E AND CHOLESTERYL ESTER TRANSFER PROTEIN

Among recent genetic discoveries, the gene coding for apolipoprotein E has been extensively studied, explaining a portion of the genetically determined risk of atherosclerosis and CHD. Apolipoprotein E (apoE) is a normal constituent of the triglyceride-rich lipoproteins and high density lipoproteins (HDL), on which it serves as a ligand for the uptake by lipoprotein receptors. It also plays a crucial role in transport and redistribution of lipids among lipoproteins.[39] Genetic variation at the apoE gene locus results from three common alleles in the population (ε3, ε2, and ε4), which code for three protein isoforms: the predominant E3 isoform and its mutant variants, E2 and E4.[40,41] Sing and Davignon[42] have reported that as much as 16% of the total variation in LDL cholesterol levels in the normal population can be attributed to the common apoE polymorphism. In most human populations, it has been found that individuals carrying the apoE4 isoform have higher plasma total and LDL cholesterol levels than those with the apoE3 isoform, whereas those with the apoE2 isoform show the opposite.[43-45] According to a meta-analysis, plasma triglycerides and HDL cholesterol levels are also modulated by apoE genotype, apoE4 carriers being associated with higher triglyceride and lower HDL cholesterol levels than apoE3/3 homozygotes.[45] As elevated levels of LDL cholesterol and low levels of HDL cholesterol predispose toward atherosclerosis, the ε4 allele may confer an increased risk for CHD. Indeed, the presence of the ε4 allele is now considered to be the most common genetic abnormality in atherosclerosis and has been demonstrated to be an important risk factor for heart disease in a number of human populations.[46-53] Several studies have shown a higher incidence and prevalence of cardiovascular disease in subjects carrying the ε4 allele than in noncarriers.[46-53] In one autopsy study involving young individuals who died of external causes, apoE4 carriers were shown to exhibit more atherosclerotic changes in vessel walls than those with other apoE phenotypes.[47] Stengard et al.[52] provided convincing evidence that carrying an apoE4 allele confers an individual's risk for future development of fatal myocardial infarction. After a 5-year follow-up of presymptomatic elderly Finnish men, the apoE4 frequency was significantly higher in men who had died because of fatal myocardial infarction than in the surviving men. The role of the ε4 allele as a risk factor is also reflected by its selective loss from aged populations, such as Finnish nonagenarians[54] and centenarians.[55]

The frequencies of apoE2, E3, and E4 in the Caucasian population is approximately 8%, 77%, and 15%, respectively.[43] Significant differences have been observed in ε4 allele frequencies among European populations, with northern countries exhibiting higher frequencies (24.4% in Finland,[56] 20.3% in Sweden[57]) than southern countries (9.4% in Italy,[58] 6.5% in Greece[59]). This suggests that the ε4 allele may, in part, account for the differences in cardiovascular disease prevalence in the two European regions, and exactly this was demonstrated by the European Atherosclerosis Research Study (EARS),[51] a multicenter study carried out in 11 European countries, showing that regions with a high apoE4 frequency present with an increased incidence of CHD.

Although the average effect of the apoE4 allele is to increase the cholesterol level in populations, this effect is clearer in populations consuming diets rich in saturated fat and cholesterol than in other populations,[56,60-62] which indicates that the influence of apoE genetic variation on plasma lipid levels is not independent of environmental and ethnic factors. It has been suggested that the higher LDL cholesterol levels observed in subjects carrying the apoE4 isoform are manifested primarily in the presence of an atherogenic diet characteristic of certain societies, and that the response to dietary fat and cholesterol may differ among individuals with different apoE phenotypes. On this basis, several investigations[63-75] have focused on the interaction between lipoprotein responsiveness to dietary manipulation and apoE genetic polymorphism. Some studies involving changes in dietary cholesterol intake, or changes in both cholesterol and fat intake, have reported greater plasma lipid responses in individuals carrying the apoE4 allele.[63-69] However, others have failed to do so.[70-75] Despite some inconsistency, an overall significant apoE gene–diet interaction has been reported in studies with men alone, which suggests a significant gene–gender interaction. A recent meta-analysis of data from nine published studies supports the concept that the apoE4 allele is associated with an increased cholesterol response to dietary manipulation, and that male subjects carrying the apoE4 allele are the most responsive to diets restricted in saturated fat and cholesterol.[69] In the study by Cobb et al.,[68] women of the apoE3/2 phenotype were shown to benefit the least from a high polyunsaturate:saturate diet because of reduction in the more "protective" HDL cholesterol, whereas men of the Apo4/3 phenotype showed the greatest improvement in the LDL:HDL ratio. Therefore, a general recommendation to increase the polyunsaturated content of the diet to reduce cholesterol level and the risk for CHD may be appropriate for men carrying the apoE4 allele but not for women with the apoE3/2 phenotype. Other studies using dietary manipulation, including type of carbohydrates and fiber rather than type and amount of dietary fat and cholesterol, resulted in apoE gene–diet interactions in which apoE3/3 homozygotes and apoE2 carriers were more responsive to these dietary modifications than apoE4 subjects.[76,77] More recently, Loktionov et al.[78] reported that tea drinking has a beneficial effect on plasma lipid levels and coagulation factors, especially in subjects carrying the apoE2 allele. These results clearly show the genetic effects on plasma lipid responses to dietary change.

Apart from the apoE gene, polymorphisms in a number of other apo-genes (e.g., apoB, apoA-IV, apoA-I) and lipid related enzymes (lipoprotein lipase-LPL, cholesteryl ester transfer protein-CETP) have also been implicated in the genetic regulation of dietary response.[79-81] Thus, specific genetic information is needed to define the optimal diet for an individual.

Another well known lipid-related risk factor for atherosclerosis and CHD is HDL. Epidemiologic studies have shown a strong inverse correlation between plasma levels of HDL cholesterol and the incidence of CHD.[82] One of the factors influencing HDL levels is plasma CETP. CETP facilitates the exchange of neutral lipids among plasma lipoproteins and induces a transfer of cholesteryl esters from the core of HDL particles to triglyceride-rich lipoproteins in exchange for triglycerides.[83] Recent data show that an increased transfer of cholesteryl esters from HDL to VLDL and LDL may characterize patients with established coronary artery disease.[84] An increased CETP activity leading to a reduction in the cholesterol content of HDL relative to VLDL and LDL could contribute to an increased risk of CHD.

Recently, a number of polymorphisms and rare variants in the human CETP gene have been identified,[85,86] some of which have been implicated in determining the levels and activity of CETP, apoAI, and HDL plasma concentrations, as well as the risk of developing CHD.[86-94] One common polymorphism is a variable *Taq*I site in the first intron of the CETP gene (CETP/*Taq*IB), which has been consistently associated with plasma HDL cholesterol levels, individuals carrying the less frequent B2 allele (absence of cutting site) having the highest levels of HDL cholesterol.[86-94]

Previous studies have confirmed a protective role of moderate alcohol intake on the incidence of CHD and on angiographic disease severity, as well as a positive association between alcohol consumption and HDL levels. Because this association may, in part, be mediated by the effects of alcohol on CETP activity, a possible interaction between the CETP/*Taq*IB polymorphism and alcohol consumption on plasma HDL cholesterol and the risk of myocardial infarction has been investigated by Fumeron et al.,[95] as part of the ECTIM study (a case-control study designed to identify genetic variants associated with myocardial infarction[33]). Very interestingly, these researchers found that the B2 allele was strongly positively associated with plasma HDL cholesterol only in alcohol drinkers ($\leq$ 25 g/day) and that the cardio-protective effect of the B2B2 genotype was restricted to subjects who consumed the highest amounts of alcohol.[94] These results provided strong evidence of a gene–diet interaction affecting HDL-C levels and the risk of CHD.

C. Lipoprotein(a) and Low Density Lipoprotein Subclass Patterns

High levels of lipoprotein(a), or Lp(a), is another genetically determined disorder that has been positively associated with atherosclerosis and the risk of CHD.[96-100] Lp(a) is a lipoprotein particle consisting of an LDL molecule in which the apolipo-protein apoB100 is linked to another large protein, apo(a), that has structural homol-ogy with plasminogen, hence with possible negative influence in fibrinolysis. The gene coding for apo(a) is highly polymorphic, each allele determining a specific number of multiple tandem repeats of a unique coding sequence known as Kringle IV. The number of these repeats correlates with the size of the Lp(a) protein. The smaller the protein, the higher the Lp(a) levels, and thus the higher the risk for heart disease.[101]

In the last 15 years, a plasma lipoprotein profile characterized by the predomi-nance of small, dense LDL particles has been described (LDL subclass pattern B); it is associated with increased levels of triglycerides and reduced levels of HDL.[102,103] The features of this metabolic trait are associated with up to a threefold increased risk for CHD. This has been demonstrated in case-control studies of myocardial infarction and of angiographically documented coronary disease.[104-107] Moreover, increased levels of small, dense LDL have been found in a majority of the familial disorders commonly associated with a risk of premature CHD in the general popu-lation, consistent with the genetic influences underlying this trait.[103]

Family studies have indicated that pattern B is under the influence of one or more major genes with genetic linkage to the region of the LDL-receptor locus and several other loci in other chromosomes.[108-110] However, estimates of heritability of LDL particle size have ranged from approximately 30 to 50%,[111] indicating the important role of nongenetic factors in influencing the expression of this trait. Variation in dietary fat and carbohydrate has been shown to strongly influence the expression of the small, dense LDL phenotype, and contribute to variations in LDL particle size distribution observed among individuals and population groups.[103] In a large dietary study[112] contrasting the effects of a high- (46%) and a low-fat (23%) diet, male subjects with LDL subclass B on the high-fat diet exhibited a twofold greater reduction in LDL cholesterol than the majority of healthy subjects without this trait (LDL subclass pattern A). Only pattern B subjects showed significant reductions in plasma apoB, and in LDL relative to HDL cholesterol levels.[112] Fur-thermore, almost half of the individuals with LDL pattern A were shown to exhibit the more atherogenic pattern B following intake of the low-fat diet.[113] Taken together, these results indicate that lowering the dietary fat intake may preferentially benefit individuals with the small-LDL trait. These findings further support the concept that the efficacy of CHD risk reduction in the general population may be improved by the application of individualized dietary guidelines.

D. HOMOCYSTEINE AND FIBRINOGEN

Among the risk factors of CHD that are not related to lipids are high homocysteine concentrations and elevated plasma fibrinogen levels. Both factors have recently been shown to have genetic determinants.

Homocysteine is a normal amino acid that, when elevated in the blood, promotes clotting everywhere. The independent association of high homocysteine concentrations with all forms of premature vascular disease has previously been confirmed.[114] Although the underlying mechanism is probably multifactorial and not yet fully elucidated, platelet activation and a prothrombotic modification in several factors in the coagulation cascade have been described.[115] High levels of homocysteine have been correlated with an increased frequency of heart attacks.[116] Homocysteine levels can be high when there is a deficiency of vitamin B_6, B_{12}, or folate. Selhub et al.[117] reported that more than 60% of patients with atherosclerosis and elevated homocysteine levels were deficient in these essential vitamins. During the last 10 years, a specific thermolabile variant of the folate related enzyme 5,10-methylenetetrahydrofolate reductase, which causes partial enzyme deficiency, has been described in 5–15% of normal populations.[118-121] This variant (mutation 677C→T) causes mild hyperhomocysteinemia and is positively associated with coronary artery disease.[119,122-124]

Increased plasma fibrinogen levels have also been identified as a risk indicator for myocardial infarction, stroke, and thrombosis.[125-126] Fibrinogen is a major component of the coagulation system. Upon the action of thrombin, fibrinogen is converted into fibrin monomers, which, in turn, polymerize into a fibrin network, leading to the formation of a blood clot. In a review on the epidemiological evidence relating fibrinogen to CHD, Ernst and Resh[127] concluded that high fibrinogen levels are an independent predictor of cardiovascular disease, with a 2.3-fold increase in risk, and a markedly enhanced cholesterol-related risk. These data were confirmed in a recent study that showed that, among patients with angina pectoris, those with low plasma fibrinogen concentration were at low risk for subsequent coronary syndromes, despite increased cholesterol levels.[128]

Both environmental and genetic factors make an important contribution to plasma fibrinogen levels in humans. Cigarette smoking, for example, has a strong influence on fibrinogen levels, smokers and ex-smokers exhibiting higher levels than non-smokers.[129,130] Studies have shown that between 15 and 50% of the variance in fibrinogen levels is genetically determined.[131,132] Fifteen percent of the variance was found in the UK,[131] while 50% is the figure among the Hawaiian population,[132] indicating significant differences between populations. Fibrinogen is composed of three pairs of nonidentical polypeptide chains that are encoded by different genes (denoted α, β, and γ).[133] The β chain appears to play a limiting role on the production of the other components of fibrinogen. Several polymorphisms of the β-fibrinogen gene have been characterized, some of which have been independently associated with plasma fibrinogen levels, as well as with the presence or severity of coronary and peripheral atherosclerosis.[134-138] One such, a β HaeIII polymorphism located in the promoter region of the gene, was found to be strongly and independently associated with plasma fibrinogen levels, this association being significant in smokers but not in non-smokers.[138] Very recently, de Maat et al.[139] reported that an A for G nucleotide substitution, 455 nucleotides upstream from the transcription start site of the β-fibrinogen gene, is positively related to the progression of coronary atherosclerosis in symptomatic men. In this study, patients carrying the –455A allele had higher mean plasma fibrinogen levels at baseline than patients with the –455GG genotype. After a 2-year follow up period, those of the –455AA genotype had more progression of coronary artery disease, as expressed by a significantly greater change in some angiographic variables. The authors hypothesized[139] that the –455A allele may promote a stronger acute-face response in fibrinogen and that the resulting higher fibrinogen levels may form the pathogenetic basis for the stronger progression of coronary atherosclerosis.

Recently, a particular polymorphism (PIA2) of the gene encoding for the IIIa-moeity of the platelet glycoprotein IIb/IIIa, which functions as a receptor for fibrinogen and von Willebrand factor, and is known to be involved in the pathogenesis of acute coronary syndromes, was shown to be associated with high risk of coronary thrombosis (6:1 in subjects who had experienced a coronary event before the age of 60 years).[140] More recently, a strong association between the PIA2 allele and the severity of CHD has been found among a group of low-risk male individuals[141] referred for angiography. These findings disclose new opportunities for identifying subjects at risk of CHD.

E. ANGIOTENSIN-CONVERTING ENZYME (ACE)

Genetic variability in the renin-angiotensin system has also been associated with the risk of CHD. Among the important components of the renin-angiotensin system is the ACE, which plays a key role in the production of angiotensin II and in the catabolism of bradykinin, two peptides involved in the modulation of vascular tone and in the proliferation of smooth muscle cells. Plasma ACE levels are strongly genetically determined.[142,143] The ACE gene is polymorphic, as a consequence of a frequent insertion(I)/deletion(D) polymorphism, due to the presence/absence of a 287bp fragment in the 16th intron of the gene.[142] The D/D genotype is associated with higher levels of circulating ACE than I/D and I/I genotypes.[143] In a study comparing patients after myocardial infarction with controls, Cambien et al.[144] explored a possible association between the ACE I/D polymorphism and CHD. They found that the DD genotype was significantly more frequent in patients with myocardial infarction than in controls, especially in a group of low-risk subjects defined by absence of hyperlipidemia and obesity. In another study, these researchers reported a higher frequency of the D allele among those subjects having a parental history of fatal myocardial infarction.[145] Recent data indicate that the increased risk of myocardial infarction in the presence of the ACE D allele is not a consequence of more-severe atherosclerosis, but may be due to plaque rupture or to vasoconstriction of coronary arteries.[33] Interestingly, the ACE D allele and another common variant of the angiotensin II type 1 receptor (AT1R) gene was found to have a strong synergistic effect on the risk of myocardial infarction,[33,146] which indicates an important gene–gene interaction in the determination of the risk of CHD.

F. Conclusion

Considerable research indicates that genetics is a predominant factor in determining an individual's risk of CHD. Some indicative studies have been discussed here. While, in most cases, the quantitative effects of the genetic variants are small, it is expected that discovery of additional genetically influenced factors as well as genes and variants involved in the development of CHD will improve our understanding of the etiology and mechanisms of this disease. Genetics also influences response to diet. Support has been building up for the concept that dietary guidelines to decrease chronic diseases, such as CHD, must consider genetic variability. Furthermore, genetic variation and ethnic differences need to be taken into consideration in the determination of nutritional requirements. In the future, simultaneous analysis of several predisposing alleles should provide the means to identify individuals at high risk and to characterize groups in which specific dietary interventions would be most effective. A joint interdisciplinary effort of geneticists and nutritionists is needed for the identification of individuals susceptible to chronic diseases and for nutritional intervention early in life.[147]

IV. EFFECTS OF THE MEDITERRANEAN DIET ON THE DEVELOPMENT OF CORONARY HEART DISEASE

A. Olive Oil

1. Introduction

In the Cretan Mediterranean Diet, as it was described in the early 1960s, fat intake accounts for 40% of the total energy intake.[1] However, 30 years ago, morbidity and mortality rates from cardiovascular disease and atherosclerosis were very low in the Cretan population, in comparison with the populations in other countries such as Finland and the Netherlands, despite the similar levels of dietary fat intake. It was then observed that the main difference in the dietary habits between the Cretans and the northern Europeans was not in the total fat intake, but in the fatty acid composition of their diet. In particular, in the traditional Cretan diet, the main source of fat was olive oil, a vegetable oil rich in monounsaturated fatty acids and especially oleic acid. Olive oil was found to have beneficial properties in the prevention of cardiovascular diseases because it reduces the rate of the atherosclerotic plaque development and also influences thrombus formation.

2. Olive Oil and Plasma Lipid Levels

Recent research suggests that the beneficial effects of olive oil on plasma lipid metabolism are partly due to its containing monounsaturated fatty acids. The main monounsaturated fatty acid in olive oil is oleic acid, which has hypocholesterolemic properties, compared with saturated fatty acids. It is already widely known that saturated fatty acids, which are present in foods of animal origin, increase blood cholesterol levels, whereas polyunsaturated fatty acids, which are present in foods of vegetable origin, decrease them. The main saturated fatty acids that have this increasing effect on plasma cholesterol levels are lauric, myristic, and palmitic acids. The latter is present in greater proportions in the habitual diets of Americans and Northern Europeans.

In a study[148] that compared the effects of saturated, monounsaturated, and poly-unsaturated fatty acids on plasma lipid levels, it was observed that monounsaturated fatty acids decreased LDL cholesterol levels to the same extent as polyunsaturated fatty acids, when compared with saturated fatty acids. However, monounsaturated fatty acids had an additional beneficial effect: They decreased HDL cholesterol levels less often than polyunsaturated fatty acids. More recently, an intervention study[149] on volunteers with family histories of CHD revealed that a diet rich in monounsat-urated fatty acids decreased plasma cholesterol and LDL cholesterol levels, and, therefore, improved the lipid profile of these volunteers, compared with a diet rich in saturated fatty acids. In the same study, it was also observed that HDL cholesterol levels were not altered, and, moreover, the LDL cholesterol: HDL cholesterol ratio was decreased.

In another study,[150] volunteers were put on diets rich in monounsaturated or polyunsaturated fatty acids, and their plasma lipid levels were compared after fol-lowing diets rich in saturated fatty acids. It was observed that the diet that was rich in monounsaturated fatty acids decreased LDL cholesterol levels by 17.9%, whereas the polyunsaturated fatty-acid-rich diet decreased LDL cholesterol levels by only 12%. The influence on HDL cholesterol levels was similar in both diets, but a small reduction was observed in males but not in females. The researchers were led to the conclusion that, with respect to plasma cholesterol levels, monounsaturated fatty-acid-rich diets are as beneficial as polyunsaturated fatty-acid-rich diets. It is, how-ever, noticeable that, in this study, oleic acid was found to be more beneficial than linoleic acid (the main polyunsaturated fatty acid in westernized societies' habitual diets) in the lowering effect on LDL cholesterol levels.

Oleic acid is probably oxidized to a different degree than saturated fat. In a recent study,[151] stable isotope tracer methodologies, in combination with indirect calorimetry, were used to determine the oxidation of dietary fat in subjects fed a monounsaturated-fat and a saturated-fat diet. The results from this study suggested that fatty acid composition of the background diet may influence the relative proportion of fat oxi-dation that is attributed to exogenous (i.e., dietary) and endogenous fat oxidation. It was reported that even a relatively small increase in saturated-fat content of a diet, compared with monounsaturated-fat, can decrease exogenous fat oxidation.

Olive oil also has beneficial properties, when compared with dietary carbohy-drates. In particular, when a diet rich in complex carbohydrates was compared with a monounsaturated fatty-acid-rich diet, the volunteer's lipid profile was improved following the latter. This was due to the fact that, on the one hand, the high-complex-carbohydrate diet decreased plasma LDL cholesterol levels but, on the other, it also decreased plasma HDL cholesterol levels.[152] Apart from the adverse effect of high carbohydrate diets on HDL cholesterol levels, it was also observed that they stimulated fatty synthesis and accumulation of palmitate-enriched, linoleate-deficient triglycerides in plasma compared with low fat diets.[153]

In conclusion, since high plasma HDL cholesterol and low LDL cholesterol levels are equally important for the prevention of CHD, olive oil is probably more beneficial than other vegetable oils, which are rich in polyunsaturated fatty acids, as well as foods rich in carbohydrates. The main reason for this beneficial effect of olive oil is its monounsaturated fatty acids content, which not only leads to a decrease in LDL cholesterol, but also to a probable increase in HDL cholesterol levels when compared with polyunsaturated fatty acids,[148] and carbohydrates.[152,154]

3. Olive Oil and LDL Oxidation

Olive oil has beneficial effects against LDL oxidation. The susceptibility of LDL to oxidation depends on the presence of unsaturated fatty acids and antioxidants in its molecule. It has been observed that polyunsaturated fatty acids increase LDL oxidation, compared with monounsaturated fatty acids.[155,156] In particular, several studies have been carried out looking at the effects of LDL oxidation on diets different in fatty acid composition. In the Jerusalem Study,[157] it was observed that a polyunsaturated fatty-acid-rich diet led to increased LDL oxidation compared with a monounsaturated fat-rich diet. In addition, in volunteers with mildly elevated plasma cholesterol levels, LDL was less susceptible to lipid peroxidation following a diet rich in monounsaturated than a diet rich in polyunsaturated fatty acids.[158]

Another factor that influences LDL oxidation is the presence of antioxidants such as vitamin E and polyphenols. Olive oil composition is unique in this respect, because, not only is it rich in monounsaturated fatty acids, which have increased resistance to oxidation, but it is also rich in vitamin E (approximately 12 mg/100 g) and phenolic compounds, such as flavonoids, which decrease even further the susceptibility of LDL to oxidation. It has already been observed that an increase in vitamin E levels in blood circulation decreases the risk for developing CHD.[159] The daily vitamin E and other antioxidant requirements seem now to be dependent on the degree of unsaturation of dietary fatty acids and their concentration in blood circulation. LDL, formed following a diet rich in monounsaturated fatty acids, tends to be resistant to lipid peroxidation.[160,161] Even though the extent by which the balance between dietary antioxidants and the degree of fatty acid unsaturation influences the risk for developing CHD is still unknown, the high concentration of vitamin E and the predominance of monounsaturated fatty acids in olive oil seem to contribute to the low prevalence of CHD that is observed in certain Mediterranean countries.

Another antioxidant that is present in increased concentration in olive oil is squalene (136–708 mg/100 g). Beneficial effects of squalene include the inhibition of the development of atherosclerosis. In general, the actions of phenols present in olive oil and contributing to its beneficial effects also include the inhibition of LDL oxidation.[162]

4. Anti-Thrombotic Properties

In addition to its anti-atherogenic properties, through the reduction of LDL cholesterol and the increase in HDL cholesterol levels, as well as the decrease in the susceptibility of LDL to oxidation, olive oil also has anti-thrombotic properties. In a recent study, it was found that a diet rich in monounsaturated fatty acids coming from olive oil reduced plasma factor VII levels, especially following the consumption of a meal, which suggests that the rate of blood clotting is reduced and, as a consequence, so is the risk for thrombogenesis.[163] Another study compared the effects of a diet rich in monounsaturated fatty acids on plasminogen activating inhibitor-1 (PAI-1) levels with the effects of a low-fat diet on the same parameter.[164] PAI-1 inactivates the function of endogenous plasminogen activator in the tissues, which leads to thrombus breakdown and, as a consequence, PAI-1 increases the risk for developing thrombosis. This study indicated that a diet rich in monounsaturated fatty acids decreased plasma PAI-1 levels and, as a result, the risk for thrombogenesis. Another study indicated that oleic acid, the main fatty acid of olive oil, decreases plasma factor VII and PAI-1 levels, compared with palmitic acid.[165] However, after comparing the response to a low-fat meal with a high-fat meal, the latter increased plasma factor VII levels, regardless of the fatty acid composition of the meal.[166]

We can therefore conclude that olive oil has beneficial effects on plasma lipid metabolism. The effects include decrease of LDL cholesterol and probable increase in HDL cholesterol levels. Apart from its effects on plasma lipid levels, olive oil, with its unique fatty acid composition and its high concentration in antioxidants, decreases LDL oxidation, rendering these lipoprotein particles less atherogenic. Finally, olive oil protects against thrombogenesis through the reduction in several plasma-clotting-factor levels.

B. Fruits, Vegetables, and Legumes

1. Introduction

Major constituents of the traditional Mediterranean Diet are fruits, vegetables, and legumes,[167,168] which also contribute to the low rates of CHD exhibited in the countries of this region. Several studies have reported a correlation between increased fruit, vegetable, and fiber consumption, and decreased incidence of CHD. A significant protective association of fruit and vegetable consumption against the development of CHD has been reported.[169] In Albania, in areas with high dietary intake of olive oil, fruit, and vegetables, the incidence of CHD was lower than the country's already low overall rate.[170]

It is noteworthy that, in people with habitual low intake of fruit and vegetables (≤ 3 servings daily) an increase of the daily intake to eight servings per day, which is similar to the intake in the Mediterranean countries, resulted in an increase in vitamin C, α-carotene, and β-carotene levels but the levels of α-tocopherol, lipids, and lipoproteins remained unchanged.[171] However, in this study, the levels of folic acid, pre- and post-intervention, were not measured.

In another study,[172] after 2 weeks on a fruit and vegetable diet (25% fat as energy), lipid risk factors (LDL cholesterol, total cholesterol:HDL cholesterol ratio, apoB:apoA-1 ratio, Lp(a)) were significantly reduced in 10 healthy volunteers. However, this diet was not similar to the traditional Mediterranean Diet since it was low in total fat intake. In another study,[173] PAI-1 activity was found to be lower in subjects who were high consumers of fruit and vegetables, indicating beneficial effects of their consumption on the fibrinolytic system, and thus a reduced risk of thromboembolic events.

The evidence supporting an inverse correlation between CHD and increased fruit and vegetable consumption comes mainly from studies that examined the effects of dietary fiber and antioxidant vitamins on risk factors for developing CHD. However, in a study that investigated the effect of fruits and vegetables on mortality and reinfarction, a decrease in cardiac end points was observed in 204 patients with acute myocardial infarction who were on a high fruit and vegetable diet for 12 weeks, compared with controls.[174] Moreover, a decrease in total mortality, including cardiac mortality, was also reported.

Legumes are a good source of dietary fiber. The high soluble-fiber content of peas and beans has been reported to decrease plasma cholesterol levels.[175] However, there are little data from epidemiologic and metabolic studies that could support conclusive evidence on the effects of legumes on CHD risk,[176] and further research is necessary.

As has already been mentioned, major constituents of fruits, vegetables, and legumes with protective effects on atherogenesis are dietary fiber and antioxidant vitamins. However, more recently, scientific interest has also emerged to examine the effects of non-nutrients and folic acid on CHD risk.

2. Dietary Fiber

It has been suggested that there is an inverse relationship between high dietary fiber consumption and CHD.[177,178] In subjects with dietary fiber intake of 16 g/24 hours or more, it was observed that the relative risk for ischemic heart disease mortality was 0.33 in men and 0.37 in women when compared with those with a daily intake of less than 16 g.[177] This effect was found to be independent of other dietary variables such as energy, fat, cholesterol, protein, carbohydrate, alcohol, calcium, and potassium. In another study,[178] it was reported that the relative risk for total myocardial infarction was 0.59 among men in the highest quintile of total dietary fiber intake (median 28.9 g/day) when compared with men in the lowest quintile (median 12.4 g/day). It was also noted that for this cohort (43,757 U.S. male health professionals), within the three main food contributors to total fiber intake (fruit, vegetables, and cereal), cereal fiber was most strongly associated with a reduced risk of total myocardial infarction.

The composition of dietary fiber ranges from insoluble substances, including cellulose, to water-soluble pectin, gels, and gums. The function of these two forms of fiber differ. In particular, insoluble dietary fiber is not absorbed in the small intestine and reaches the colon, where it is fermented to various degrees by resident bacteria. On the other hand, the main function of soluble dietary fiber occurs in the small intestine, where it interacts with the digestion and absorption of other nutrients. The main effect of insoluble dietary fiber is the prevention of constipation, but it is the soluble fiber that is correlated with decreased plasma cholesterol levels. In general, plant foods and wheat bran are good sources of insoluble fiber, whereas dried beans, oat products, and fruits and vegetables are good sources of soluble fiber.[179]

Pectin was the first type of soluble dietary fiber reported to lower plasma cholesterol levels.[180] Pectin constitutes approximately 1% of the net weight of fruits and vegetables,[181] and it has been suggested that one of the mechanisms of its hypocholesterolemic effect is the decrease of bile acid reabsorption in the ileum.[182] Another possible mechanism is the increase in volatile fatty acids from pectin fermentation in the large intestine, which then are absorbed in the portal vein and possibly suppress cholesterol synthesis in the liver.[183]

Oat bran also decreases plasma cholesterol levels but its effect is small and can be masked by other influences that affect the variability of plasma cholesterol.[183] However, its main effect is on total- and LDL- and not on HDL-cholesterol.

Another soluble fiber that lowers plasma cholesterol levels is guar gum. Guar gum is used as a thickening agent and is a natural product from the leguminous plant *Cyamopsis tetragonoloba*. Apart from its hypocholesterolemic effects, guar gum also lowers plasma glucose response to a meal and it can be useful in the treatment of diabetes. However, it is viscous and unpalatable and has to be taken with meals.[184]

It must be mentioned that it is very difficult to isolate the effects of dietary fiber on CHD risk factors from the effects of other nutrients in high-fiber diets. In particular, fiber-rich foods contain phytochemicals and antioxidants and some are good sources of complex carbohydrates.[185] Therefore, the effects of these nutrients should also be considered when assessing the benefits of foods rich in dietary fiber.

3. Antioxidants

Several observational and metabolic studies have been carried out looking at the effects of antioxidants, and, in particular, vitamins C and E as well as carotenoids and polyphenols, on risk factors for developing CHD. Cross-cultural, prospective, and interventional studies suggest that α-tocopherol, the most active form of vitamin E, could act synergistically with vitamin C against LDL oxidation.

In the Seven Countries Study,[186] associations between the intake of food groups and 25-year mortality from CHD were investigated. Eighteen different food groups and combinations were considered for comparison and it was observed that vegetable food groups (except potatoes) were inversely correlated with CHD mortality.

A large cross-cultural study,[187] which was part of the WHO/MONICA Project (initiated as the International Collaborative Study on the Fatty Acid Antioxidant Hypothesis of Atherosclerosis) investigated 12 populations with "common" plasma cholesterol (220–240 mg/dl) and blood pressure. Both classical risk factors lacked significant correlations to ischemic heart disease, whereas absolute levels of α-tocopherol showed a strong inverse correlation. In addition, a synergism between vitamins E and C was also suggested.

In the Established Populations for Epidemiologic Studies of the Elderly,[188] 11,178 subjects between 67 and 105 years of age participated. It was observed that the use of vitamin E supplements reduced all-cause mortality, and the effects were even stronger for CHD mortality. Simultaneous use of vitamins E and C was associated with an even lower risk of total mortality and CHD mortality. The results of this study suggest that vitamin E supplements can be protective in the elderly.

However, the dose was unknown since the supplements users in this study were defined as subjects who reported individual vitamin E or vitamin C use.

In the U.S. Male Health Professionals Study,[189] 39,910 subjects completed detailed dietary questionnaires that assessed their vitamin C, carotene, and vitamin E intake. In this study, an inverse correlation was observed between vitamin E intake and CHD risk. Carotene intake was also associated with a lower risk of CHD, but this protective effect was limited only to smokers. On the other hand, vitamin C was not associated with a lower risk of CHD. The investigators concluded that the data from this study did not prove a causal relation, but provided evidence on the association between high intakes of vitamin E and lower risk for CHD. Similar are the results from the Nurses Health Study.[190] A protective effect of vitamin E was observed, but only in subjects who were on supplements for more than 2 years. In contrast, the Cambridge Heart Antioxidant Study[191] (CHAOS) investigated the effects of vitamin E supplementation (400–800 IU of vitamin E per day) in 2,000 patients with angiographically proven coronary atherosclerosis. The supplementation resulted in fewer non-fatal myocardial infarctions (14 vs. 41 $p < 0.0001$) but an adverse trend towards more cardiovascular deaths was also reported. However, the results of the study were limited by the small sample size of the trial and it was terminated prematurely.

The antioxidant hypothesis has been questioned recently by Elinder and Walldius.[192] In their review, they reported conflicting evidence on the atherogenicity of oxidized LDL and the antioxidant potential, mainly of vitamin E. In particular, several studies have reported that: (a) LDL extracted from human atherosclerotic aortic intima showed only modest signs of oxidation, less than required for scavenger receptor uptake, (b) oxidation resistance may be related to LDL particle size and not to its content of vitamin E and polyunsaturated fatty acids, and (c) in white rabbits, a high dose of vitamin E impaired vasodilator function and stimulated smooth muscle cell proliferation, despite reducing LDL oxidation *in vitro*. The authors suggested that vitamin E has other effects on cellular functions that may reduce the risk of CHD, as (a) the inhibition of interleukin-1 secretion from monocytes, which is involved in smooth muscle cell proliferation and monocyte differentiation, by inhibiting protein kinase C, (b) the reduction of platelet reactivity, (c) the maintenance of endothelial membrane integrity, and (d) the modulation of the release of prostacyclin.

It has also been reported that, to achieve some potential preventive effect of vitamin E against the development of CHD, plasma levels should be > 10.8 mg/dl (25 μM), representing daily vitamin E intake of 30 IU. However, after taking into account the present recommendations for increasing dietary polyunsaturated fatty acid intake, a more likely prudent dose of vitamin E should be at a range of 60–100 IU.[193] However, since the traditional Cretan Mediterranean Diet was poor in polyunsaturated fatty acids, the daily intake of vitamin E was not needed to be as high. Moreover, if the dietary fat is reduced to provide 25% of energy, as some recommend, the actual intake of vitamin E could be as low as 15 IU, which can be considered deficient.

Vitamin C and carotenoids are not as potent antioxidants as vitamin E. As has already been indicated, vitamin C could act synergistically with vitamin E to protect

LDL from the attack of free radicals. Citrus fruit supplementation, rich in vitamin C, was found to decrease *in vitro* the susceptibility of lipoproteins to oxidation, although vitamin E concentration remained unchanged.[194] In contrast, a daily intake of 500 mg of vitamin C for 6 weeks has also been reported to cause DNA damage through some pro-oxidant action.[195] However, these are high doses that can be ingested only with the use of supplements. In the U.S. Health Professionals Study, the effects of β-carotene supplementation were also investigated.[196] After 12 years of follow-up, no difference in cardiovascular disease was observed between the placebo and the treatment groups.

Another group of antioxidants present in fruits and vegetables is the flavonoids. Flavonoids are polyphenols that occur in foods of plant origin. Variation in the heterocyclic ring C forms flavonols, flavones, catechins, flavanones, anthocyanidins, and isoflavonoids.[197] A major component of vegetables is the antioxidant quercetin, which is a polyphenol. Tomatoes are rich in lycopene, a carotenoid that is fairly stable to storage and cooking and thus is present in cooked tomatoes, which are often consumed in the Mediterranean countries.[198,199] Moreover, garlic and onions, which are also rich sources of various antioxidants are frequently consumed in the Mediterranean countries. In the Seven Countries Study,[200] the average flavonol and flavone intake was inversely correlated with mortality rates of CHD after 25 years of follow-up. In a prospective study, the Zutphen Elderly Study,[201] CHD mortality was also strongly associated with flavonol and flavone intake. In particular, a 50% reduction in the mortality risk was observed in the highest tertile of flavonol intake (42 mg/day). However, in the U.S. Male Health Professionals Study,[202] a modest but not significant inverse association was reported between flavonols and flavones intake, and coronary mortality rates. In this study, mean flavonol intake in the highest quartile was 43 mg/day and 14 mg/day in the lowest. Several mechanisms have been proposed for the protective effect of flavonoids. They bind to LDL and inhibit its oxidation, and decrease its susceptibility to aggregate. In addition, they inhibit macrophage-mediated LDL oxidation by increasing cellular glutathione transferase content, and inhibiting cellular enzymes that are involved in cell-mediated LDL oxidation.[203]

Another constituent of fruits and vegetables that is associated with decreased risk of CHD is folic acid. Folic acid decreases plasma homocysteine levels, which is a risk factor for developing CHD. Interest in folic acid intake has emerged since it was observed that, in the U.S., fruits and vegetables provide only about 20% of daily α-tocopherol intake and, therefore, this vitamin could not be the major component contributing to fruits' and vegetables' antiatherogenic effect.[204] Folic acid, together with vitamins B_6 and B_{12}, are involved in the synthesis of homocysteine from methionine. In particular, an increase in folic acid intake from fruits and vegetables results in a decrease in plasma homocysteine levels.[205] It has been proposed that, even the French Paradox, characterized by high dietary saturated fat intake and low CHD prevalence, should be redefined, taking into consideration the fact that hyperhomocysteinemia may explain CHD development in normocholesterolemic patients.[206] A cross-cultural study would be very useful in evaluating the effect of folic acid and homocysteine levels on CHD risk and mortality, and would probably strengthen even more the differences between north and south, in dietary terms.

The evidence is still conflicting so far as the antioxidants and their effect on CHD are concerned. Even the well known hypothesis of LDL oxidation and its contribution to foam cell formation and atherogenesis process has been questioned recently. Epidemiological studies seem to suggest that vitamin E has the most protective effect and it could act synergistically with vitamin C. Therefore, randomized controlled trials are still necessary to investigate the mechanisms of action of these substances. However, the presence of dietary fiber, vitamins C, E, B_6, B_{12}, folic acid, β-carotene, and others, in fruits and vegetables, seem to make them unique and although the use of antioxidant supplements should still be discouraged, the inclusion of fruit and vegetables in the daily diet, as well as whole grain cereals and olive oil, should be strongly encouraged.

C. MEAT AND MEAT PRODUCTS

1. Epidemiological Studies

In the Mediterranean countries, consumption of beef, pork, and lamb has traditionally been low.[207] Meat contains no fiber and very few antioxidant nutrients. Moreover, its energy displaces that from plant foods, which are rich in these nutrients.[208] In particular, increased meat intake, expressed in quintiles and adjusted for energy, was found to be associated with decreased intakes of poultry, fish, fruits, bread, cereals, and cheese in both genders.[209] Therefore, the positive association reported between meat and CHD might not be directly linked to meat components.

As has already been mentioned, in the Seven Countries Study,[186] animal food groups were directly correlated with CHD mortality. In particular, univariate analysis showed significant positive correlation — among others — for meat (r = 0.645) consumption. In addition, combined animal foods (excluding fish) were directly correlated (r = 0.798) with CHD mortality rates.

Epidemiological studies have linked the frequent consumption of red meat with increased risk for CHD.[207] Evidence that supports the above suggestion probably comes from a study that compared Seventh-Day Adventists who frequently consumed red meat with others from the same group who consumed it less often.[210] In this study, men and women who consumed red meat daily had a 60% greater chance of dying from CHD than those who consumed red meat less than once per week.

The CARDIA Study[211] reported that people who ate red meat and poultry less than once per week consumed diets higher in carbohydrates, starch, fiber, vitamins A and C, and calcium, and lower in energy, fat, and protein than people who consumed meat more frequently. Similar findings derived from the Bogalusa Heart Study,[212] which showed that persons in the < 25th percentile for meat consumption had higher intakes of carbohydrates and calcium, and lower intakes of fat and protein than persons in the > 75th percentile.

Another study indicated that, after adjusting for the standard risk factors, saturated fat, and cholesterol intake, that the relative risk of myocardial infarction for men consuming beef four or more times per week was 1.38 (95% CI, 0.77, 2.29), compared with men consuming beef once per month or less. However, a meat score — calculated as the sum in grams per day of beef (main dish or sandwich), hamburger, hot dog, chicken, liver, and other processed meat intake — was only weakly, and not significantly, associated with an increased risk of myocardial infarction; the relative risk for the top quintile (median intake, 145 g/day) compared with the bottom quintile (median intake, 16 g/day) was 1.18 (95% CI, 0.78, 1.80).[213]

Another study combined data from five prospective studies to compare the death rates from common diseases of vegetarians with those of non-vegetarians with similar life-style.[214] Mortality from ischemic heart disease was found to be 24% lower in vegetarians than in non-vegetarians. This lower mortality among vegetarians was greater at young ages and was restricted to those who had followed their current diet for at least 5 years. It was observed that, comparing with regular meat eaters, mortality rates from ischemic heart disease were 20% lower in occasional meat eaters, 34% lower in fish eaters, 34% lower in lacto-ovovegetarians, and 26% lower in vegans.

2. Blood Lipid Levels

Atherosclerotic effects of red meat have generally been attributed to its relatively high content of cholesterol and long-chain saturated fatty acids, which both elevate cholesterol levels, a known risk factor for CHD and atherosclerosis.[207] Prospective studies confirm the association of dietary cholesterol with the risk for CHD.[215]

It has been observed that saturated fatty acids and cholesterol intakes were significantly higher, and polyunsaturated fatty acids intake was significantly lower in meat eaters than vegetarians.[216] Data on young adults in the CARDIA study[211] showed that people who consumed red meat and poultry less than once per week had lower concentrations of total serum cholesterol, LDL cholesterol, and triglycerides than those who consumed meat more frequently. Nevertheless, regular consumption of beef, when added to a vegetarian diet, has been demonstrated to increase blood cholesterol, especially LDL cholesterol, and to increase blood pressure.[217]

3. Heme Iron and Risk for CHD

In addition to the effects on blood cholesterol, red meat intake may also have additional effects on other parameters of CHD risk. Associations were observed between body iron stores,[218,219] dietary consumption of heme iron, and increased CHD risk. An association was not observed in the case of non-heme iron.[213] However, epidemiological evidence on the role of iron, a lipid peroxidation catalyst, in CHD is inconsistent. It is noteworthy that studies looking at iron status and its effects on heart disease have yielded conflicting results, with claims ranging from positive to negative associations. It has been suggested[220] that the discrepancy may be largely a result of the vast biological and measurement variabilities in methods used to assess body iron stores. Results from a systematic meta-analysis concluded that published prospective studies do not provide good evidence to support the existence of strong epidemiological associations between iron status and CHD.[221] Furthermore, in a study that investigated whether increased body iron stores and dietary iron intake are associated with an increased risk of CHD mortality,[222] no relationship was reported between total iron-binding capacity and coronary mortality in men, while in women, an inverse but not significant association was found. No association was noted on dietary iron intake and coronary mortality.

In a prospective study,[213] no significant association between total iron intake and risk of CHD was identified. In particular, dietary intake of heme iron, mainly from red meat, was not significantly associated with risk of CHD. However, incidence of fatal coronary disease or nonfatal myocardial infarction was higher among men in the top quintile of heme iron intake than in men in the lowest quintile. Therefore, the results of this study do not support the hypothesis that dietary iron increases coronary risk in men. They are consistent, however, with an increased risk of myocardial infarction among men with higher intake of heme iron, which is itself positively associated with iron stores. Moreover, it was noticed that the association between heme iron intake and risk of myocardial infarction was limited to men who were not taking vitamin E or multiple vitamin supplements. This is consistent with the hypothesis that iron may adversely affect coronary risk only in the presence of oxidative stress from other sources.[116]

In another prospective study[223] among 1932 Finnish men, it was concluded that serum ferritin and total iron intake were both strongly and positively associated with the risk of myocardial infarction. The reported increase in risk of myocardial infarction was 5% for each 1 mg increase of daily iron intake.

A prospective case-control study[220] investigating the association of the concentration of serum transferrin receptor to serum ferritin (TfR/ferritin) with the risk of acute myocardial infarction, reported an association between increased body iron stores and excess risk of acute myocardial infarction, confirming previous epidemiological findings. The results from this study suggested that men with high iron stores (low TfR/ferritin ratio) are at a twofold to threefold increased risk for the first acute myocardial infarction. The association between TfR/ferritin ratio and of acute myocardial infarction risk was stronger among men who did not use either antioxidant vitamins or aspirin.

4. Meat Intake and Homocysteine Levels

It is well known that red meat, apart from being the primary source of heme iron — contributing to almost all of it,[213] — is also a major source of methionine in the diet, the direct metabolic precursor of homocysteine. Homocysteine is derived from the amino acid methionine, which is more common in animal protein than in vegetable protein, and can be converted back into methionine with the help of folic acid and vitamin B_{12}.[224] Therefore, increased consumption of red meat is likely to elevate plasma homocysteine concentrations,[207] not only through increased intake of methionine, but also through decreased intake of folic acid and vitamin B_6 as a result of a decrease in the consumption of vegetables and cereals due to the increased meat intake. According to the results of the Nurses' Health Study[225] folic acid and B_6 are much more important than vitamin B_{12} in controlling homocysteine levels.

Homocysteine plays an important role in the etiology of heart disease through its role in the development of atherosclerosis. Elevated plasma homocysteine levels are an independent risk factor for vascular disease, in particular myocardial infarction,[226] or peripheral arterial disease in older men and women.[227]

A prospective study showed that moderately elevated levels of plasma homocysteine could be an independent risk factor for CHD through their association with the risk of myocardial infarction, independent of other coronary risk factors.[116] In this study, individuals in the top 5% of the distribution had a threefold higher risk of developing myocardial infarction than did those in the bottom 95% of the distribution, but only a small association between homocysteine levels and other coronary risk factors was observed.

Recommendations from the U.S. Department of Agriculture suggest that the daily consumption of red meat should vary between 140–196g[228] despite the evidence for the contrary. The consumption of moderate amounts of lean meat, along with healthier choices in other food groups, may be necessary to meet the current dietary recommendations.[212] The traditional model of the Mediterranean Diet suggests the rare intake of red meat in small portions.

D. FISH

1. Epidemiology

The amount of fish consumed in the Mediterranean Diet depends on geographic regions, e.g., very high fish consumption in the northern Basque province of Spain compared with the rest of Spain.[229] The same is more or less valid in Greece, with fish constituting a major part of the food consumed by the Cretan population. The average fish consumption in Crete in 1960 was 18 g per day per person and was almost doubled by the year 1988.[230]

Epidemiological evidence shows that persons consuming diets rich in fish have better cardiovascular health than those consuming meat and other animal foods rich in saturated fatty acids.[231] Daviglus et al.[232] mention that the suggestion that the consumption of fish reduces the risk of CHD is supported by data from at least five epidemiological studies, two case-control studies, and one secondary-prevention trial, while the results from other studies are apparently inconsistent with these findings. This apparent inconsistency may be due to different methods of assessing diet and categorizing fish consumption, different distributions of reported fish consumption, differences in study sites and times, with associated dietary differences (e.g., levels of intake of cholesterol, saturated fatty acids, antioxidants, and fiber) that might have influenced the relation between fish consumption and the risk of CHD; and different periods of follow-up, ranging from 4 years to several decades.[232]

To assess the consistency of findings of numerous prospective cohort studies, Markmann et al.[233] gave a scientific quality score to these studies, dividing them into categories of high, intermediate, or insufficient quality. The conclusion of this systematic review was that individuals at low risk of CHD and with healthy lifestyles gain no additional protection against CHD from eating fish. On the other hand, high-risk individuals appear to benefit in a dose-dependent manner from increasing their fish consumption up to an optimum of 40–60 g/day. At the optimal fish intake, risk of CHD mortality may be approximately half the risk of individuals not consuming fish at all.

The Chicago Western Electric Study[232] showed a significant, independent inverse association between baseline fish consumption and the 30-year risk of fatal myocardial infarction, particularly non sudden death from myocardial infarction. This relation accounted for the lower rates of death from all causes, and all cardiovascular causes in association with higher fish consumption, which persisted throughout the 30-year duration of the study and in analyses adjusted for potentially confounding demographic, biomedical, and dietary factors.

Kromhout et al.[231] reported that, over a 20-year period, heart attack rates were significantly lower in men reporting daily fish intakes of about 30 g than in men reporting no fish consumption.

Fatty fish and fish oil reduced mortality in men after myocardial infarction by about 29% during the first 2 years.[234] It was suggested that fatty acids are necessary for the human body, especially the n-3 fatty acids that are related to CHD reduction if consumed regularly on a daily or weekly basis.[234] In addition, the study of Tornaritis et al.[230] reaffirms the belief that the eight species of Mediterranean fish studied are a good source of n-3 fatty acids.[230] The magnitude of the n-6:n-3 ratio and the percentage of the saturated fatty acids, as well as the total fat content of these fish, classifies them as highly nutritional food.

The available epidemiological data, although limited, suggest that a dietetic recommendation on the consumption of one or two servings per week (200–300 g) of cold-water marine fish could lead to a reduction of the CHD risk. With the same levels of intake, a small reduction in blood pressure in men with coronary disease was observed.[235] However, Garcia-Closes et al.[236] reported that fish consumption is not positively correlated with ischemic heart disease mortality. This suggests that dietary factors other than fish, such as the lower meat consumption associated with the higher fish intake, or other differences of life-style have perhaps intervened, possibly explaining the healthy nature of the Mediterranean Diet.[236]

2. Metabolic Studies

The most profound effect of fish oils is the lowering of plasma triglyceride levels in both fasting and postprandial states.[237–239] The probable mechanism for this effect is the decrease of hepatic triglyceride synthesis and the suppression of VLDL production or secretion,[240] as well as the increase in postprandial activity in lipoprotein lipase, which is the enzyme responsible for chylomicron- and VLDL-triglyceride hydrolysis in the adipose tissue and skeletal muscle.[241] The theory of increased catabolism via lipoprotein lipase is still somewhat controversial because, on one hand, there is some evidence to suggest that fish oils, and not their catabolism, may reduce the rate at which chylomicrons are produced and secreted.[242] On the other hand, there is evidence suggesting that fish oils may not influence lipoprotein lipase and hepatic lipase activities regardless of the observed decrease in plasma triglyceride levels.[243]

Fish oils may induce different qualitative effects on VLDL particles from those of n-6 polyunsaturated fatty acids by shifting the distribution of VLDL subclasses toward predominantly small $VLDL_2$ and not large $VLDL_1$.[244] As a consequence, since $VLDL_2$ is a better precursor of LDL formation than $VLDL_1$, it could be suggested that fish oils would increase plasma LDL levels. However, this LDL-raising effect that occurs through increased conversion of VLDL[245] or competition between VLDL and LDL for the LDL receptor[246] may be associated with the use of supplements and not with an increase in dietary fish intake. In addition, it has been observed that fish oils may increase LDL particle size, rendering them less atherogenic.[247]

The decrease in plasma triglyceride levels could suggest a decrease in neutral lipid transfer between lipoprotein fractions. As a result, HDL would not be enriched with triglycerides and would remain as large, cholesterol ester-containing particles. This accumulation of large HDL_2 has been previously reported in healthy volunteers on fish oil supplements[248] and would suggest a decreased atherogenicity.

Moderately increased triglyceride levels in the fasting and postprandial states, predominance of small and dense LDL and HDL particles, as well as low levels of HDL, describe the atherogenic lipoprotein phenotype (ALP) which confers an increased risk for CHD.[249] The reported observation that, in North America, between 30–35% of middle-aged men may be affected by these sub-clinical symptoms,[250] promotes the recommendation for the adoption of the Mediterranean Diet as a way toward the decrease of these lipoprotein abnormalities and the prevalence of ALP.

E. MILK AND MILK PRODUCTS

Cheese and yogurt have been a basic component in most Mediterranean Diet patterns, contributing to their flavor and variety. On the contrary, milk, butter, and creams were traditionally not widely consumed.[168] Dietary recommendations advocate two to three servings of dairy products daily, mainly because they are important sources of calcium and high-quality protein.[251] In contrast, the fat contained in dairy products is high in saturated fatty acids,[252] which are responsible for the increased risk of CHD and other occlusive cardiovascular diseases.[253]

The term "milk fat" applies to fat from any of the full range of dairy foods (i.e., milk, cheese, ice cream, yogurt, butter, etc., with all their accompanying nutrients), whereas "butter" refers to one specific food.[254] The fatty acid content of dairy products is higher in saturated fatty acids than other animal foods (50–60%; 38–49% in beef fat). Myristic acid (C14:0) is one of the principal fatty acids in dairy products, and it appears to have a more pronounced adverse effect on blood lipids than the longer-chain saturated fatty acids[255] or palmitic acid (C16:0).[254] Moreover, the increased risk for thrombosis associated with high consumption of dairy products could be partly due to the displacement of unsaturated — which have an antithrombotic effect — by saturated fatty acids.

In the Seven Countries Study, it was observed that, in Finland, which had the highest CHD rates, the intake of milk and other dairy products was high.[1] Although there was no case control study that examined the association between the consumption of dairy products and the risk for the development of CHD, there are indications that a causal association does exist. It is noteworthy that animal food groups were directly correlated with CHD mortality.[186] In particular, as far as dairy products are concerned, univariate analysis showed significant positive correlation coefficients, among others, for butter (r = 0.887) and milk (r = 0.600) consumption.[186]

Human metabolic studies[254] in which butter intake is increased showed that butter is hypercholesterolemic compared with many other fat sources such as vegetables oils. Few studies have assessed the impact of butter, or other sources of milk fat, on serum cholesterol in free mixed-fat diets.

Except for the correlation mentioned above between milk fat and CHD, Grant[224] presented ecological statistical results to support strong evidence for dietary non-fat milk compounds playing an important role in the etiology of heart disease. In a study that investigated associations with ischemic heart disease and CHD, milk carbohydrates were found to have the highest association for males aged 45+ and females aged 65+ for ischemic heart disease, while for females 35–64, sugar was found to have the highest association.[224] In the case of CHD, non-fat milk was found to have the highest association for males aged 45+ and females aged 75+, while for females ages 65–74, milk carbohydrates and sugar had the highest associations, and for females 45–64, sugar had the highest association.

One of the most prominent theories is that animal proteins contribute to homocysteine production; in addition, milk lacks more than meat in adequate B vitamins to convert homocysteine to useful products.[224] Moreover, high protein intake is correlated with an increased prevalence of CHD as well as bone loss and fracture risk.[168]

Seely[256] made the case that excess dietary calcium in Western counties is a major cause of arterial disease. A possible action of calcium in the cardiovascular system could be the calcification of the soft tissues, which leads to increased hypertension and a greater burden on the heart.[224] Nevertheless, Ganong[257] argues that lactose increases calcium absorption, which, in combination with the statement that lactose is the important factor in plaque formation,[258] may lead to the hypothesis that non fat milk — with lactose and calcium — contributes significantly to increased calcification of the arteries. To avoid this, either a reduced intake of calcium or an increased intake of phytic acid is proposed as the best antagonist of calcium, by converting it into insoluble phosphates.[256]

High calcium intake is believed to reduce, among others, the risk of high blood pressure. However, the National Dairy Council in the U.K.[251] states that, although there is some suggestive but rather weak evidence of an influence of calcium intake on blood pressure, the case is unproven.

In early studies, attention has been directed to unfermented milk proteins, namely the protein content of all dairy products, with the only important exception of cheese, as a possible important atherogenic influence.[259,260] Similar results were derived by the same investigator in another study,[261] where the highest correlations for coronary mortality were found, among others, also for milk proteins (other than the protein content of cheese).

The past consumption of cheese and yogurt, instead of milk, in Mediterranean cultures was mainly due to the lack of refrigeration. Whether saturated fat in the form of yogurt and cheese shares the same adverse effects on blood lipids as saturated fat in butter or milk is uncertain.[168] However, there is evidence that there is a correlation between high intake of milk, butter, and other, rich-in-fat dairy products and increased risk for development of CHD. Therefore, the relatively low consumption of dairy products among the Mediterranean populations has undoubtedly contributed to their health.

F. ALCOHOL

In the Mediterranean countries, except for the Muslim ones, wine has been moderately consumed with meals. High consumption of alcohol has undoubtedly adverse effects, while moderate consumption has been shown to have both positive and negative effects.

The inverse association among moderate alcohol consumption, reduced morbidity, and mortality from CHD is well established.[262-264] Evidence for a causal interpretation comes from over 60 ecological, case-control, and cohort studies.[262] Alcohol intake is causally related to a lower risk of CHD through changes in lipids and hemostatic factors.[265] Reviews concluded that men and women who drink one to two drinks a day have the lowest risk of CHD.[263,266,267] Epidemiological data show that moderate consumption of alcohol reduces the risk of CHD, with two drinks daily, 20–30 g of alcohol, leading to a reduction of 30–40%.[266]

On the other hand, another study denied the strong relationship between alcohol consumption and mortality from CHD after adjustment was made for potential confounding factors, and claimed that there is no clear evidence of any protective effect for men drinking moderate amounts of alcohol.[268]

In addition, mortality rates are slightly lower in individuals with a moderate alcohol intake than in those with none.[263,269] This was concluded from studies carried out in Western populations and have also been reconfirmed in Asians.[270,271]

In several prospective studies, it was observed that men and women who consumed one to three drinks daily had the same or lower risk of CHD as abstainers or those who drank substantially more.[272] In particular, the association between alcohol and CHD in studies is generally U-shaped, with the nadir occurring among individuals who consume one to three drinks daily. A review of nine follow-up cohort studies reporting mortality data from 1986 to 1992 demonstrated that, in all studies, at least some alcohol consumption was associated with a lower total mortality rate in comparison to abstainers.[273]

The biological mechanisms by which alcohol reduces coronary risk have been previously reviewed.[274] High-density lipoprotein (HDL) cholesterol has consistently been found to be inversely associated with CHD and positively associated with alcohol consumption.[275] More recently, it has been shown that both HDL_2 and HDL_3 are related positively to alcohol consumption and inversely to CHD rates.[276] From epidemiological studies for which data are available on both alcohol intake and HDL cholesterol, results suggest that the association between alcohol and HDL cholesterol explains 30–50% of the overall reduction in CHD that is attributable to alcohol.[276,277] The above may also affect hemostatic mechanisms by reducing platelet aggregation, by decreasing fibrinogen, and antithrombin activity.[278]

Part of the inverse association between moderate alcohol consumption and a reduced risk of CHD may be explained by its effects on HDL. Paraoxonase, an HDL-associated enzyme, has been suggested to protect against LDL oxidation. Data from a study[279] examining the effects on paraoxonase activity in serum of moderate consumption of red wine, beer, and spirits in comparison with mineral water, suggest that increased serum paraoxonase may be one of the biological mechanisms underlying the reduced CHD risk in moderate alcohol consumers. The increases in paraoxonase activity were strongly correlated with coincident increases in concentrations of HDL cholesterol and apoA-I (r = 0.60, r< 0.05 and r = 0.70, r< 0.05).

Another study suggested that ethanol may reduce cardiovascular risk by modulating vascular muscle cell growth during the postprandial period.[280] Considering the amount of time humans spend in the postprandial state during their lifetimes, these findings may be of great importance in the pathogenesis of atherosclerosis.

The anti-aggregatory effects of alcohol on platelets may not be so important in reducing CHD rates in Mediterranean populations that characteristically consume a diet that is high in mono- and polyunsaturated fatty acids. Reduction of the risk of coronary disease is observed in diets rich in saturated fatty acids.[48]

Several phenols and flavonoids that possess antioxidant characteristics have been identified in the skins of grapes. The catechin compounds and phenolic acids present in red wine display similar antioxidant activities, while catechins exhibit a greater antioxidant activity than flavonols and polymeric anthocyanidins.[281] Resveratrol, a naturally occurring phytoalexin found in grapes and wine, regulates many biological activities.[282] Resveratrol has been reported to give protection against atherosclerosis-exerting antioxidant activity, to inhibit platelet aggregation[283] and production of atherogenic eicosanoids by human platelets and neutrophils,[283] and to modulate the synthesis of hepatic apolipoprotein and lipids.[284] Since red wine represents the main resveratrol source,[282] one can assume that some of the beneficial effects of a moderate red wine intake on CHD are due to the presence of this phytoalexin in the beverage.

However, an attempt to determine whether phenolic compounds present in red wine and grape juice modulate plasma lipid and lipoprotein concentrations in healthy human subjects revealed that the favorable effects of wines to the above are probably due to their alcohol content and cannot be reproduced by grape juices.[285] These favorable effects were similar for red and white wine, modulating plasma lipids and lipoproteins toward a pattern associated with reduced risk of CHD, since red wine showed no advantage over white.[285] A prospective study of coronary disease hospitalizations concluded that drinking ethyl alcohol apparently protects against coronary disease, and that there may be minor additional benefits associated with drinking both beer and wine, but not especially red wine.[286]

On the other hand, Seigneur et al.[278] found that protective effects on platelet function were much greater for red wine than for white wine or ethanol itself, suggesting that there may be additional protection from red wine due to nonethanol components. Red wine has been shown *in vitro* to inhibit LDL oxidation,[287,288] increase antioxidant capacity in humans,[289] reduce the susceptibility of human plasma to lipid peroxidation,[290] and raise plasma levels of HDL cholesterol and apolipoproteins A-I and A-II.[285,291] In some of the above studies, the administration of pure alcohol[289] or of white wine with the same alcohol content,[289,290] failed to show any protective effect. In addition, another prospective cohort study resulted in findings wherein no association between intake of beer or spirits on risk of stroke could be established, while the intake of wine (on a monthly, weekly, or daily basis) was associated with a lower risk of stroke compared with no wine intake.[292]

The Male Health Professional Study[202] did not report a strong inverse association between intake of flavonoids and total heart disease in healthy men. However, the data do not exclude the possibility that flavonoids have a protective effect in men with established CHD.

An alternative explanation for a potential superiority of wine over other alcoholic beverages is that, because wine is mostly consumed during meals, as it is in Greece, it is absorbed slowly, and thus has a prolonged effect on, for example, blood platelets, at a time when they are under the influence of dietary lipids that are known to increase their reactivity.[293] The fact that wine is mostly taken with food, slowly, and with regularity is also being mentioned in a large prospective population study.[294]

An excellent protection of red wine to the risk of CHD, over and above that due to ethanol itself, but due to phenolic components and other micronutrients with which red wines are richly endowed, is supported by several studies.[283,288-290,292,295] However, any overall cardioprotective advantage to humans of wine over other beverages containing alcohol is still speculative.

A study examining the effects of beer, spirits, and wine drinking on CHD events (fatal and nonfatal) resulted in findings that suggest that regular intake of all alcoholic drinks is associated with a lower risk of CHD than occasional drinking.[296] A large part of the greater benefit seen for wine drinkers relative to other drinkers in that study can be attributed to advantageous life-style characteristics: They were predominantly non-manual workers, had the lowest rate of current smoking and obesity, and were more likely to be physically active and to be light drinkers.[296] Nevertheless, Serafini et al.[297] have demonstrated that the nonalcoholic fraction of red wine (alcohol-free red wine) does significantly raise total plasma antioxidant capacity and that this increase is paralleled by a concomitant increase in plasma concentrations of phenolic compounds. The above led them to speculate that the changes in plasma antioxidant potential may be entirely attributable to the phenolic fraction of red wine. Added to that, red wine lost its antioxidant activity after being stripped of phenols and did not inhibit LDL oxidation.[284]

From the ten cohort studies that Rimm et al.[262] have examined, with data collected from more that 305,000 men and women followed up for over 1.8 million person-years, it is concluded that, if any type of drink does provide extra cardiovascular benefit apart from alcohol content, the benefit is likely to be modest at best, or possibly restricted to certain sub-populations.

According to the above, no single type of drink provides all or most of the cardiovascular benefit. However, results from several individual cohort studies suggest a stronger association for one particular type of drink. Rimm et al.[262] explained that the variations between studies might be due to different drinking patterns or aspects of lifestyle correlated with the choice of drink in certain populations. In the studies where only one type of drink was significantly associated with reduced risk of CHD, that drink was usually consumed by most of the population, typically at levels of one or two glasses daily. This pattern of widespread "healthy" drinking is more likely to take place with meals than is heavy or episodic drinking by a small percentage of the population.

Rimm et al.[262] added that, in the health professionals follow up study in which spirits were the most commonly consumed type of drink and were the most strongly protective, total alcohol consumption was strongly correlated with total numbers of days in which alcohol was consumed (r = 0.89).[267] This suggests that spirits were consumed most days of the week and were not restricted to heavy weekend consumption. Conversely, in the Copenhagen City Heart Study,[295] in which consumption of spirits did not reduce CHD, only 8.5% of the men and 4% of the women reported drinking spirits on average once a day or more. Rimm et al.[262] suggested that, because this small sample of consumers of spirits may have had different drinking habits (and other life-style characteristics) from the rest of the population in Copenhagen, it may explain the absence of a cardioprotective effect of spirits in this population.

In conclusion, it seems that wine has been beneficial not only for meal enjoyment around the Mediterranean, but also for reducing the risk of coronary disease in the area, even if equivalent inverse outcomes have been demonstrated with other alcoholic beverages. Moderate consumption of alcohol — as a part of meals— should be considered more as an additional, rather than a primary, component of a Mediterranean Diet.

REFERENCES

1. Keys, A., Coronary heart disease in seven countries, *Circulation*, 41(Suppl 1), 1, 1970.
2. Christakis, G., Severinghaus, E.L., Maldonado, Z., Kafatos, F.C., and Hashim, S.A., Crete: A study in the metabolic epidemiology of coronary heart disease, *Am. J. Cardiol.*, 15, 320, 1965.
3. Kromhout, D., Menotti, A., Bloemberg, B., Aravanis, C., Blackburn, H., Buzina, R., Dontas, A.S., Fidanza, F., Glampaoli, S., Jansen, A., Karvonen, M., Katan, M., Nissinen, A., Nedeljkovic, S., Pekkanen, J., Pekkarinen, M., Punsar, S., Rasanen, L., Simic, B., and Toshima, H., Dietary saturated and *trans* fatty acids and cholesterol and 25-year mortality from coronary heart disease: The Seven Countries Study., *Prev. Med.*, 24, 308, 1995.
4. Verschuren, W.M., Jacobs, D.R., Bloemberg, B.P., Kromhout, D., Menotti, A., Aravanis, C., Blackburn, H., Buzina, R., Dontas, A.S., Fidanza, F., et al., Serum total cholesterol and long-term coronary heart disease mortality in different cultures. Twenty-five-year follow-up of the Seven Countries Study, *J. Am. Med. Assoc.*, 274, 131, 1995.
5. Menotti, A., Cross-cultural relationship of dietary habits and coronary heart disease in the Seven Countries Study, *Atherosclerosis*, 144 (Suppl 1), 169A, 1999.
6. Hertog, M.G., Kromhout, D., Aravanis, C., Blackburn, H., Buzina, R., Fidanza, F., Giampaoli, S., Jansen, A., Menotti, A., Nedeljkovic, S., Pekkarinen, M., Simic, B.S., Toshima, H., Feskens, E.J.M., Hollman, P.C.H., and Katan, M.B., Flavonoid intake and long-term risk of coronary heart disease and cancer in the Seven Countries Study, *Arch. Intern. Med.*, 155, 381, 1995.
7. De Longeril, M., Renaud, S., Mamelle, N., Salen, P., Martin, J.L., Monjaud, I., Guidollet, J., Toubol, P., Delaye, J., Mediterranean alpha-linolenic acid-rich diet in secondary prevention of coronary heart disease, *Lancet*, 343, 1454, 1994.
8. Renaud, S., de Longeril, M., Delaye, J., Guidollet, J., Jacquard, F., Mamelle, N., Martin, J.L., Monjaud, I., Salen, P., and Toubol, P., Cretan Mediterranean Diet for prevention of coronary heart disease, *Am. J. Clin. Nutr.*, 61 (6 Suppl), 1360S, 1995.

9. De Longeril, M., Salen, P., Martin, J.L., Mamelle, N., Monjaud, I., Touboul, P., and Delaye, J., Effect of a Mediterranean type of diet on the rate of cardiovascular complications on patients with coronary artery disease. Insights into the cardioprotective effect of certain nutriments, *J. Am. Coll. Cardiol.*, 28, 1103, 1996.

10. De Longeril, M., Salen, P., Martin, J.L., Monjaud, I., Boucher, P., and Mamelle, N., Mediterranean dietary pattern in a randomized trial: prolonged survival and possible reduced cancer rate, *Arch. Intern. Med.*, 158, 1181, 1998.

11. De Longeril, M., Salen, P., Martin, J.L., Monjaud, I., Delaye, J., and Mamelle, N., Mediterranean diet, traditional risk factors, and the rate of cardiovascular complications after myocardial infarction: final report of the Lyon Diet Heart Study, *Circulation*, 99, 779, 1999.

12. Kannel, W.B., Overview of atherosclerosis, *Clin. Ther.*, 20 (Suppl B), B2, 1998.

13. Boyle, E.M. Jr., Lille, S.T., Allaire, E., Clowes, A.W., and Verrier, E.D., Endothelial cell injury in cardiovascular surgery: atherosclerosis, *Ann. Thorac. Surg.*, 63, 885, 1997.

14. Kottke, B.A., Current understanding of the mechanisms of atherogenesis, *Am. J. Cardiol.*, 72, 48C, 1993.

15. De Meyer, G.R. and Herman, A.G., Vascular endothelial dysfunction, *Prog. Cardiovasc. Dis.*, 39, 325, 1997.

16. Sanders, M., Molecular and cellular concepts in atherosclerosis, *Pharmacol. Ther.*, 61, 109, 1994.

17. Steinberg, D., Parthasarathy, S., Carew, T.E., Khoo, J.C., and Witztum, J.L., Beyond cholesterol. Modifications of low-density lipoprotein that increase its atherogenicity, *N. Eng. J. Med.*, 320, 915, 1989.

18. Miller, G.J., Lipoproteins and the hemostatic system in atherothrombotic disorders, *Baillieres Clin. Hematol.*, 7, 713, 1994.

19. Fisher, A., Gutstein, D.E., and Fuster, V., Thrombosis and coagulation abnormalities in the acute coronary syndromes, *Cardiol. Clin.*, 17, 283, 1999.

20. Davies, M.J., Pathology of arterial thrombosis, *Br. Med. Bull.*, 50, 789, 1994.

21. Libby, P., The interface of atherosclerosis and thrombosis: basic mechanisms, *Vasc. Med.*, 3, 225, 1998.

22. Shah, P.K., Plaque disruption and thrombosis. Potential role of inflammation and infection, *Cardiol. Clin.*, 17, 271, 1999.

23. Gronholdt, M.L., Dalager-Pedersen, S., and Falk, E., Coronary atherosclerosis: determinants of plaque rupture, *Eur. Heart J.*, 19 (Suppl C), C24, 1998.

24. Hennig, B., Diana, J.N., Toborek, M., McChain, C.J., Influence of nutrients and cytokines on endothelial cell metabolism, *J. Am. Coll. Nutr.*, 13, 224, 1994.

25. Cooke, J.P., Is atherosclerosis an arginine deficiency disease? *J. Investig. Med.*, 46, 377, 1998.

26. De Jong, S.C., van den Berg, M., Rauwerda, J.A., and Stehouwer, C.D., Hyperhomocysteinemia and atherothrombotic disease, *Semin. Thromb. Hemost.*, 24, 381, 1998.

27. Verhoef, P., Stampfer, M., and Buring, J., Homocysteine metabolism and risk of myocardial infarction. Relation with vitamins B6, B12 and folate, *Am. J. Epidemiol.*, 143, 845, 1996.

28. Ubbink, J., Vermaak, W.J., and van der Merwe, A., Vitamin B12, vitamin B6 and folate nutritional status in men with hyperhomocysteinemia, *Am. J. Clin. Nutr.*, 57, 47, 1993.

29. Simopoulos, A.P., and Childs, B., Eds., *Genetic Variation and Nutrition*, World Rev. Nutr. Diet., vol. 63, Basel, Karger, 1990.

30. Nora, J.J., Berg, K., and Nora, A.H., *Cardiovascular Diseases: Genetics, Epidemiology, and Prevention*, Oxford University Press, New York, 1991.

31. Berg, K., Genetic variability of risk factors for coronary heart disease (CHD), in *Proc. IUNS. Nutrition in a Sustainable Environment,* Wahlqvist, M.L., Truswell, A.S., Smith, R., Nestel, P.J., Eds., Smith-Gordon, London, 1994, 437.

32. Goldbourt, U., de Faire, U., and Berg, K., *Genetic Factors in Coronary Heart Disease*, Kluwer, Dordrecht, 1994.

33. Cambien, F., Insight into the genetic epidemiology of coronary heart disease, *Ann. Med.*, 28, 465, 1996.

34. National Heart, Lung, and Blood Institute report of the Task Force on Research in Atherosclerosis: US Department of Health and Human Services, September, 1991.

35. Mongeau, J. G., Heredity and blood pressure, *Semin. Nephrol.*, 9, 208, 1989.

36. Kobberling, J., and Tillil, H., Genetic and nutritional factors in the etiology and pathogenesis of diabetes mellitus, in *Genetic Variation and Nutrition*, World Rev. Nutr. Diet., vol. 63, Simopoulos, A.P. and Childs, B., Eds., Karger, Basel, 1990, 102.

37. Bouchard, C., Genetic factors in obesity, *Med. Clin. N. Am.*, 73, 67, 1989.

38. Goldstein, J.L. and Brown, M.S., Familial hypercholesterolemia, in *The Metabolic Basis of Inherited Disease* , vol. 1, Scriver, C.R., Beaudet, A.L., Sly, W.S. and Valle, D., Eds., McGraw-Hill, New York, 1989,1215.

39. Mahley, R.W., Apolipoprotein E: Cholesterol transport protein with expanding role in cell biology, *Science*, 240, 622,1988.

40. Utermann, G., Langenbeck, U., Beisiegel, U., and Weber, W., Genetics of the apolipoprotein E system in man, *Am. J. Hum. Genet.*, 32, 339, 1980.

41. Zannis, V.I., Just, P.W., and Breslow, J.L., Human apolipoprotein E isoprotein subclasses are genetically determined, *Am. J. Hum. Genet.*, 33, 11, 1981.

42. Sing, C.F. and Davignon, J., Role of the apolipoprotein E polymorphism in determining normal plasma lipid and lipoprotein variation, *Am. J. Hum. Genet.*, 37, 268, 1985.

43. Davignon, J., Gregg, R.E., and Sing C.F., Apolipoprotein E polymorphism and atherosclerosis, *Arteriosclerosis*, 8, 1, 1988.

44. Hallman, D.M., Boerwinkle, E., Saha, N., Sandholzer, C., Menzel, H.J., Csazar, A., and Utermann, G., The apolipoprotein E polymorphism: A comparison of allele frequencies and effects in nine populations, *Am. J. Hum. Genet.,* 49, 338, 1991.

45. Dallongeville, J., Lussier-Cacan, S., and Davignon, J., Modulation of plasma triglyceride levels by apoE phenotype: a meta-analysis, *J. Lipid. Res.*, 33, 447, 1992.

46. Kuusi, T., Nieminen, M.S., Ehnholm, C., Yki, J.H., Valle, M., Nikkila, E.A., and Taskinen, M.R., Apoprotein E polymorphism and coronary artery disease. Increased prevalence of apolipoprotein E-4 in angiographically verified coronary patients, *Arteriosclerosis,* 9, 237, 1989.

47. Hixson, J. E., Apolipoprotein E polymorphisms affect atherosclerosis in young males: pathobiological determinants of atherosclerosis in youth (PDAY) research group, *Arterioscler. Thromb.*, 11, 1237, 1991.

48. van Bockxmeer, F.M. and Mamotte, C.D.S., Apolipoprotein epsilon-4 homozygosity in young men with coronary heart disease, *Lancet*, 340, 879, 1992.

49. Eichner, J.E., Kuller, L.H., Orchard, T.J., Grandits, G.A., McCallum, L.M., Ferrell, R.E., and Neaton, J.D., Relation of apolipoprotein E phenotype to myocardial infarction and mortality from coronary artery disease, *Am. J. Cardiol.*, 71, 160, 1993.

50. Wilson, P., Myers, R.H., Larson, M.G., Ordovas, J.M., Wolt, P.A., and Schaefer, E.J., Apolipoprotein E alleles, dyslipidemia and coronary heart disease: The Framingham Offspring Study, *J. Am. Med. Assoc.,* 272, 1666,1994.

51. Tiret, L., de Knijff, P., Menzel, H.J., Ehnholm, C., Nicaud, V., and Havekes, L., Apo E polymorphism and predisposition to coronary heart disease in youths of different European populations. The EARS study. European Atherosclerosis Research Study, *Arterioscler. Thromb.,*14, 1617, 1994.

52. Stengard, J.H., Zerba, K.E., Pekkanen, J., Ehnholm, C., Nissinen, A., and Sing, C.F., Apolipoprotein E polymorphism predicts death from coronary heart disease in a longitudinal study of elderly Finnish men, *Circulation,* 91, 265, 1995.

53. de Knijff, P., and Havekes, L.M., Apolipoprotein E as a risk factor for coronary heart disease: a genetic and molecular biology approach, *Cur. Opin. Lipidol.,* 7, 59, 1996.

54. Kervinen, K., Savolainen, M.J., Salokannen, J., Hynninen, A., Heikkinen, J., Ehnholm, C., Koistinen, M.J., and Kesäniemi, Y.A., Apolipoprotein E and B polymorphisms – longevity factors assesed in nonangenarians, *Atherosclerosis,* 105, 89, 1994.

55. Louhija, J., Miettinen, H.E., Kontula, K., Tikkanen, M.J., Miettinen, T.A., and Tilvis, R.S., Aging and genetic variation of plasma apolipoproteins: Relative loss of the apolipoprotein E4 phenotype in centenarians, *Arterioscler. Tromb.,* 14, 1084, 1994.

56. Ehnholm, C., Lukka, M., Kuusi, T., Nikkila, E., and Utermann, G., Apolipoprotein E polymorphism in the Finnish population: gene frequencies and relation to lipoprotein concentrations, *J. Lipid Res.,* 27, 227, 1986.

57. Eggertsen, G., Tegelman, R., Ericsson S., Angelin B., and Berglund, L., Apolipoprotein E polymorphism in a healthy Swedish population. Variation of allele frequency with age and relation to serum lipid concentrations, *Clin. Chem.,* 39, 2125, 1993.

58. James, R.W., Boemi, M., Giansanti, R., Fumelli, P., and Pometta D., Underexpression of the apolipoprotein E4 isoform in an Italian population, *Arterioscler. Thromb.,* 13, 1456, 1993.

59. Sklavounou, E., Economou-Petersen, E., Karadima, G., Panas, M., Avramopoulos, D., Varsou, A., Vassilopoulos, D., and Petersen, M.B., Apolipoprotein E polymorphism in the Greek population, *Clin. Genet.,* 52, 216, 1997.

60. Tikkanen, M.J., Huttunen, J.K., Ehnholm, C., and Pietinen, P., Apolipoprotein E4 homozygosity predisposes to serum cholesterol elevation during high fat diet. *Arteriosclerosis,* 10, 285, 1990.

61. Sepehrnia, B., Kamboh, M.I., Adams, C.L., Bunkner, C.H., Nwankwo, M., Majumder, P.P., and Ferrell, R.E., Genetic studies of human apolipoproteins. X. The effect of the apolipoprotein E polymorphism on quantitative levels of lipoproteins in Nigerian blacks. *Am. J. Hum. Genet.,* 45, 586, 1989.

62. Tikkanen, M.J., Apolipoprotein E polymorphism and plasma cholesterol response to dietary change, in *Genetic Variation and Dietary Response*, World Rev. Nutr. Diet., vol. 80, Simopoulos, A.P. and Nestel, P.J., Eds., Basel, Karger, 1997,15.

63. Miettinen, T.A., Gylling, H., and Vanhaven, H., Serum cholesterol response to dietary cholesterol and apolipoprotein E phenotype, *Lancet,* II,1261, 1988.

64. Miettinen, T.A. and Kesäniemi, Y.A., Cholesterol absorption: regulation of cholesterol synthesis and elimination and within-population variation of serum cholesterol levels, *Am. J. Clin. Nutr.,* 49, 629, 1989.

65. Mänttäri, M., Koskinen, P., Ehnholm, C., Huttunen, J.K., and Mannine, V., Apolipoprotein E polymorphism influences the serum cholesterol response to dietary intervention, *Metabolism,* 40, 217, 1991.

66. Miettinen, T.A., Gylling, H., Vanhaven, H., and Ollus, A., Cholesterol absorption, elimination, and synthesis related to LDL kinetics during varying fat intake in men with different apoprotein E phenotypes, *Arterioscler. Thromb.*, 12, 1044, 1992.

67. Lehtimäki, T., Moilanen, T., Solakivi, T., Laippala, P., and Ehnholm, C., Cholesterol-rich diet induced changes in plasma lipids in relation to apolipoprotein E phenotype in healthy students, *Ann. Med.*, 24, 61, 1992.

68. Cobb, M.M., Teitelbaum, H.S., Risch, N., Jekel, J.J., and Ostfeld, A.M., Influence of dietary fat, apolipoprotein E phenotype and sex on plasma lipoprotein levels. *Circulation*, 86, 849, 1992.

69. Lopez-Miranda, J., Ordovas, J.M., Mata, P., Lichtestein A.H., Cleridence, B., Judd, J.T., and Schaefer, E.J., Effect of apolipoprotein E phenotype on diet induced lowering of plasma low density lipoprotein cholesterol. *J. Lipid Res.*, 35, 1965, 1994.

70. Boerwinkle, E., Brown, S.A., Rohrbach, K., Gotto, A.M., and Patsch, N., Role of apolipoprotein E and B gene variation in determining responce of lipid, lipoprotein and apolipoprotein levels to increased dietary cholesterol. *Am. J. Hum. Genet.*, 49, 1145, 1991.

71. Glatz, J.F.C., Demacker, P.N.M., Turner, P.R., and Katan, M.B., Response of serum cholesterol to dietary cholesterol in relation to apolipoprotein E phenotype. *Nutr. Metab. Cardiovas. Dis.*, 1, 13,1991.

72. Savolainen, J.M., Rantala, M., Kervinen, K., Jarvi, L., Suvanto, K., Rantala, T., and Kesaniemi, Y.A., Magnitude of dietary effects on plasma cholesterol concentration: role of sex and apolipoprotein E phenotype, *Atherosclerosis*, 86, 145, 1991.

73. Cobb, M.M., and Risch, N., Low-density lipoprotein cholesterol responsiveness to diet in normolipidemic subjects, *Metabolism*, 42, 7, 1993.

74. Sarkkinen, E.S., Uusitupa, M.I.J., Pietinen, P., Aro, A., Ahola, I., Penttila, I., Kervinen, K., and Kesaniemi, Y.A., Long term effects of three fat-modified diets in hypercholesterolemic subjects, *Atherosclerosis*, 105, 9, 1994.

75. Zambon, D., Ros, E., Casals, E., Sanllehy, C., Bertomeu, A., and Campero, I., Effect of apolipoprotein E polymophism on the serum lipid response to a hypolipidemic diet rich in monounsaturated fatty acids in patients with hypercholesterolemia and combined hyperlipidemia, *Am. J. Clin. Nutr.*, 61, 141, 1995.

76. Uusitupa, M.I.J., Ruuskanen, E., Makinen, E., Laitinen, J., Toskala, E., Kervinen, K., and Kesäniemi, Y.A., A controlled study on the effect of beta-glycan-rich oat bran on serum lipids in hypercholesterolemic subjects: relation to apolipoprotein E phenotype, *J. Am. Coll. Nutr.*, 11, 651, 1992.

77. Jenkins, D.J.A., Hegele, R.A., Jenkins, A.L., Connely, P.W., Hallak, K., Bracci, P., Kashtan, H., Corey, P., Pintilia, M., Stern, H., and Bruce, R., The apolipoprotein E gene and the serum low-density lipoprotein cholesterol response to dietary fiber, *Metabolism*, 42, 585, 1993.

78. Loctionov, A., Bingham, S.A., Vorster, H., Jerling, J. C., Runswick, S.A., and Cummings, J.H., Apolipoprotein E genotype modulates the effect of black tea drinking on blood lipids and blood coagulation factors: a pilot study, *Br. J. Nutr.*, 79, 133, 1998.

79. Dreon, D.M. and Krauss, R.M., Diet-gene interactions in human lipoprotein metabolism, *J. Am. Coll. Nutr.*, 16, 313, 1997.

80. Ordovas, J.M., The genetics of serum lipid responsiveness to dietary interventions. *Proc. Nutrition Society*, 58, 171, 1999.

81. Simopoulos, A.P. and Nestel, P., Eds., *Genetic Variation and Dietary Response.* World Rev. Nutr. Diet., vol 80, Basel, Karger, 1997.

82. Tall, A.R., Plasma high density lipoproteins. Metabolism and relationship to atherogenesis. *J. Clin. Invest.*, 86, 379, 1990.

83. Tall, A.R., Plasma cholesteryl transfer protein. *J. Lipid Res.,* 34,1255, 1993.

84. Bhatnagar, D., Durrington, P.N., Channon, K.M., Prais, H., and Mackness, M.I., Increased transfer of cholesteryl esters from high density lipoproteins to low density and very low density lipoproteins in patients with angiographic evidence of coronary artery disease, *Atherosclerosis*, 98, 25, 1993.

85. Drayna, D., and Lawn, R., Multiple RFLPs at the human cholesteryl ester transfer protein (CETP) locus, *Nucleic Acids Res.*, 15, 4698, 1987.

86. Inazu, A., Brown, M.L., Hesler, C.B., Agellon, L.B., Koizumi, J., Takata, K., Maruhama, Y., Mabuchi, H., and Tall, A.R. Increased high-density lipoprotein levels caused by a common cholesteryl-ester transfer protein gene mutation. *N. Engl. J. Med.*, 323, 1234, 1990.

87. Inazu, A., Jiang, X.C., Haraki, T., Yagi, K., Kamon, N., Koizumi, J., Mabuchi, H., Takeda, R., Takata, K., Moriyama, Y., Doi, M., and Tall, A.R., Genetic cholesteryl ester transfer protein deficiency caused by two prevalent mutations as a major determinant of increased levels of high density lipoprotein cholesterol, *J. Clin. Invest.*, 94, 1872, 1994.

88. Freeman, D.J., Packard, C.J., Shepherd, J., and Gaffney, D., Polymorphisms in the gene coding for cholesteryl transfer protein are related to plasma high-density lipoprotein cholesterol and transfer protein activity, *Clin. Sci. Colch.*, 79, 575, 1990.

89. Freeman, D.J., Griffin, B.A., Holmes, A.P., Lindsay, G.M., Gaffney, D., Packard, C.J., and Shepherd, J., Regulation of plasma HDL cholesterol and subfraction distribution by genetic and evnironmental factors: Associations between the TaqI B RFLP in the CETP gene and smoking and obesity, *Arterioscler. Thromb.*, 14, 336, 1994.

90. Hannuksela, M.L., Liinamaa, M.J., Kesaniemi, Y.A., and Savolainen, M.J., Relation of polymorphisms in the cholesteryl ester transfer protein gene to transfer protein activity and plasma lipoprotein levels in alcohol drinkers, *Atherosclerosis*, 110, 35, 1994.

91. Kondo, I., Berg, K., Drayna, D., and Lawn, R., DNA polymorphism at the locus for human cholesteryl ester transfer protein (CETP) is associated with high density lipoprotein cholesterol and apolipoprotein levels, *Clin. Gent.*, 35, 49, 1989.

92. Mendis, S., Shepherd, J., Packard, C.J., and Gaffney, D., Genetic variation in the cholesteryl ester transfer protein and apolipoprotein A-I genes and its relation to coronary heart disease in a Sri Lankan population, *Atherosclerosis*, 83, 21, 1990.

93. Zhong, S., Sharp, D.S., Grove, J.S., Bruce, C., Yano, K., Curb, J.D., and Tall, A.R., Increased coronary heart disease in Japanese-American men with mutation in the cholesteryl ester transfer protein gene despite increased HDL levels, *J. Clin. Invest.*, 97, 2917, 1996.

94. Gudnason, V., Kakko, S., Nicaud, V., Savolainen, M.J., Kesaniemi, Y.A., Tahvanainen, E., and Humphries, S., on behalf of the EARS group, Cholesteryl ester transfer protein gene effect on CETP activity and plasma high-density lipoprotein in European populations, *Eur. J. Clin. Invest.*, 29,116, 1999.

95. Fumeron, F., Betoulle, D., Luc, G., Behague, I., Ricard, S., Poirier, O., Jemaa, R., Evans A., Arveiler, D., Marques-Vidal P., Bard, J.M., Fruchart, J.C., Ducimetiere P., Apfelbaum M.,and Cambien F., Alcohol intake modulates the effect of a polymorphism of the cholesteryl ester transfer protein gene on plasma high density lipoprotein and the risk of myocardial infarction, *J. Clin. Invest.*, 96,1664, 1995.

96. Scanou, A.M., Lawn, R.M., and Berg, K., Lipoprotein(a) and atherosclerosis. *Ann. Intern. Med.*, 115, 209, 1991.

97. Kostner, G.M., and Krempler, F., Lipoprotein(a). *Curr. Opin. Lipidol.*, 3, 279, 1992.

98. Dahlen, G.H., Lp(a) lipoprotein in cardiovascular disease, *Atherosclerosis*, 108, 111, 1994.

99. Djurovic, S., and Berg, K., Epidemiology of Lp(a) lipoprotein: its role in atherosclerotic /thrombotic disease, *Clin. Genet.*, 52, 281,1997.

100. Harris, E.D., Lipoprotein[a]: a predictor of atherosclerotic disease, *Nutr. Rev.*, 55, 61, 1997.

101. Kraft, H.G., Lingenhel, A., Kochl, S., Hoppichler, F., Kronenberg, F., Abe, A., Muhlberger, V., Schonitzer, D., and Utermann, G., Apolipoprotein(a) Kringle IV repeat number predicts risk for coronary heart disease. *Arterioscler. Thromb. Vasc. Biol.*, 16, 713, 1996.

102. Chait, A., Brazg, R.L., Tribble, D.L., and Krauss, R.M., Susceptibility of small, dense, low-density lipoproteins to oxidative modification in subjects with the atherogenic lipoprotein phenotype, pattern B. *Am. J. Med.*, 94, 350, 1993.

103. Krauss, R.M., Genetic, metabolic and dietary influences on the atherogenic lipoprotein phenotype, in *Genetic Variation and Dietary Response*, World Rev. Nutr. Diet., vol 80, Simopoulos, A.P., and Nestel, P.J., Eds., Basel, Karger, 1997, 22.

104. Austin, M.A., Breslow, J.L., Hennekens, C.H., Buring, J.E., Willett, W.C., and Krauss, R.M., Low-density lipoprotein subclass patterns and risk of myocardial infarction, *J. Am. Med. Assoc.*, 260, 1917, 1988.

105. Crouse, J.R., Parks, J.S., Schey, H.M., and Kohl, F.R., Studies of low density lipoprotein molecular weight in human beings with coronary artery disease, *J. Lipid. Res.*, 26, 566, 1985.

106. Campos, H., Genest, J.J., Jr., Blijlevens, E., McNamara, J.R., Jenner, J.L., Ordovas, J.M., Wilson, P.W.F., and Scaefer, E.J., Low density lipoprotein particle size and coronary artery disease, *Arterioscler. Tromb.*, 12, 187, 1992.

107. Coresh, J., Kwiterovich, P.O.Jr., Smith, H.H., and Bachorik, P.S., Association of plasma triglyceride concentration and LDL particle diameter, density, and chemical composition with premature coronary artery disease in men and women, *J. Lipid Res.*, 34, 1687, 1993.

108. Austin, M.A., King, M.C., Vranizan, K.M., Newman, B., and Krauss, R.M., Inheritance of low-density lipoprotein subclass paterns: results of complex segregation analysis, *Am. J. Hum. Genet.*, 43, 838, 1988.

109. Austin, M.A., Genetic epidemiology of low-density lipoprotein subclass phenotypes, *Ann. Med.*, 24, 477, 1992.

110. Rotter, J.I., Bu, X., Cantor, R., Warden, C.H., Brown, J., Gray, R.J., Blanche, P.J., Krauss, R.M., and Lusis, A.J., Multilocus genetic determinants of LDL particle size in coronary artery disease families, *Am. J. Hum. Gent.*, 58, 585, 1996.

111. Austin, M.A., Newman, B., Selby, J.V., Edwards, K., Mayer, E.J., and Krauss, R.M., Genetics of LDL subclass phenotypes in women twins: Concordance, heritability, and commingling analysis, *Arterioscl. Tromb.*, 13, 687, 1993.

112. Krauss, R.M. and Dreon, D.M., Low density lipoprotein subclasses and response to a low-fat diet in healthy men, *Am. J. Clin. Nutr.*, 62, 478S, 1995.

113. Dreon, D.M., Fernstrom, H.A., Miller, B., and Krauss, R.M., Low-density lipoprotein subclass patterns and lipoprotein response to a reduced-fat diet in men. *FASEB J.*, 8, 121, 1994.

114. Graham, I.M., Homocysteinaemia and vascular disease, in *Epidemiology*, Luxembourg: Commission of the European Community, Vuylsteek, K., and Hallen, M., Eds., Ios Press, 1994, 332.

115. Mayer, H., Jacobsen, D.W., and Robinson, K., Homocystein and coronary atherosclerosis, *J. Am. Coll. Cardiol.*, 27, 517, 1996.

116. Stampfer, M.J., Malinow, M.R., Willlett, W.C., Newcomer, L.M., Upson, B., Ullmann, D., Tishler, P.V., and Hennekens, C.H., A prospective study of plasma homocyst(e)ine and risk for myocardial infarction in US physicians, *J. Am. Med. Assoc.*, 268, 877, 1992.

117. Selhub, J., Jacques, P.F., Wilson, P.W., Rush, D., and Rosemberg, I.H., Vitamin status and intake as primary determinants of homocysteinemia in an elderly population, *J. Am. Med. Assoc.*, 270, 2693, 1993.

118. Kang, S.S., Wong, P.W.K., Susman, A., Sora, J., Norusis, M., and Ruggie, N., Thermolibile methylenetetrahydrofolate reductase: An inherited risk factor for coronary heart disease, *Am. J. Hum. Genet.*, 48, 538, 1991.

119. Frost, P., Blom, H.J., Milos, R., Goyette, P., Sheppard C.A., Matthews, R.G., Boers, G.J., den Heijer, M., Kluuijtmans, L.A., van den Heuvel, L.P., et al., A candidate genetic risk factor for vascular disease: A common mutation in methylenetetrahydrofolate reductase, *Nat. Genet.*, 10, 111, 1995.

120. De Franchis, R., Sebastio, G., Mandato, C., Andria, G., and Mastroiacovo, P., Spina bifida, 667→C mutation and role of folate, *Lancet,* 346, 1703, 1995.

121. Kirke, P.N., Mills, J.L., Whitehead, A.S., Molloy, A., and Scott, J.M., Methylenetetrahydrofolate reductase mutation and neural tube defects, *Lancet,* 348, 1037, 1996.

122. Kang, S.S., Passen, E.L., Ruggie, N., Wong, P.W.K., and Sora, H., Thermolibile defect of methylenetetrahydrofolate reductase in coronary artery disease, *Circulation*, 88, 1463, 1993.

123. Engbersen, A.M.T., Franken, D.G., Boers, G.H.J., Stevens, E.M.B., Trijbels, F.J.M., and Blom, H.J., Thermolibile 5,10-methylenetetrahydrofolate reductase as a cause of mild hyperhomocycteinemia, *Am. J. Hum. Gen.*, 56, 142, 1995.

124. Kluijtmans, L.A.J., van den Heuval, L.P.W., Boers, G.H.J., Frosst, P., Stevens, E.M., van Dost, B.A., den Heijer, M., Trijbels, F.J., Rozen, R., and Blom, H.J., Molecular genetic analysis in mild hyperhomocycteinemia: A common mutation in the methylenetetrahydrofolate reductase gene is a genetic risk factor for cardiovascular disease, *Am. J. Hum. Genet.*, 58, 35, 1996.

125. Wilhemsen, L., Svardsudd, K., Korsan-Bengtsen, K., Larsson, B., Welin, L., and Tibblin, G., Fibrinogen as a risk factor for stroke and myocardial iunfraction, *N. Engl. J. Med.*, 311, 501, 1984.

126. Yarnell, J.W., Baker, I.A., Sweetnam, P.M., Bainton, D., O'Brien, J.R., Whitehead, P.J., and Elwood, P.C., Fibrinogen, viscosity and white blood cell count are major risk factors for ishaemic heart disease. The Caerphilly and Speedwell Collaborative Heart disease Studies, *Circulation*, 83, 836, 1991.

127. Ernst, E. and Resh, K.L., Fibrinogen as a cardiovascular risk factor: a meta-analysis and review of the literature, *Ann. Inter. Med.*, 118, 956, 1993.

128. Thompson, S.G., Kienast, J.K., Pyke, S.D.M., Havberkate, F., and van de Loo, C.W., for the European Concerted Action on Thrombosis and Disabilities Angina Pectoris Study Group, Hemostatic factors and the risk of myocardial infarction or sudden death in patients with angina pectoris, *N. Engl. J. Med.*, 332, 635, 1995.

129. Balleisen, L., Schulte, H., Assman, G., Epping, P.H., and van de Loo, J., Coagulation factors and the progress of coronary heart disease, *Lancet*, II 461, 1987.

130. Kannel, W.B., Wolf, P.A., Castelli, W.P., and D'Agostino, R.P., Fibrinogen and risk of cardiovascular disease. The Framingham Study, *J. Am. Med. Assoc.*, 258, 1183, 1987.

131. Humphries, S.E., Cook, M., Dubowitz, M., Stirling, Y., and Meade, T.W., Role of genetic variation at the fibrinogen locus in determination of plasma fibrinogen concentrations, *Lancet*, i,1452, 1987.

132. Hamsten, A., Iselius, L., de Faire, U., and Blomback, M., Genetic and cultural inheritance of plasma fibrinogen concentration, *Lancet*, i, 988, 1987.

133. Chung, D.W., Harris, J.E., and Davie, E.W., Nucleotide sequence of the 3 genes coding for human fibrinogen, in *Thrombosis, Coagulation and Fibrinolysis*, Liu, C.Y., and Chien, S., Eds., New York, Plenum, 1990, 39.

134. Fowkes, F.G.R., Connor, J.M., Smith, F.B., Wood, J., Donnan, P.T., and Lowe, G.D.O., Fibrinogen genotype and the risk of peripheral atherosclerosis, *Lancet*, 339, 693, 1992.

135. Heinrich, J., Funke, H., Rust, S., Schulte, H., Schonfeld, R., Kohler, E., and Assmann, G., Impact of polymorphisms in the alpha- and beta-fibrinogen gene on plasma fibrinogen concentrations of coronary heart disease patients, *Thromb. Res.*, 77, 209, 1995.

136. Yu, Q., Safavi, F., Roberts, R., and Marian, A.J., A variant of beta fibrinogen is a genetic risk factor for coronary artery disease and myocardial infarction, *J. Invest. Med.*, 44, 154, 1996.

137. Lee, A.J., Fowkes, F.G., Lowe, G.D., Connor, J.M., and Rumley, A., Fibrinogen, factor VII and PAI-1 genotypes and the risk of coronary and peripheral atherosclerosis: Edinburgh Artery Study, *Thromb. Haemost.*, 81, 553,1999.

138. Behague, I., Poirier, O., Nicaud, V., Evans, A., Arveiler, D., Luc, G., Cambou, J.P., Scarabin, P.Y., Bara, L., Green, F., and Cambien, F., Beta fibrinogen gene polymorphisms are associated with plasma fibrinogen and coronary artery disease in patients with myocardial infarction. The ECTIM Study. Etude Cas-Temoins sur l'Infarctus du Myocarde, *Circulation*, 93, 440, 1996.

139. de Maat, M.P., Kastelein, J.J., Jukema, J.W., Zwinderman, A.H., Jansen, H., Groenemeier, B., Bruschke, A.V., and Kluft, C., -455G/A polymorphism of the beta-fibrinogen gene is associated with the progression of coronary atherosclerosis in symptomatic men: proposed role for an acute-phase reaction pattern of fibrinogen. REGRESS group, *Arterioscler. Thromb. Vasc. Biol.*, 18, 265, 1998.

140. Weiss, E.J., Bray, P.F., Tayback, M., Schulman, S.P., Kickler, T.S., Becker, L.C., Weiss, J.L., Gerstenblith, G., and Goldschmidt-Clermont, P.J., A polymorphism of a platelet glycoprotein receptor as an inherited risk factor for coronary thrombosis, *New Engl. J. Med.*, 334, 1090, 1996.

141. Gardemann, A., Humme, J., Stricker, J., Nguyen, Q.D., Katz, N., Phillip, M., Tillmanns, H., Hehrlein, F.W., Rau, M., and Haberbosch, W., Association of the platelet glycoprotein IIIa PIA1/A2 gene polymorphism to coronary artery disease but not to nonfatal myocardial infarction in low risk patients, *Thromb. Haemost.*, 80, 214, 1998.

142. Cambien, F. and Soubrier, F., The angiotensin-converting enzyme: molecular biology and implication of the gene polymorphism in cardiovascular diseases, in *Hypertension: Physiology, Diagnosis and Management*, 2nd ed., Laragh, J.H. and Brenner, B.M., Eds., New York., Raven Press, 1995, 1667.

143. Rigat, B., Hubert, C., Alhenc-Gelas, F., Cambien, F., Corvol, P., and Soubrier, F., An insertion-deletiuon polymorphism in the angiotensin-converting enzyme gene accounting for half the variance of serum enzyme levels, *J. Clin. Invest.*, 86, 1343, 1990.

144. Cambien, F., Poirier, O., Lecerf, L., Evans, A., Cambou, J.P., Arveiler, D., Luc, G., Bard, J.M., Bara, L., Ricard, S., et al., Deletion polymorphism in the gene for angiotensin-converting enzyme is a potent risk factor for myocardial infarction, *Nature*, 359, 641, 1992.

145. Tiret, L., Kee, F., Poirier, O., Nicaud, V., Lecerf, L., Evans, A., Cambou, J.P., Arveiler, D., Luc, G., Amouyel, P., et al., Deletion polymorphism in the angiotensin-converting enzyme gene is associated with a parental history of myocardial infarction, *Lancet*, 341, 991, 1993.

146. Tiret, L., Bonnardeaux, A., Poirier, O., Ricard, S., Marques-Vidal, P., Evans, A., Arveiler, D., Luc, G., Kee, F., Ducimetiere, P., et al., Synergistic effect of angiotensin-converting enzyme gene and angiotensin-II type 1 receptor gene polymorphisms on the risk of myocardial infarction, *Lancet*, 334, 910, 1994.

147. Simopoulos, A.P., Ed., *Evolutionary Aspects of Nutrition and Health. Diet, Exercise, Genetics and Chronic Disease*, World Rev. Nutr. Diet., vol. 84, Basel, Karger, 1999.

148. Mattson, F. and Grundy, S., Comparison of effects of dietary saturated, monounsaturated and polyunsaturated fatty acids on plasma lipids and lipoprotein in man, *J. Lipid. Res.*, 26, 194, 1985.

149. Williams, C.M., Knapper, J.M.E., Webb, D., Zampelas, A., Tredger, J.A., Wright, J., Meijer, G., Calder, P.C., Yaqoob, P., Roche, H., and Gibney, M.J., Cholesterol reduction using manufactured foods high in monounsaturated fatty acids, a randomized crossover study, *Br. J. Nutr.*, 81, 439, 1999.

150. Mensink, R. and Katan, M., Effect of a diet enriched with monounsaturated fatty acids on levels of LDL- and HDL-cholesterol in healthy women and men, *New Engl. J. Med.*, 321, 436, 1989.

151. Jones, A.E., Smith, R.D., Kelly, C., Williams, C.M., and Wootton, S.A., Oxidation of dietary fat is decreased on an isocaloric saturated fat diet compared with a monounsaturated fat diet, *Atherosclerosis*, 144 (Suppl 1), 171A, 1999.

152. Mensink, R., de Groot, M., van den Broeke, L.T., Severijnen-Nobels, A.P., Demacker, P.N., and Katan, M.B., Effects of monounsaturated fatty acids vs complex carbohydrates on serum lipoproteins and apoproteins in healthy men and women, *Metabolism*, 38, 172, 1989.

153. Hudgins, L.C., Hellerstein, M., Seidman, C., Neese, R., Diakun, J., Hirsch, J., Human fatty acid synthesis is stimulated by a eucaloric low fat, high carbohydrate diet, *J. Clin. Invest.*, 97, 2081, 1996

154. Mensink, R., and Katan, M., Effect of monosaturated fatty acid versys complex carbohydrates on high density lipoproteins in healthy men and women, *Lancet*, 1, 122, 1987.

155. Reaven, P., Parthasarathym, S., Grasse, B.J., Miller, E., Steinberg, D., Witztum, J.L., Effects of oleate-rich and linoleate-rich diets on the susceptibility of low density lipoprotein to oxidative modifiacation modification in midly hypercholesterolemic subjects, *J. Clin. Invest.*, 91, 668, 1993.

156. Khoo, J.C., Steinberg, D., and Witztum, J.L., Feasibility of using oleate-rich diet to reduce the susceptibility of LDL to oxidative modification in humans, *Am. J. Clin. Nutr.*, 54, 701, 1991.

157. Berry, E.M., Eisenberg, S., Haratz, D., Friedlander, Y., Norman, Y., Kaufmann, N.A., and Stein, Y., Effects of diets rich in monounsaturated fatty acids on plasma lipoproteins-the Jerusalem Nutrition Study: high MUFAs vs. high PUFAs, *Am. J. Clin. Nutr.*, 53, 899, 1991.

158. Reaven, P.D., Parthasarathy, S., Grasse, B.J., Miller, E., Steinberg, D., and Witztum, J.L., Effects of oleate-rich and linoleate-rich diets on the susceptibility of low density lipoprotein to oxidative modification in mildly hypercholesterolemic subjects, *J. Clin. Invest.*, 91, 668, 1993.

159. Stampfer, M., Hennekens, C., Manson, J.E., Colditz, G.A., Rosner, B., and Willett, W.C., Vitamin E consumption and the risk of coronary disease in women, *New Engl. J. Med.*, 328, 1444, 1993.

160. Steinberg, D. and Witztum, J., Lipoproteins and atherogenesis: current concepts, *J. Am. Med. Assoc.*, 264, 3047, 1990.

161. Mata, P., Varela, O., Alonso, R., Lahoz, C., de Oya, M., and Badimon, L., Monounsaturated and polyunsaturated n-6 fatty-acid-enriched diets modify LDL oxidation and decrease human coronary smooth muscle cell DNA synthesis, *Arterioscler. Thromb. Vasc. Biol.*, 17, 2088, 1997.

162. Visioli, F. and Galli, C., The effect of minor constituents of olive oil on cardiovascular disease: new findings, *Nutr. Rev.*, 56, 142, 1998.

163. Roche, H., Zampelas, A., Knapper, J.M., Webb, D., Brooks, C., Jackson, K.G., Wright, J., Gould, B.J., Kafatos, A., Gibney, M.J., and Williams, C.M., Effect of long-term olive oil dietary intervention on postprandial triacylglycerol and factor VII metabolism, *Am. J. Clin. Nutr.*, 68, 552, 1998.

164. Lopez-Segura, F., Velasco, F., Lopez-Miranda, J., Castro, P., Lopez-Pedrera, R., Blanco, A., Jimenez-Pereperez, J., Torres, A., Trujillo, J., Ordovas, J.M., and Perez-Jimenez, F., Monounsaturated fatty-acid enriched diet decreases plasma plasminogen activator inhibitor type 1, *Arterioscler. Thromb. Vasc. Biol.*, 16, 82, 1996.

165. Temme, E.H., Mensink, R.P., and Hornstra, G., Effects of diets enriched in lauric, palmitic or oleic acids on blood coagulation and fibrinolysis, *Thromb. Hemost.*, 81, 259, 1999.

166. Oakley, F.R., Sanders, T.A., and Miller, G.J., Postprandial effects of an oleic acid-rich oil compared with butter on clotting factor VII and fibrinolysis in healthy men, *Am. J. Clin. Nutr.*, 68, 1202, 1998.

167. Trichopoulou, A., Lagiou, P., and Trichopoulos, D., Traditional Greek diet and coronary heart disease, *J. Cardiovasc. Risk*, 1, 9, 1994.

168. Kushi, L.H., Lenart, E.B., and Willett, W.C., Health implications of Mediterranean diets in light of contemporary knowledge. 1. Plant foods and dairy products, *Am. J. Clin. Nutr.*, 61(Suppl), 1407S, 1995.

169. Ness, A.R. and Powles, J.W., Fruit and vegetables, and cardiovascular disease: a review, *Int. J. Epidemiol.*, 26, 1, 1997.

170. Gjonca, A. and Bobak, M., Albanian paradox, another example of protective effect of Mediterranean lifestyle? *Lancet*, 350, 1815, 1997.

171. Zino, S., Skeaff, M., Williams, S., and Mann J., Randomised controlled trial of effect of fruit and vegetable consumption on plasma concentrations of lipids and antioxidants, *Br. Med. J.*, 314, 1787, 1997.

172. Jenkins, D.J., Popovich, D.G., Kendall, C.W., Vidgen, E., Tariq, N., Ransom, T.P., Wolever, T.M., Vuksan, V., Mehling, C.C., Boctor, D.L., Bolognesi, C., Huang, J., and Patten R., Effect of a diet high in vegetables, fruit and nuts on serum lipids, *Metabolism*, 46, 530, 1997.

173. Nilsson, T.K., Sundell, I.B., Hellsten, G., and Hallmans, G., Reduced plasminogen activator inhibitor activity in high consumers of fruits, vegetables and root vegetables, *J. Intern. Med.*, 227, 267, 1990.

174. Singh, R.B., Niaz, M.A., Ghosh, S., Singh, R., and Rastogi, S.S., Effect on mortality and reinfarction of adding fruits and vegetables to a prudent diet in the Indian experiment of infarct survival (IEIS), *J. Am. Coll. Nutr.*, 12, 255, 1993.

175. Anderson, J. W., Johnstone, B.M., and Cook-Newell, M.E., Meta-analysis of the effects of soy protein intake on serum lipids, *New Eng. J. Med.*, 333, 276, 1995.

176. Kushi, L.H., Meyer, K.A., and Jacobs, D.R., Cereals, legumes, and chronic disease risk reduction: evidence from epidemiologic studies, *Am. J. Clin. Nutr.,* 70(Suppl): 451S, 1999.
177. Khaw, K.T. and Barrett-Connor, E., Dietary fiber and reduced ischemic heart disease mortality rates in men and women: a 12-year prospective study, *Am. J. Epidemiol.,* 126, 1093, 1987.
178. Rimm, E. B., Ascherio, A., Giovannucci, E., Spiegelman, D., Stampfer, M.J., and Willett, W.C., Vegetable, fruit and cereal fiber intake and risk of coronary heart disease among men, *J. Am. Med. Assoc.,* 275, 447, 1996
179. Anderson, J.W., Smith, B.M., and Gustafson, N.J., Health benefits and practical aspects of high fiber diets, *Am. J. Clin. Nutr.,* 59(Suppl), 1242S, 1994.
180. Keys, A., Grande, F., and Anderson, J.T., Fiber and pectin in the diet and serum cholesterol in man, *Proc. Soc. Exp. Biol. Med.,* 106, 555, 1961.
181. Truswell, A.S., Dietary fiber and blood lipids, *Curr. Opinion Lipidol.,* 6, 14, 1995.
182. Kay, R.M. and Truswell, A.S., Effect of citrus pectin on blood lipids and fecal steroids in man, *Am. J. Clin. Nutr.,* 30, 171, 1977.
183. Anderson, J.M. and Chen, W-J.L., Plant fiber, carbohydrate and lipid metabolism, *Am. J. Clin. Nutr.,* 32, 346, 1979.
184. Truswell, A.S. and Beynen, A.C., Prevention and treatment of hyperlipidemias, in *Dietary Fiber. A Company of Food,* Schweizer, T.F., and Edwards, C.A., Eds., Springer-Verlag, London, 1992, 295.
185. Anderson, J.W. and Hanna, T.J., Impact of nondigestible carbohydrates on serum lipoproteins and risk for cardiovascular disease, *J. Nutr.,* 129(Suppl 7), 1457S, 1999.
186. Menotti, A., Kromhout, D., Blackburn, H., Fidanza, F., Buzina, R., and Nissinen, A., Food intake patterns and 25-year mortality from coronary heart disease: cross-cultural correlations in the Seven Countries Study, *Eur. J. Epidemiol.,* 15, 507, 1999.
187. Gey, K.F., Puska, P., Jordan, P., and Moser, U.K, Inverse correlation between plasma vitamin E and mortality from ischemic heart disease in cross-cultural epidemiology, *Am. J. Clin. Nutr.,* 53, 326S, 1991.
188. Losonczy, K.G., Harris, T.B., and Havlik, R.J., Vitamin E and vitamin C supplement use and risk of all-cause and coronary heart disease mortality in older persons: the Established Populations for Epidemiologic Studies of the Elderly, *Am. J. Clin. Nutr.,* 64, 190, 1996.
189. Rimm, E.B., Stampfer, M.J., Ascheiro, A., Giovannucci, E., Colditz, G.A., and Willett, W.C., Vitamin E consumption and the risk of coronary heart disease in men, *New Eng. J. Med.,* 328, 1450, 1993.
190. Stampfer, M., Hennekens, C.H., Manson, J.E., Colditz, G.A., Rosner, B., and Willett, W.C. Vitamin E consumption and the risk of coronary heart disease in women. *New Eng. J. Med.,* 328, 1444, 1993.
191. Stephens, N.G., Parsons, A., Schonfield, P.A., Kelly, F., Cheeseman, K., and Mitchinson, M.J., Randomized control trial of vitamin E in patients with coronary disease: Cambridge Heart AntiOxidant Study (CHAOS), *Lancet,* 347, 781, 1996.
192. Elinder, L.S. and Walldius, G., Antioxidants and atheroscerosis progression: unresolved questions. *Curr. Opin. Lipidol.,* 5, 265, 1994.
193. Gey, K.F., Brubacher, G.B., and Stähelin, H.B., Plasma levels of antioxidant vitamins in relation to ischemic heart disease and cancer. *Am. J. Clin. Nutr.,* 45, 1368, 1987.
194. Harats, D., Chevion, S., Nahir, M., Norman, Y., Sagee, O., and Berry, E.M., Citrus fruit supplementation reduces lipoprotein oxidation in young men ingesting a diet high in saturated fat: presumptive evidence for an interaction between vitamins C and E *in vivo, Am. J. Clin. Nutr.,* 67, 240, 1998.

195. Podmore, I. D., Griffiths, H.R., Herbert, K.E., Mistry, N., Mistry, P., and Lunec, J., Vitamin C exhibits pro-oxidant properties, *Nature*, 392, 1998.
196. Hennekens, C. H., Buring, J.E., Manson, J.E., Stampfer, M., Rosner, B., Cook, N.R., Belanger, C., Lamotte, F. et al., Lack of effect of long-term supplementation with beta carotene on the incidence of malignant neoplasms and cardiovascular disease, *New Eng. J. Med.,* 334, 1145, 1996.
197. Hollman, P.C.H. and Katan, M.B., Dietary flavonoids: Intake, Health Effects and Bioavailability, *Food Chem. Toxicol.*, 37, 937, 1999.
198. Weisburger, J.H., Mechanisms of action of antioxidants as exemplified in vegetables, tomatoes and tea, *Food Chem. Toxicol.*, 37, 943, 1999.
199. Weisenberg, J.H., Evaluation of the evidence on the role of tomato products in disease prevention, *Proc. Soc. Exp. Biol. Med.*, 218, 140, 1998.
200. Hertog, M.G., Kromhout, D., Aravanis, C., Blackburn, H., Buzina, R., Fidanza, F., Giampaoli, S., Jansen, A., Menotti, A., Nedeljkovic, S., Pekkarinen, M., Simic, B.S., Toshima, H., Feskens, E.J.M., Hollman, P.C.H., and Katan, M.B., Flavonoid intake and long-term risk of coronary heart disease and cancer in the Seven Countries Study, *Arch. Intern. Med.*, 155, 381, 1995.
201. Hertog, M.G.L., Feskens, E.J.M., Hollman, P.C.H., Katan, M.B., and Kromhout, D., Dietary antioxidant flavonoids and risk of coronary heart disease: the Zutphen Elderly Study, *Lancet*, 342, 1007, 1993.
202. Rimm, E.B., Katan, M.B., Ascherio, A., Stampfer, M.J., and Willett, W.C., Relation between intake of flavonoids and risk for coronary heart disease in male health professionals, *Ann. Intern. Med.*, 125, 384, 1996.
203. Aviram, M. and Fuhrman, B., Polyphenolic flavonoids inhibit macrophage-mediated oxidation of LDL and attenuate atherogenesis, *Atherosclerosis*, 137 (Suppl), S45, 1998.
204. Murphy, S.P. Subar, A.F., and Block, G., Vitamin E intakes and sources in the United States, *Am. J. Clin. Nutr.,* 52, 361, 1990.
205. Brouwer, I. A., van Dusseldorp, M., West, C.E., Meyboom, S., Thomas, C.M.G., Duran M., van het Hof, K.H., Eskes, T.K.A.B., Hautvast, J.G.A.J., and Steegers-Theunissen, R.P.M., Dietary folate from vegetables and citrus fruit decreases plasma homocysteine concentrations in humans in a dietary controlled trial, *J. Nutr.*, 129, 1135, 1999.
206. Parodi, P.W., The French paradox unmasked: the role of folate. *Med. Hypoth.*, 49, 313, 1997.
207. Kushi, L., Lenart, E., and Willet, W., Health implications of Mediterranean diets in light of contemporary knowledge. 2. Meat, wine, fats, and oils, *Am. J. Clin. Nutr.,* 61(suppl.)1416S, 1995.
208. Willett, W., Sacks F, Trichopoulou A, Drescher G., Ferro-Luzzi A., Helsing E., and Trichopoulos D., Mediterranean diet pyramid: a cultural model for healthy eating, *Am. J. Clin. Nutr.,* 61(suppl.), 1402S, 1995.
209. Elmstahl, S., Holmqvist, O., Gullberg B., Johansson U., and Berglund G., Dietary patterns in high and low consumers of meat in a Swedish cohort study, *Appetite*, 32, 191, 1999.
210. Phillips, R., Lemon F, Beeson W., and Kuzma J., Coronary heart disease mortality among Seventh-day Adventists with differing dietary habits: a preliminary report, *Am. J. Clin. Nutr.,* 31(suppl.), 191S, 1978.

211. Slattery, M.L., Jacobs D.R., Hilner J.E., Caan B.J., Van Horn L., Bragg C., Manolio T.A., Kushi L.H., and Liv K., Meat consumption and its association with other diet and health factors in young adults: The CARDIA Study, *Am. J. Clin. Nutr.*, 54, 930, 1991.

212. Nicklas, T.A., Farris R.P., Myers L., and Berenson G.S., Impact of meat consumption on nutritional quality and cardiovascular risk factors in young adults: The Bogalusa Heart Study, *J. Am. Diet. Assoc.*, 95, 887, 1995.

213. Ascherio, A., Willett W., Rimm E., Giovannucci E., and Stampfer M, Dietary iron intake and risk of coronary disease among men, *Circulation*, 89, 969, 1994.

214. Key, T., Fraser G., Thorogood M., Appleby P., Beral V., Reeves G., Burr M., Chang-Claude J, Frentzel-Beyne R., Kuzma J., Mann J., and McPherson K., Mortality in vegetarians and non vegetarians: detailed findings from a collaborative analysis of% prospective studies, *Am. J. Clin. Nutr.*, 70(suppl.), 516S, 1999.

215. Kushi, L., Lew, R., Stare, F., Ellison, C., Lozy, M., Bourke, G., Daly, L., Graham, I., Hickey, N., Mulcahy, R., and Kevaney, J., Diet and 20-year mortality from coronary heart disease: the Ireland-Boston Diet-Heart Study. *New Eng. J. Med.*, 312, 811, 1985.

216. Li, D., Sinclair, A., Mann, N., Turner, A., Ball, M., Kelly, F, Abedin, L., and Wilson, A., The association of diet and thrombotic risk factors in healthy male vegetarians and meat-eaters, *Eur. J. Clin. Nutr.*, 53, 612, 1999.

217. Sacks, F.M. and Donner, A., Effects of ingestion of meat on plasma cholesterol of vegetarians, *J. Am. Med. Assoc.*, 246, 640, 1981.

218. Sullival, J., Iron and the sex difference in heart disease risk, *Lancet*, 1, 1293, 1981.

219. Gillum, R., Body iron stores and atherosclerosis, *Circulation*, 96, 3261, 1997.

220. Tuomainen, T.P., Punnonen, K., Nyyssoenen, K., and Salonen, J., Association between body iron stores and the risk of acute myocardial infarction in men, *Circulation*, 97, 1461, 1998.

221. Danesh, J. and Appleby, P., Coronary heart disease and iron status, meta-analysis of prospective studies, *Circulation*, 99, 852, 1999.

222. Reunanen, A., Takkunen, H., Knekt, P., Seppanen, R., and Aromaa, A., Body iron stores, dietary iron intake and coronary heart disease mortality, *J. Intern. Med.*, 238, 223, 1995.

223. Salonen, J.T., Nyyssonen, K., Korpela, H., Tuomolehto, J., Seppanen, R., and Salonen, R., High stored iron levels are associated with excess risk of myocardial infarction in Eastern Finnish men, *Circulation*, 86, 803, 1992.

224. Grant, W.B., Milk and other dietary influences on coronary heart disease, *Altern Med Rev*, 3(4), 281, 1998.

225. Rimm, E.B., Willett, W.C., Hu, F.B., Sampson, l., Colditz, G.A.., Manson, J.E., Hennekens, C., and Stampfer, M.J., Folate and vitamin B6 from diet and supplements in relation to risk of coronary heart disease among women. *J. Am. Med. Assoc.*, 279, 359, 1998.

226. Giles, W.H., Croft, J.B., Greenlund, K.J., Ford, E.S., and Kittner, S.J., Association between total homocyst(e)ine and the likelihood for a history of acute myocardial infarction by race and ethnicity: Results from the Third National Health and Nutrition Examination Survey. *Am. Heart. J.*, 139, 446, 2000.

227. Aronow, W.S. and Ahn, C., Association between plasma homocysteine and peripheral arterial disease in older persons. *Coron. Artery Dis.*, 9, 49, 1998.

228. U.S. Department of Agriculture. The food pyramid. Hyattsville, MD: Human Nutrition Information Service, 1992.

229. Gibney, M.J., Fish and the Mediterranean diet, *Atherosclerosis*, 144(Suppl.1),170A, 1999.

230. Tornaritis, M., Peraki, E., Georguli, M., Kafatos, A., Charalambakis, G., Divanack, P., Kentouri, M., Yiannopoulos, S., Frenaritou, H., and Argyrides, R., Fatty acid composition and total fat content of eight species of Mediterranean fish, *Intern. J. Food Sci. Nutr.*, 45, 135,1995.

231. Kromhout, D., Bosschieter, E.B., and Coulnader, C.L., The inverse relation between fish consumption and 20-year mortality from coronary heart disease, *New Eng. J. Med.*, 312, 1205, 1985.

232. Daviglus, M., Stamler, J., Orencia, A., Dyer, A., Liu, K., Greenland, P., Walsh, M., Morris, D., and Shekelle, R., Fish consumption and the 30-year risk of fatal myocardial infarction, *New Eng. J. Med.*, 336(15), 1046, 1997.

233. Markmann, P. and Gronbek, M., Fish consumption and coronary heart disease mortality. A systematic review of prospective cohort studies, *Eur. J. Clin. Nutr.*, 53, 585, 1999.

234. Burr, M., Gilbert, J, Holliday, R., Elwood, P., Fehily, A., Rogers, S., Sweetnam, P., and Deadman, N., Effects of changes in fat, fish, and fibre intakes on death and myocardial reinfarction: Diet And Reinfarction Trial (DART), *Lancet*, 8666, 757, 1989.

235. Ness, A., Whitley, E., Burr, M., Elwood, P., Smith, GD., and Ebrahim, S., The long-term effect of advice to eat more fish on blood pressure in men with coronary disease: from the diet and reinfarction trial, *J. Mun. Hypertens.*, 13, 729, 1999.

236. Garcia-Closas, R., Serra-Majem, L., and Segura, R., Fish consumption, omega-3 fatty acids and the Mediterranean diet, *Eur. J. Clin. Nutr.*, 47(suppl.1), S85, 1993.

237. Sullivan, D.R., Sanders, T.A.B., Trayner, I.M., and Thompson G.R , Paradoxical elevation of LDL apolipoprotein B levels in hypertriglyceridemic patients and normal subjects ingesting fish oil, *Atherosclerosis*, 61, 129, 1986.

238. Williams, C.M., Moore, F., Morgan, L.M., and Wright, J., Effect of n-3 fatty acids on postprandial triacylglycerol and hormone concentrations in normal subjects, *Br. J. Nutr.*, 69, 63, 1992.

239. Polyunsaturated fatty acids of the n-6 and n-3 series: effects on postprandial lipid and apolipoprotein levels in healthy men, *Eur. J. Clin. Nutr.*, 48, 842, 1994.

240. Nestel, P.J., Connor, W.E., Reardon, M.F., Connor S., Wong, S., and Boston, R., Suppression by diets rich in fish oil of very low density lipoprotein production in man, *J. Clin. Invest.*, 74, 82, 1984.

241. Zampelas, A., Murphy, M., Morgan, L.M., and Williams, C.M., Postprandial lipoprotein lipase, insulin and gastric inhibitory polypeptide responses to test meals of different fatty acid composition: comparison of saturated, n-6 and n-3 polyunsaturated fatty acids, *Eur. J. Clin. Nutr.*, 48, 849, 1994.

242. Harris, W.S. and Muzio, F., Fish oil reduces postprandial triglyceride concentrations without accelerating lipid-emulsion removal rates, *Am. J. Clin. Nutr.*, 58, 68, 1993.

243. Nozaki, S., Garg, A., Vega, G.L., and Grundy, S.M., Postheparin lipolytic activity and plasma lipoprotein response to ?-3 polyunsaturated fatty acids in patients with primary hypertriglyceridemia, *Am. J. Clin. Nutr.*, 53, 638, 1991.

244. Harris, W.S., Fish oils and plasma lipid and lipoprotein metabolism in humans: a critical review, *J. Lipid Res.*, 30, 785, 1989.

245. Huff, M.W. and Telford, D.E., Dietary fish oil increases conversion of very low density lipoprotein apolipoprotein B to low density lipoprotein, *Arteriosclerosis*, 9, 58, 1989.

246. Gianturco, S.H. and Bradley, W.A., A cellular basis for the atherogenicity of triglyceride-rich lipoproteins, *Atheroscler. Rev.*, 22, 9, 1991.

247. Contacos, C., Barter, P.J., and Sullivan, D.R., Effect of pravastatin and ω-3 fatty acids on plasma lipids and lipoproteins in patients with combined hyperlipidemia, *Arterioscler. Thromb.*, 13, 1755, 1993.

248. Blonk, M.C., Bilo, H.J.G., Nauta, J.J.P., Popp-Snijders, C., Mulder, C., and Donker, A.J.M., M., Dose-response effects of fish-oil supplementation in healthy volunteers, *Am. J. Clin. Nutr.*, 52, 120, 1990.

249. Griffin, B.A. and Zampelas, A., Influence of dietary fatty acids on the atherogenic lipoprotein phenotype, *Nutr. Res. Rev.*, 8, 1, 1995.

250. Austin, M.A., King, M.C., Vranizan, K.M., Krauss, R.M., Atherogenic lipoprotein phenotype. A proposed genetic marker for coronary heart disease risk, *Circulation*, 82, 495, 1990.

251. Calcium and Health, Fact File n.1. Nutrition Service, National Dietary Council, UK, 1992.

252. Ney, D., Symposium: The role of the nutritional and health benefits in the marketing of dairy products; Potential for enhancing the nutritional properties of milk fat, *J. Dairy Sci.*, 74, 4002, 1991.

253. Report on Health and Social Subjects 46. *Nutritional Aspects of Cardiovascular Disease. Department of Health*, UK, 1995.

254. Berner, L.A., Roundtable discussion on milkfat, dairy foods, and coronary heart disease, *J. Nutr.*, 123, 1175, 1993.

255. Artaud-Wild, S., Connor S., Sexton G., and Connor W., Differences in coronary mortality can be explained by differences in cholesterol and saturated fat intakes in 40 countries but not in France and Finland, a paradox, *Circulation*, 88, 2771, 1993.

256. Seely, S., Is calcium excess in Western diet a major cause of arterial disease? *Int. J. Cardiol.*, 33, 191, 1991.

257. Ganong, W.F., *Review of Medical Physiology*, 10th ed., Los Altos, CA, Lange Medical Pub, 1981.

258. Segall, J.J., Why is cheese safe for coronary arteries?, Int. J. Cardiol., 35, 281, 1992.

259. Seely, S., Diet and coronary heart disease: a survey of female mortality rates and food consumption statistics of 21 countries, *Med. Hypotheses*, 7, 1133, 1981.

260. Seely, S., Diet and coronary disease: a survey of mortality rates and food consumption statistics of 24 countries. *Med. Hypotheses*, 7, 907, 1981.

261. Seely, S., Diet and coronary arterial disease: a statistical study, *Int. J. Cardiol.*, 20, 183, 1988.

262. Rimm, E., Klatsky, A., Grobbee, D., and Stampfer, M., Review of moderate alcohol consumption and reduced risk of coronary heart disease: is the effect due to beer, wine, or spirits?, *Br. Med. J.*, 312, 731, 1996.

263. Rimm, E. and Ellison, C., Alcohol in the Mediterranean diet, *Am. J. Clin. Nutr.*, 61(suppl.), 1378S, 1996.

264. Kanel, W. and Ellison, C., Alcohol and coronary heart disease: the evidence for a protective effect, *Clin. Chim. Acta*, 246, 59, 1996.

265. Rimm, E., Williams, P., Fosher, K., Criqui, M., and Stampfer, M., Moderate alcohol intake and lower risk of coronary heart disease: meta-analysis of effects on lipids and hemostatic factors, *Br. Med. J.*, 319, 1523, 1999.

266. Rimm, E., Giovannucci, E., Willett, W., Colditz, G., Ascherio, A., Rosner, B., and Stampfer, M., Prospective study of alcohol consumption and risk of coronary disease in men, *Lancet*, 331, 464, 1991.

267. MacLure, M., A demonstration of deductive meta-analysis: ethanol intake and risk of myocardial infarction, *Epidemiol. Rev.*, 15, 328, 1993.

268. Hart, C.L., Smith, G.D., Hole, D.J., and Hawthorne, V.M., Alcohol consumption and mortality from all causes, coronary heart disease, and stroke: results from a prospective cohort study of Scottish men with 21 years of follow-up, *Br. Med. J.*, 318, 1725, 1999.

269. Gronbek, M., Deis, A., Sorensen, T., Becker, U., Borch-Johnsen, K., Muller, C., Schnor, P., and Jensen, G., Influence of sex, age, body mass index, and smoking on alcohol intake and mortality, *Br. Med. J.*, 308, 302, 1994.

270. Yuan, J. M., Ross, R., Gao, Y.T., Henderson, B., and Yu, M., Follow up study of moderate alcohol intake and mortality among middle aged men in Shanghai, China, *Br. Med. J.*, 314, 18, 1997.

271. Tsugane, S., Ueda, R., Hino, Y., and Yoshimura, T., Alcohol consumption and all-cause and cancer mortality among middle-aged Japanese men: seven-year follow-up of the JPHC Study Cohort I., *Am. J. Epidemiol.*, 150, 1201, 1999

272. Stampfer, M., Colditz, G., Willett, W., Speizer, F., and Hennekens, C., A prospective study of moderate alcohol consumption and the risk of coronary disease and stroke in women, *N. Eng. J. Med.*, 319, 26, 1988.

273. Ellison, R.C., Does moderate alcohol consumption prolong life?, New York: American Council on Science and Health, 1,1993.

274. Meade, T., Vickers, M., Thompson, S., Stirling, Y., Haines, A., and Miller, G., Epidemiologic characteristics of platelet aggregability, *Br. Med. J.*, 290, 428, 1985.

275. Moore, R. and Pearson, T., Moderate alcohol consumption and coronary artery disease: a review, *Medicine*, 65, 242, 1986.

276. Gaziano, J., Buring, J., Breslow, G., Goldhaber, S., Rosner, B., van de Burgh, M., Willett, W., and Hennekens, C., Moderate alcohol intake, increased levels of HDL and its subfractions and decreased risk of myocardial infarction, *N. Eng. J. Med.*, 329, 1829, 1993.

277. Suh, I., Shaten, J., Cutler, J.A., and Kuller, L., Alcohol use and mortality from coronary heart disease: the role of high density lipoprotein cholesterol, *Ann. Intern. Med.*, 116, 881, 1992.

278. Seignreur, M., Bannet, J., and Darian, B., Effect of the consumption of alcohol, white wine and red wine on platelet function and serum lipids, *J. Appl. Cardiol.*, 5, 215,1990.

279. van der Gaag, M.S., van Tol, A., Scheek, L.M., James, R.W., Urgert, R., Schaafsma, G., and Hendriks, H.F., Daily moderate alcohol consumption increases serum paraoxonase activity; a diet-controlled, randomized intervention study in middle-aged men, *Atherosclerosis*, 47, 405,1999.

280. Locher, R., Suter, P., and Vetter, W., Ethanol suppresses smooth muscle cell proliferation in the postprandial state: a new antiatherosclerotic mechanism of ethanol?, *Am. J. Clin. Nutr.*, 67, 338, 1998.

281. Kerry, N. and Abbey, M., Red wine and fractioned phenolic compounds prepared from red wine inhibit low-density lipoprotein oxidation *in vitro*, *Atherosclerosis*, 135, 93, 1997.

282. Ragione, F., Cucciola, V., Borriello, A., Pietra, V., Racioppi, L., Soldati, G., Manna, C., Galletti, P., and Zappia, V., Resveratrol arrests the cell division cycle at S/G2 phase transition, *Chem. Biochem. Res. Com.*, 250, 53, 1998.

283. Pace Asciak, C., Hahn, S., Diamandis, E., Soleas, G., and Goldberg, D., The red wine phenolics trans-resveratrol and quercetin block human platelet aggregation and eicosanoid synthesis: implication for protection against coronary heart disease, *Clin. Chim. Acta*, 235, 207, 1995.

284. Franted, E., Waterhouse, A., and Kinsella, J., Inhibition of human LDL oxidation by resveratrol, *Lancet*, 341, 1103, 1993.

285. Goldberg, D., Garovic-Kocic, V., Diamandis, E., and Pace-Asciak, C , Wine: does the colour count?, *Clin. Chim. Acta*, 246, 183, 1996.
286. Klatsky, A., Armstrong, M., and Friedman, G., Red wine, white wine, liquor, beer, and risk for coronary artery disease hospitalization, *Am. J. Cardiol.*, 80(4), 416, 1997.
287. Kondo, K., Matsumoto, A., Kurata, H., Tanahashi, H., Koda, H., Amachi, T., and Itakura, H., Inhibition of oxidation of low-density lipoprotein with red wine, *Lancet*, 344, 1152, 1994.
288. Frankel, E., Kanner, J., German, J., Parks, E., and Kinsella, J., Inhibition of oxidation of human low-density lipoprotein by phenolic substances in red wine, *Lancet*, 341, 454, 1993.
289. Whitehead, T., Robinson D., Allaway S., Syms J, and Hale A., Effect of red wine ingestion on the antioxidant capacity of serum, *Clin. Chem.*, 41, 32, 1995.
290. Fuhrman, B., Lavy, A., and Aviram, M., Consumption of red wine with meals reduces the susceptibility of human plasma and low-density lipoprotein to lipid peroxidation, *Am. J. Clin. Nutr.*, 61, 549, 1995.
291. Gottrand, F., Beghin, L., Duhal, N., Lacroix, B., Bonte, J.P., Fruchart, J.C., and Luc, G., Moderate red wine consumption in healthy volunteers reduced plasma clearance of apolipoprotein AII, *Eur. J. Clin. Invest.*, 29, 387, 1999.
292. Truelsen, T., Gronbaek, M., Schnor, P., and Boysen, G., Intake of beer, wine, and spirits and risk of stroke, The Copenhagen Study, *Stroke*, 29, 2467, 1998.
293. Renaud, S. and de Lorgeril, M., Wine, alcohol, platelets, and the French paradox for coronary heart disease, *Epidemiology*, 339, 1523, 1992.
294. Klatsky, A. and Armstrong, M., Alcoholic beverage choice and risk of coronary artery disease mortality: Do red wine drinkers fare best?, *Am. J. Cardiol.*, 71, 467, 1993.
295. Gronbek, M., Deis, A., Sorensen, T., Becker, U., Schnor, P., and Jensen, G., Mortality associated with moderate intakes of wine, beer, or spirits, *Br. Med. J.*, 310, 1165, 1995.
296. Wannamethee, S. and Shaper, G., Type of alcoholic drink and risk of major coronary heart disease events and all-cause mortality, *Am. J. Public Health*, 89, 685, 1999.
297. Serafini, M., Maiani, G., and Fero-Luzzi, A., Alcohol-free red wine enhances plasma antioxidant capacity in humans, *J. Nutr.*, 128, 1003, 1998.

12 Cancer and the Mediterranean Diet

Constantina Papoutsakis-Tsarouhas and Ira Wolinsky

CONTENTS

I. INTRODUCTION

The Mediterranean Diet is well known for its contribution to reducing rates of cardio-vascular disease and other chronic conditions.[1-5] Recently, there has been tremendous scientific interest in identifying its possible cancer-protective properties.[6-17]

Cancer is a chronic disease that is considered a major cause of death. In 1996, more than 10 million cases of cancer were diagnosed around the world and approximately 7 million deaths occurred due to cancer.[18] Statistical projections have estimated that about 35% of cancer deaths may be diet-related, with acceptable ranges varying from 10% to as much as 70% by location.[19] Several environmental studies have reported similar contributions of diet to cancer.[20-22] For example, in 1977, Wynder and Gori[20] published a study on the environmental contribution to cancer incidence and concluded that diet may be responsible for as much as 60% of female cancers and 40% of male cancers. The most frequent types of cancer around the world (lung, stomach, breast, colon and rectum, mouth and pharynx, liver, cervix, esophagus, prostate, bladder, ovary, and endometrium) are thought to be affected by diet.[23] Furthermore, cancer studies in recent years have increasingly demonstrated striking associations between the risk for various cancer types and dietary patterns.[24-27] The vast majority of research strongly supports the premise that diets rich in fruits, vegetables, and whole-grain products are related to decreased risks for cancers at various locations, most notably epithelial cancers.[24-29] Because the Mediterranean Diet, as typified by its Greek version, is indeed heavily plant-based, it serves as an appropriate model for study of its effect on cancer risk.[30]

The Greek diet has become widely accepted as the prototype of the traditional Mediterranean Diet because the earliest studies on the significant health-promoting qualities of the Mediterranean Diet were conducted in Greece in the 1950s and the 1960s.[31] Olive oil is the major source of fat and a central element of the Greek diet. Thus, the term Mediterranean Diet is commonly used to refer to all diets similar to those of Greece and other olive-growing regions of the Mediterranean, where olive oil is the principle dietary fat.[32] Besides the high use of olive oil, the Mediterranean Diet is rich in fruit, vegetables, legumes, grains, nuts, and seeds, moderate in milk and dairy products, moderate in alcohol intake (usually consumed as wine with meals), and low in meat products and saturated fat.[32] Total fat intake tends to be high in the Mediterranean (ranging from 30% of total calories in Italy to more than 40% in Greece) yet the ratio of monounsaturated fat to saturated is exceptionally high when compared with other geographic areas including northern Europe and the U.S.[33,34]

Although there are at least 16 Mediterranean countries, this chapter will concentrate on cancer and diet epidemiological evidence from southern European Mediterranean countries, namely Greece, Italy, Spain, and France.

II. COMPARATIVE CANCER AND DIETARY PATTERNS OF SELECTED MEDITERRANEAN COUNTRIES AND THE U.S.

A. CANCER AND DIET: RELEVANT BACKGROUND INFORMATION

Despite high levels of smoking and lower quality of health care in Mediterranean countries, respective mortality data indicate that death rates were, and continue to be, lower when compared with economically developed countries such as the U.S.[35-38] Specifically, statistics from the World Health Organization Databank[39] demonstrate that Mediterranean populations experience lower levels of cancer than people in the U.S., especially for cancers of the colon, breast, ovary, and prostate (Table 1). Also, 1990s data from the European Network of Cancer Registries (ENCR)[40] show that overall incidence rates in male and female cancers for Greece and Spain are below average rates for the European Union.

TABLE 1
Average Standardized[a] Cancer Mortality Rates in Selected Mediterranean Countries and the U.S. up to 1993 (per 100,000)[39]

Country	Colon Cancer	(Female) Breast Cancer	Ovary Cancer	Prostate Cancer
Greece	10	12	3	7
Spain	14	11	3	11
Italy	16	17	4	10
France	27	17	6	15
U.S.A.	25	22	6	15

[a] Rates are age-adjusted to the world standard

The progression of cancer-diet studies in Mediterranean areas has paralleled the intensity of global cancer-diet research. Systematic study of cancer patterns around the world became possible in the early 1950s, when cancer registries were formally instituted.[23] Although the increase in the number of documented cancer cases was partly attributed to aging populations and improved methods of diagnosis,[23] epidemiological studies showed that cancer occurrence and rates of specific cancer types varied greatly between countries and that diet might be an eminent contributing factor in such variations.[41,42] Also, epidemiological investigations demonstrated that degree of urbanization, a driving force for dietary change, might be a significant environmental influence on cancer rates.[43,44] In Mediterranean populations, the lower rates of various cancer types (e.g., breast, prostate, colon, rectum, and bladder) have been associated with dietary practices.[45,46] An ecological correlation study conducted in ten European countries (circa 1990s) by Lagiou et al.[47] reported a correlation coefficient between diet and age-adjusted mortality (of the respective disease) of +0.51 (p about 0.14) for colorectal cancer and +0.72 (p about 0.07) for breast cancer in females. In a comparison between Italy and the U.S., geographic and temporal variations of cancer rates as a function of life-style factors (tobacco use, alcohol intake, and diet) were studied by La Vecchia, Harris and Wynder.[48] They proposed that, as differences in diet diminish between the two countries, cancer patterns are expected to converge accordingly, particularly for cancers of the breast, ovary, intestines, and probably prostate.[48] Their prediction, at least in part, appears to be confirmed in a recent report on global breast cancer statistics that places Greece, Italy, and Spain among the few countries whose breast cancer mortality, even though at lower rates, continues to rise.[49] On the other hand, breast cancer mortality in the U.S. and other economically developed countries such as the U.K., Germany, Austria, and Canada is declining.[49]

The relationship between diet and cancer is complex and at times puzzling, especially when carcinogenesis is perceived to be the result of a specific carcinogen.[50] It is more likely that the excess of dietary components may act as potential procarcinogens or promoters of cancer. Also, sufficient amounts of beneficial dietary components may act in ways to prevent the development of cancer.[50] Upon thorough review of the relationship between cancer and diet, the World Cancer Research Fund and the American Institute for Cancer Research[51] underlined the importance of maintaining and promoting' known healthy dietary patterns as a whole without labeling isolated dietary constituents as cures for cancer prevention. The same panel pointed to the traditional Mediterranean Diet as an example of a favorable dietary model when compared with the diets of more economically developed countries such as the U.S.

Although diet alone may not account for the lower levels of chronic disease observed in the Mediterranean, it has been suggested that the traditional dietary pattern of Mediterranean populations plays a significant disease-preventive role that has not been explored or appreciated adequately.[34] Recent economic development and urbanization have negatively affected the integrity of the traditional Mediterranean Diet.[52] Thus, there is a unique opportunity to examine how dietary changes, or evidence of nutrition transition in the Mediterranean, relate to evolving cancer rates. In this section, a comparison of cancer and diet between selected Mediterranean countries and the U.S. is presented. Such a comparison should be treated with caution. It is meant as a simple snapshot between two periods of time: the early 1960s, when the traditional Mediterranean Diet was originally described, and the 1990s, as a reflection of the present. Such a comparison is general and descriptive by nature. It is not meant to imply that changing dietary patterns cause changes in cancer. This type of evidence is circumstantial and constitutes an empirical assessment.

B. COMPARISON OF TOTAL CANCER MORTALITY IN THE EARLY 1960s AND 1990s: DISTINCT CHANGES

Mortality comparisons of specific cancer types would reveal detailed developments. However, it has been documented that Mediterranean populations exhibited low levels for various cancers in the 1960s.[11] Also, an increase in the mortality of many cancers has been reported for the last 30 years in southern European countries, which justifies an all-cancer approach for the present comparison.[11,53]

During the early 1960s, Greece and Spain had the lowest cancer mortality in comparison with Italy, France, and the U.S., with Greece exhibiting the lowest mortality among compared countries (Figure 1). In the 1990s, Greece still remained the country with the lowest cancer mortality, while Spain presented comparable mortality to that of Italy. As seen in Figure 1, for both time periods, France and the U.S. demonstrated the highest mortality for cancer. The mortality in Italy remained virtually unchanged. When examining the percentage change in cancer mortality between the two periods, the mortality in Greece and Spain climbed by an alarming 15%, with the U.S. showing the second-highest increase, 7%. The sharper rise in cancer mortality seen in Greece and Spain may be related to the concurrent rapid rate of urbanization and economic development, forces perceived to affect dietary habits. France (1% mortality increase) and Italy (0 % increase), which, on average, have always been more economically developed than Greece and Spain, have not experienced as intense a change in urbanization, which may be related to the smaller rise in mortality increases. Also, in the case of France and Italy, it is important to recognize that there are differences in trends of cancer mortality between northern and southern regions that possibly affect the total mortality of each country as a whole. Nevertheless, given the common geographic vicinity, such a comparison among Mediterranean countries is valid. In terms of the U.S., the environmental forces there are probably different, yet progressive urbanization may partly explain the observed increase in cancer mortality there as well.

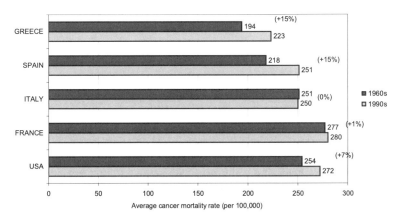

FIGURE 1   Comparative average cancer mortality between selected Mediterranean countries and the U.S. during the 1960s and 1990s.[39] Cancer mortality rates are age-adjusted to the world standard. Figures in parentheses represent percent changes in cancer between the two periods. *Note*: Annual mortality data are published by the World Health Organization (WHO) on behalf of its members. WHO mortality data have been used elsewhere[8,45,49] to examine cancer trends and will be the main source of cancer statistics in this chapter as well.

C. COMPARISON OF DIETARY PATTERNS IN THE EARLY 1960s AND 1990s: DISTINCT CHANGES

The examination of dietary patterns aims to determine how well the integrity of the Mediterranean Diet has been maintained since the 1960s among selected Mediterranean countries (Greece, Italy, France, and Spain). Also, these countries are contrasted against the U.S., an example of an economically developed country.

The source of data for the present comparison of dietary patterns among countries are the Food Balance Sheets made available by the Food and Agriculture Organization (FAO).[54] Annual Food Balance Sheets of a country show the available foods per person (produced plus imported minus exported). The data do not account for waste of foods or foods not obtained through the market (e.g., home-grown food products or hunted game). Thus, the food supply provided in these sheets represents indirect and approximate information on actual food intake. Food Balance Sheets offer a pooled estimate of food availability for a country as a whole. They do not differentiate availability within regions of a country where distinct dietary patterns may exist. Such is the case in France and Italy, whose northern populations are more industrialized than their traditional rural counterparts in the south. Despite these well-known limitations of Food Balance Sheets, if used cautiously, they are a useful medium for the assessment of dietary patterns.[8,48,55]

A common dietary feature among countries of the Mediterranean is the elevated fat consumption mainly due to olive oil. Also, the diet of these countries is rich in fruit, vegetables, and cereals, with animal foods used as an accompaniment. With this in mind, food data have been grouped as follows: cereals (grains), fruit, vegetables (including starchy vegetables such as potatoes), meat and meat products (excluding milk and dairy), milk and dairy products, olive oil, all other vegetable oils and fats, and added animal fats (such as butter and cream).

1. Cereals

During the early 1960s, cereals were a central source of energy in Mediterranean countries. Figure 2 shows that food availability of cereals decreased in all four Mediterranean countries from the 1960s to the 1990s, while the opposite occurred in the U.S. Still, the current consumption of cereals in the U.S. is, on average, lower than that of Mediterranean countries, especially when compared with Greece. The decrease of cereal consumption in the selected Mediterranean countries follows the overall theme of an increasingly uniform "Westernized" diet characterized by a lessening of carbohydrate-rich staples with concurrent increases in animal foods such as meats and dairy products.[8]

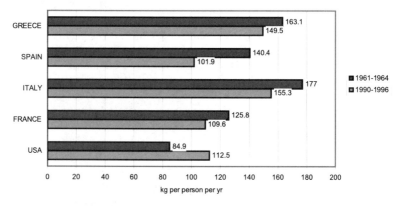

FIGURE 2   The average supply of cereals in selected Mediterranean countries and the U.S in 1961–1964 and 1990–1996.[54]

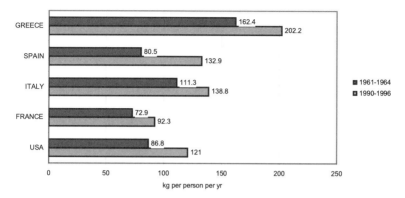

FIGURE 3 The average supply of fruit in selected Mediterranean countries and the U.S. in 1961–1964 and 1990–1996.[54]

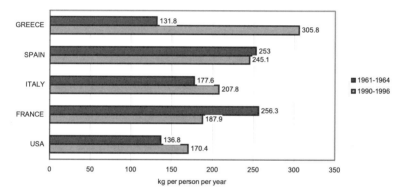

FIGURE 4 The average supply of vegetables (including starchy vegetables) in selected Mediterranean countries and the U.S. in 1961–1964 and 1990–1996.[54]

2. Fruit and Vegetables

A comparison of the Food Balance Sheet data indicates that the fruit supply increased in all countries from the 1960s to the 1990s (Figure 3). During both time periods, the availability of fruit was on average greater in the selected Mediterranean countries than the U.S. The highest availability was seen in Greece (in the 1960s: 162.4 kg per person per year; in the 1990s: 202.2 kg per person per year). During the 1960s, the availability of vegetables among Mediterranean countries showed marked differences (Figure 4). This may be because Food Balance Sheets indicate availability via market channels. In countries, such as Greece, that were mainly rural during the 1960s, the vegetable availability may appear deceivingly lower. Thus, vegetable availability during the 1960s seems similar between Greece (131.8 kg per person per year) and the U.S. (136.8 kg per person per year). In the 1990s, however, there is distinct difference in vegetable availability between Greece (305.8 kg per person per year) and the U.S. (170.4 kg per person per year). The superior availability of vegetables in Greece during the 1990s is probably a more accurate representation of Greeks' preference for vegetable consumption, since Greeks in the 1990s are more likely to acquire their foods through markets when compared with the 1960s. Overall, the average Mediterranean availability of vegetables in both periods exceeds that of the U.S. (Figure 4). The Food Balance Sheet data show that fruit and vegetables played, and continue to play, a significant role in the plant-based nature of the Mediterranean Diet. The U.S. also shows an increase in these foods. The uniform increasing trend of fruit and vegetables has also been linked to improved refrigeration systems available throughout the world.[23]

3. Meats, Milk, and Dairy Products

Figure 5 shows an overwhelming increase in meat and meat products in all countries when comparing the early 1960s with the 1990s. In both periods, the U.S. presents the highest availability (1960s: 122.5 kg per person per yr, 1990s: 152.1 kg per person per yr). During the early 1960s, the availability of meats was modest in the selected Mediterranean countries, with the exception of France. Again, Greece is the country that demonstrates in both time periods the most Mediterranean "character," meaning, in this instance, the lowest amount of meats (1960s: 50.8 kg per person per yr, 1990s: 108.7 kg per person per yr) . On the other hand, the sharpest increase in meat availability is seen in Greece, Italy, and Spain (over 100% increase) (Figure 5).

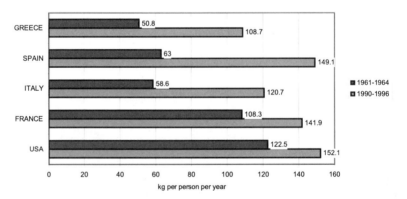

FIGURE 5   The average supply of meat and meat products (excluding milk and dairy products) in selected Mediterranean countries and the U.S. in 1961–1964 and 1990–1996.[54]

The picture of milk and dairy products is similar to that of meats, at least for the Mediterranean countries, since availability in the U.S. seems unchanged (Figure 6). This is expected, because an increase in meat availability is bound to be accompanied by an increase in its related products, such as milk and dairy products. Therefore, a notable increase in milk and dairy has occurred in all Mediterranean countries since the early 1960s. The highest increases are seen in Greece, Italy, and Spain, where the availability of milk and dairy has almost doubled.

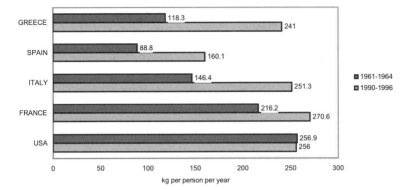

FIGURE 6   The average supply of milk and dairy products (excluding butter) in selected Mediterranean countries and the U.S. in 1961–1964 and 1990–1996. [54]

Overall, such increasing preferences for animal foods in the Mediterranean imply a change in the consumption of types of fats, with animal fats becoming more important. This finding suggests that one of the salient characteristics of the Mediterranean Diet, its modest consumption of animal products, is being challenged.

4. Olive Oil

Olive oil is the predominant source of fat for most Mediterranean populations. It is important, therefore, to examine its availability separately without grouping it with other vegetable oils and fats. Figure 7 shows the profound difference of olive oil availability between the U.S. and Mediterranean countries during both periods; the higher consumption of olive oil among Mediterranean countries is not surprising. The highest availability of olive oil is always observed in Greece. Despite the low olive oil levels in the U.S., it is interesting that the availability quadrupled in the 1990s. The Food Balance Sheet data confirm that olive oil remains a significant choice of fat in the Mediterranean, despite the passage of time.

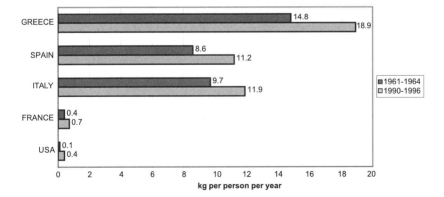

FIGURE 7   The average supply of olive oil in selected Mediterranean countries and the U.S. in 1961–1964 and 1990–1996.[54]

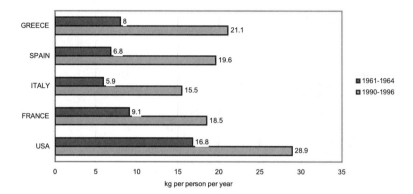

FIGURE 8   The average supply of all vegetable oils and fats (excluding olive oil) in selected Mediterranean countries and the U.S. in 1961–1964 and 1990–1996.[54]

5. Other Vegetable Oils and Fats

Although olive oil is still important in the Mediterranean Diet (Figure 7), all other vegetable oils and fats have gained great significance in all countries, including the U.S., since the 1960s (Figure 8). This increase in vegetable oils and fats that exclude olive oil is probably important because it represents a shift in the balance among types of fats. Also, this increase may imply a tendency for increase in the intake of trans fatty acids in Mediterranean countries: an unfavorable change. It should be noted though, that the TRANSFAIR Study,[56] which assessed the intake of trans fatty acids in 14 European countries, showed that Mediterranean countries still consume the lowest quantities of trans fatty acids (0.5–0.8% of total energy).

In summary, the increase in other vegetable oils and fat is another indication toward a more unified dietary Westernized pattern, one that progressively deviates from traditional diets.

6. Added Animal Fats

Except for the U.S., where the supply of added fats is almost half in the 1990s (5.9 kg per person per year) compared with the supply during the early 1960s (11 kg per person per year), all Mediterranean countries have increased their supply of added fats since the 1960s (Figure 9). This trend is consistent with the tendency of Mediterranean countries to incorporate more foods of animal origin into their diet.

D. SUMMARY AND COMMENTS

The comparison of cancer mortality rates between the 1960s and 1990s shows that total cancer mortality rates accelerated at rather high rates in the Mediterranean, despite the absolute lower levels, when compared with the U.S. (Figure 1). These findings are consistent with other comparative epidemiological studies and reports.[11,48,49]

The comparison of food supply between Mediterranean countries and the U.S. during the 1960s and 1990s indicates that the relative differences are still maintained

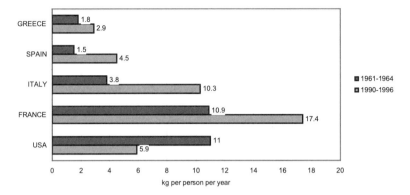

FIGURE 9   The average supply of added animal fats in selected Mediterranean countries and the U.S. in 1961–1964 and 1990–1996.[54]

but have lessened. Such a conclusion has also been reached in a follow-up study of food consumption patterns among the seven countries (Finland, Greece, Italy, Japan, the Netherlands, U.S., and Yugoslavia) originally researched to evaluate the relations between diet and cardiovascular disease (Seven Countries Study).[57]

The contrast in Mediterranean Dietary patterns during the 1960s and 1990s may be summarized as follows: There is a decrease in cereal consumption, and a sharp increase in animal foods and vegetable oils and fats (other than olive oil). These are the observed features that compromise the integrity of the Mediterranean Diet. On the other hand, the comparison between the two time periods shows that the high consumption of olive oil, fruit, and vegetables is maintained. The lasting consumption of olive oil by Mediterraneans has been reported by other authors as well.[21,57-62] Since olive oil consumption is strong, but consumption of animal foods and other vegetable fats has also increased, it can be inferred that the consumption of fat, especially animal fat, has increased in Mediterranean populations. Using national food survey data, Moreiras-Varela[62] showed that, in Spain, there has been an increase in fat consumption from 30% to about 40% of energy. In a study of trends in nutrition, Zilidis[63] reported that, in Greece, calories derived from animal sources increased by 106%, lipid intake rose by 62.2%, while animal fats specifically increased by 114.3% during the period 1961–86. In a follow-up dietary study of two Italian cohorts of the Seven Countries Study, Alberti-Fidanza et al.[64] reported that the subjects of these two cohorts have been "abandoning the traditional Mediterranean Diet" with notable increases in meat and milk. Also, in a comparison of mortality trends and past and current dietary factors of breast cancer in Spain, Prieto-Ramos et al.[65] showed significant changes in food consumption patterns (increased consumption of beef and total meat) that were associated with increased breast cancer mortality. Indeed, animal fat has been characterized as a significant dietary influence on cancer risk.[10,36,44]

Overall, it is noteworthy that in the present comparison between the 1960s and 1990s, the upward trend in total cancer mortality in the Mediterranean is paralleled by features of nutritional transition and westernization of the diet. It seems likely that at least Mediterranean populations would benefit from actively preserving and promoting their own traditional Mediterranean eating pattern.[34]

III. WEIGHING THE EVIDENCE: DOES THE MEDITERRANEAN DIET CONTAIN CANCER-FIGHTING COMPONENTS?

A. SIGNIFICANT NUTRIENT AND NON-NUTRIENT COMPONENTS

1. Dietary Fat

High consumption of fat in Western societies has been associated with increased risk of many common cancers such as colon and rectum, prostate, breast, endometrium, and lung.[66-70] Epidemiological and experimental research suggests that total fat, as well as the types of fats, may play a significant role in the development and occurrence of various types of cancer.[11,46,71-79] Thus, the majority of public health groups recommend a diet modest in fat for the purpose of cancer prevention.[80-82]

The role of fat in cancer, however, is an issue of ongoing scientific debate. Limitations in the precision of dietary intake measurements and the difficulty of obtaining a wide range of fat intake within relatively homogeneous populations are some reasons for the limited success in resolving the fat–cancer issue.[67]

It is intriguing that, in both Greece and the U.S., consumption of fat is generous, about 44%[33] and about 35% of total calories[83], respectively, yet Greece and other Mediterranean countries with similar fat consumption, exhibit a lower risk for various cancers than economically developed countries such as the U.S (Table 1). A number of investigations addressing the significance of fat consumption in have taken place in Mediterranean areas.[7,84-106] The predominant emerging theme from this research is that the types of fat, and their respective food sources, may be more important than the total amount of fat consumed. It appears that increased consumption of unsaturated fat and low consumption of saturated fat may be associated with reduced cancer risk in Mediterranean populations.[107] For example, in an Italian study, risk for breast and colorectal cancer was reduced when 5% of total energy as saturated fat was substituted by unsaturated fat.[108] Ecological research has suggested a positive correlation between cancer and animal fat and saturated fat.[44,48] In Italy, another ecological study that compared diet and tumor mortality rates showed strong positive correlations between animal proteins and saturated fatty acids, while oleic acid was negatively associated with cancer risk.[109] The same study projected that, for every gram of increase in animal fat consumption within the Italian population, there will be a 1% increase in the number of cancer cases.[109]

a. Breast cancer

The association between risk of breast cancer and dietary fat is controversial. The increasing number of relevant studies including Mediterranean populations suggests that the potential of the Mediterranean Diet to reduce breast cancer risk has not been fully explored. Descriptive epidemiological evidence indicates that patterns of fat consumption are strongly correlated with breast cancer occurrence.[21] Taioli and coworkers[110] examined dietary habits and breast cancer in the U.S. and Italy. Their study showed that, in 1981, southern Italy experienced the lowest breast cancer mortality (19.1 deaths in 100,000), while the highest mortality for breast cancer was seen in the U.S. (27.1 in 100,000). In terms of types of fat, consumption of saturated fat and linoleic acid was higher and consumption of monounsaturated fat was lower in the U.S. than in southern Italy.[110]

In Greece, two noteworthy breast cancer case-control studies have been conducted.[98,105] The earlier case-control study,[105] which included 120 cases and 120 control participants, assessed the role of diet in the occurrence of breast cancer by use of a food-frequency questionnaire. It was observed that a high intake of dietary fat did not increase the risk of breast cancer. The authors acknowledged that the small size of study participants limited the strength of the findings. The subsequent Greek case-control study led by the same scientific team included a larger number of subjects: 820 breast-cancer cases and 1,548 controls.[98] The results of this Greek case-control study regarding fat were as follows: total intake of fat or types of fat were not associated with breast cancer risk.[98]

Two Italian case-control studies[93,111,112] have also contributed significantly to elucidating the breast cancer–dietary fat question. The first Italian case-control study[111] included data from 250 women with breast cancer and 499 age-matched population controls. A dietary-history questionnaire was used to assess diet. Multivariate analyses showed a relative risk for breast cancer of 3.0 (95% confidence interval, 1.9–4.7) for subjects in the highest quintile of saturated fat intake.[111] The second Italian multicentric case-control[93,112] studied 2,569 women with breast cancer and 2588 control women. Diet was evaluated by using a food-frequency questionnaire. Increasing total fat intake was associated with a decrease in breast cancer risk (odds ratio = 0.81). Also, increased consumption of polyunsaturated and unsaturated fatty acids was significantly associated with a decreased risk for breast cancer (odds ratio = about 0.7). The protection of high consumption of polyunsaturated fat was mainly attributed to consumption of olive oil and seed oils.[112] The protection conferred by unsaturated fatty acids was stronger in postmenopausal and elderly participants.[90] High polyunsaturated to saturated fat (P/S) (odds ratio = 0.71) and unsaturated to saturated fat (U/S) (odds ratio = 0.78) ratios indicated protection against breast cancer as well.[93] The authors estimated that if Italian women increased their consumption of unsaturated fatty acids to the level of the highest quintile in their study (more than 48 g/d), a 16% reduction of breast cancer could be observed in the respective population.[93] Indeed, the results of this major case-control study showed the need to evaluate the effect of different types of fat separately in relation to cancer risk. In subsequent data analysis of the same case-control study, La Vecchia et al.[113] evaluated the role of different types of fat on breast cancer. They reported the following multivariate odds ratios: 1.10 (95% confidence interval 0.99–1.23) for an increase of 10 g in daily saturated fat consumption, 0.99 (0.94–1.04) for an increase of 10 g in daily monounsaturated fat intake, and 0.91 (0.87–0.96) for an increase of 5 g in daily polyunsaturated fat intake. Their results support the premise that saturated fat may be directly associated with increased risk for breast cancer and that mono- and polyunsaturated fats may not increase the same risk.[113]

The findings of two Spanish case-control studies are interesting as well. Landa, Frago, and Tres[99] evaluated the role of diet in the causation of breast cancer in a case-control study of 100 female breast cancer patients and 100 hospital female controls. Breast cancer subjects reported a significantly lower consumption of monounsaturated fat and the respective relative risk was calculated to be 0.30 (confidence limit = 0.1–1.08). Consumption of total fat did not affect breast cancer risk. Martin-Moreno et al.[100] carried out a larger case-control study in Spain that assessed 762 breast cancer patients against 988 controls. They used the same food-frequency questionnaire as in the previous Spanish study.[99] Neither total fat consumption nor types of fat were significant in affecting breast cancer risk.

An exception to the previous Mediterranean studies is a case-control study that took place in southern France.[114] The study was composed of 409 cases of breast cancer and 515 control subjects. Risk for breast cancer increased with consumption of total fat (odds ratio = 1.6), animal fat (odds ratio = 1.6), saturated fat (odds ratio = 1.9), and monounsaturated fat (odds ratio = 1.7). Saturated fat was strongly associated with increasing breast cancer risk, especially in postmenopausal women (odds ratio = 3.3).

Mediterranean case-control studies provide valuable information in terms of the role of dietary fat and types of fat in breast carcinogenesis. Still, the available evidence is not adequate to reach conclusions. It is also very important to note that the cancer-preventive potential of a true low fat diet (10–15% kcal from fat) cannot be evaluated by observation or studies in the Mediterranean, where such populations typically consume large quantities of fat. To obtain definitive answers, large prospective intervention trials would be necessary. Such trials should address the pattern of fat intake that is characteristic of Mediterranean populations.

b. Colorectal cancer

Rates of colorectal cancer are high in North America and northern Europe, and lower in southern Europe.[115] It has long been accepted that diet, including fat intake, plays an important role in the development of this cancer. A plausible hypothesis is that a high intake of fat enhances the production of cholesterol and bile acids. These are resynthesized into secondary bile acids by colonic flora.[11] It is believed that secondary bile acids are implicated in tumor promotion and that monounsaturated fat contributes less to this process than other types of fat.[11] The scientific panel of the World Cancer Research Fund and the American Institute for Cancer Research[115] concluded that diets high in total and saturated fat possibly increase the risk of colorectal cancer. Mediterranean studies show that the type of fat consumed may be more influential on colorectal cancer incidence, whereas total dietary fat may not increase risk appreciably.[116-121]

In Greece, one case-control study has investigated the role of diet in colorectal cancer.[116] The study included 100 cases of colorectal cancer and 100 controls. In this study, saturated fat and dietary cholesterol were higher in cases than in controls but a statistically significant association was not identified. A large case-control study (1953 colorectal cancer cases vs. 4154 controls) that investigated macronutrient intake in relation to colorectal cancer in Italy[112,116] concluded that saturated fat was mildly associated with risk of rectal cancer, monounsaturated fat was found to be neutral, whereas increased intake of polyunsaturated fat was negatively associated with colon cancer risk. Elevated consumption of polyunsaturated fat was primarily due to consumption of olive oil and seed oils.[112]

Benito et al.[118,119] carried out two case-control studies in Majorca. The first[118] investigated nutritional factors in colorectal cancer risk. The sample of the study included 286 cases of colorectal cancer, 295 population controls, and 203 hospital controls. The second[119] examined the relationship between diet and colorectal adenomas. In this study, 101 cases of colorectal adenomas were contrasted against 242 control subjects. In both these Spanish studies, increased consumption of fat or saturated fat was not associated with risk for colorectal cancer. For monounsaturated fat, the odds ratio for colorectal cancer was 0.72 when comparing subjects in the upper quartile (> 49.4 g/d) with the lowest quartile (< 27.2 g/d).[117] The odds ratio for colorectal adenomas was similar: 0.74 when comparing individuals in the upper quartile of monounsaturated intake (> 42.6 g/d) with the lower quartile (< 25.5 g/d).[118] In both studies, however, the protective effects of monounsaturated fat were not statistically significant.

Similar to Spain, two case-control studies have taken place in France.[120,121] One study assessed the role of diet in colorectal cancer[120] and the other in colorectal polyps.[121] The study on colorectal cancer[120] reported no association with fat whereas the study on colorectal polyps[121] suggested that a higher intake of saturated fat increased risk, although the result was not significant.

The Mediterranean evidence on diet and colorectal cancer suggests that increased intake of saturated fat may be implicated in increasing risk of colorectal cancer, while monounsaturated may be protective or uninfluential. At this time, though, the available Mediterranean data on fat and colorectal cancer is limited. Further studies are needed to definitively state the importance of the Mediterranean fat-intake pattern to the lower levels of colorectal cancer observed in these regions.

c. Cancer of the oral cavity, pharynx, and esophagus

Mediterranean studies on the oral cavity, pharynx, and esophagus in relation to dietary fat are sparse. Franceschi et al.[123] examined the role of diet in cancers of the oral cavity and pharynx in 754 subjects with these types of cancer and 1775 controls. Even though participants were recruited from two Italian regions and one Swiss, the results on different types of fat are worth noting. Monounsaturated fat was found to be protective (odds ratio = 0.80) while saturated fat was positively associated with oral cancer risk (odds ratio = 1.4).[123] In Greece, Tzonou et al.[124] conducted a hospital-based case-control study to investigate diet in relation to esophageal cancer. Forty-three patients with esophageal squamous-cell carcinoma, 56 patients with esophageal adenocarcinoma, and 200 control subjects participated. The study showed that added oils and fats and consumption of polyunsaturated fat increased risk of adenocarcinoma but not of squamous cell carcinoma.[124] The odds ratio for the highest quintile of monounsaturated fat intake, although statistically nonsignificant, showed a positive association for adenocarcinoma (odds ratio = 1.31) and a negative association for squamous-cell carcinoma (odds ratio = 0.31).[124]

The available Mediterranean evidence is not adequate to support clear conclusions on the significance of fat intake in relation to cancers of the oral cavity, pharynx, and esophagus. Because rates of these cancers are notably lower in Greece (especially for esophageal cancer),[39] further research is needed to clarify if dietary fat is in any way responsible for this protection.

d. Endometrial cancer

Cancer of the endometrium is generally higher in economically developed countries such as the U.S. and Canada, which present the highest rates in the world.[39] Endometrial cancer has been associated with breast, ovarian, and colorectal cancer.[125] From a dietary perspective, saturated/animal fat possibly increases risk of endometrial cancer, whereas the evidence on total fat and cholesterol is considered insufficient at this time.[115] Also, there is adequate convincing data that increased body weight increases risk of endometrial cancer.[115] In a Greek case-control study, however, weight, adjusted for height, was not correlated with increased risk of endometrial cancer.[126]

Dietary factors and the risk of endometrial cancer were assessed in a Greek hospital-based case-control study.[94] The study included 145 women with endometrial cancer and 298 controls. A validated semi-quantitative food frequency questionnaire was utilized to calculate nutrient intakes. Relative to fat, a significant protective result was noted only for monounsaturated fat intake, mostly in the form of olive oil. It was estimated that increasing intake of monounsaturated fat by one standard deviation would result in a 26% reduction of risk (odds ratio = 0.74; 95% confidence interval 0.54–1.03). Because the number of subjects was rather small and the dietary variability within the examined sample was not substantial, the results of the study should be viewed with caution.

e. Ovarian cancer

Cancer of the ovary may be affected by dietary fat intake.[115] International comparisons have exhibited that increased ovarian cancer mortality rates are associated with increased consumption of total fat ($r = 0.67$), largely due to animal fats ($r = 0.78$) and not necessarily due to vegetable fats ($r = 0.18$).[46] Recently, a study[11] that examined changes in diet and mortality from cancer in southern Mediterranean countries identified Greece and Spain as the countries with the lowest ovarian cancer mortality. These low rates were associated with the respective lowest consumption of animal fat and highest consumption of olive oil observed in Greece and Spain.

In Greece, a case-control study was conducted to examine the contribution of diet to ovarian cancer.[103] 189 cases of epithelial ovarian cancer were compared with 200 controls (hospital visitors). The study participants were interviewed using a semi-quantitative food-frequency questionnaire. The results of the study, adjusted for total energy intake, showed a significant protective effect for monounsaturated fat, with an odds ratio of 0.80 (95% confidence interval 0.65–0.99). No significant association was identified for saturated or polyunsaturated fat. The authors suggested that the identified favorable association of monounsaturated fat against ovarian cancer may explain the overall lower rates of ovarian cancer in Greece, and the concurrent increasing rates are possibly related to recent dietary changes. Another case-control study[122] that took place in northern Italy, assessed 455 subjects with histologically confirmed epithelial ovarian cancer and 1,385 controls. Although the data was not adjusted for total energy, fat intake, largely due to butter intake, was associated with increased risk of ovarian cancer (relative risk = 2.1 for highest compared with lowest reported fat intake).

The limited evidence on dietary fat and ovarian cancer does not permit comprehensive conclusions. More research is needed to clarify the potential protection of the Mediterranean Diet in relation to the lower rates of ovarian cancer exhibited in southern Mediterranean countries like Greece and Spain.

e. Prostate cancer

Prostate cancer is the fourth most frequent cancer in males and the ninth most common cancer in the world.[115] Its rates are higher in economically developed countries, partly attributed to more advanced screening and diagnostic methods.[11,115] Available evidence indicates that total fat, and especially saturated or animal fat,[46] possibly increase the risk of prostate cancer, but the evidence is scanty.[21,115,127] It is of interest that in countries with high olive oil consumption, such as Greece and Italy, mortality rates for prostate cancer were[128] and are lower when compared with more affluent countries like the U.S. (Table 1).

One Greek case-control study has reported results on the influence of dietary fat on prostate cancer.[84] This investigation included 320 prostate cancer patients and 246 controls. Only polyunsaturated fat was found to significantly increase prostate cancer risk (odds ratio = 1.79, 95% confidence interval 1.13–2.84).[84] In addition, Lagiou et al.[85] conducted a case-control study (184 patients vs. 246 control subjects) to assess the role of diet in benign prostatic hyperplasia. An increased risk was found for saturated and polyunsaturated fat, yet these findings were statistically nonsignificant.[85]

Given the lower levels of prostate cancer in the Mediterranean when compared with more economically developed societies, further studies are warranted to clarify the potential influence of dietary fat or other dietary components of the Mediterranean Diet in this common cancer of affluent populations.[11]

1. Dietary Fiber

Diets high in fiber may decrease the risk of pancreatic, colorectal, and breast cancer.[129] Available research also suggests that fiber-rich eating patterns may decrease the risk of stomach cancer, but the amount of international evidence is insufficient.[129] The Mediterranean Diet has long been recognized for its abundance of plant foods, a dietary feature that promotes the consumption of fiber. Several studies assessing Mediterranean populations have examined the role of dietary fiber in cancer prevention.[93,102,105,118-121,130-136]

A Greek hospital-based case-control study evaluated the relationship of nutrient intake and cancer of the pancreas.[102] The study contrasted 181 patients with pancreatic cancer to hospital-patient controls and hospital-visitor controls in a ratio of 1:1:1. The data was controlled for smoking, total energy intake, and confounding relationships among nutrients. With reference to crude fiber, when pancreatic cancer patients were compared with patient controls and visitor controls, the adjusted odds ratios (OR) and 95% confidence intervals (CI) were respectively: OR = 0.80 (CI =

0.64–1.00) and OR = 0.65 (CI = 0.50–0.86), suggesting a protective effect of fiber against pancreatic cancer in both instances.[102]

In the case of colorectal cancer, fiber has received appreciable scientific attention as a potential preventive agent.[26] Mechanisms by which dietary fiber may reduce risk of colorectal cancer include alteration of bile acid metabolism, increase in fecal bulk, and decrease in gastrointestinal transit time.[137] Recently, the Seven Countries Study Research Group[130] conducted an ecological study using data from the Seven Countries Study to assess the contribution of fiber to cross-cultural differences in 25-year male colorectal cancer mortality. Consumption of fiber was negatively associated with mortality of colorectal cancer (energy adjusted rate ratio = 0.89, 95% confidence interval 0.80-0.97). Also, for every additional 10 grams of fiber intake per day, a 33% reduction in 25-year colorectal cancer mortality risk was observed. The authors supported that fiber consumption in their population study may function as an indicator for the portion of plant foods that is associated with protection against colorectal cancer in men.[130] In an Italian case-control study 131 of 1225 colon cancer patients, 728 rectal cancer patients and 4,154 control participants, fiber again was found to decrease the risk for colorectal cancer. Various types of fiber were assessed according to chemical composition and food source. In almost all types of fiber, the odds ratio was less than 1. Specifically, the odds ratios for colorectal cancer were 0.68 for total fiber, 0.67 for soluble noncellulose polysaccharides (NCP), 0.71 for total insoluble fiber, 0.67 for cellulose, 0.82 for insoluble NCP, and 0.88 for lignin. For fiber classified according to food source, the following odds ratios were reported: 0.75 for vegetable fiber, 0.85 for fruit fiber, and 1.09 for cereal fiber. A case-control study[118] that was conducted in Majorca evaluated the relationship between nutrients and colorectal cancer. The protection of fiber against colorectal cancer was limited to fiber derived from legumes (relative risk for the highest consumption quartile = 0.40, p < 0.01). Legumes are a good source of soluble fiber, a fiber type that was also found to offer strong protection against colorectal cancer in the large Italian case-control[131] study on fiber. A French investigation[120] on diet and colorectal cancer concluded that no appreciable benefit was conferred by higher intake of fiber from cereals. In two Mediterranean case-control studies[119,121], fiber was reported as a possible protective factor in decreasing the risk for colorectal adenomatous polyps. Overall, studies that have included Mediterranean populations seem to support the beneficial properties of dietary fiber in reducing colorectal cancer risk.[118,130,131]

Five Mediterranean breast cancer case-control studies have reported on dietary fiber intake, one Greek,[105] three Italian,[93,132,133] and one French.[134] Three of these studies[93,105,132] did not identify a significant relationship between dietary fiber and breast cancer. However, two of these case-control studies[133,134] did report a possible protection of fiber against breast cancer, with an emphasis on the potential benefits of cellulose and soluble fiber.[133] Mediterranean data, therefore, suggest that fiber-rich foods may convey some protection against breast cancer specifically, while a clear association has not been established.

The role of dietary fiber on stomach cancer has been investigated in four Mediterranean case-control studies.[135,136,138,139] Two of the studies[135,136] identified an inverse relationship between fiber intake and risk for stomach cancer, while the other two[138,139] reported no statistically significant associations.

More scientific information is required to evaluate thoroughly the contribution of dietary fiber and types of fiber on cancer risk. Mediterranean populations should be ideal for such studies in light of the traditional high consumption of plant foods.

3. Antioxidants

A multitude of antioxidant compounds predominantly found in plant foods, and consequently in the plant-rich Mediterranean Diet, may have an anticancer effect.[9,26,35,84,140] Besides the antioxidant nutrients: vitamin C, vitamin E, selenium, and vitamin A (including β-carotene), there are many non-nutrient components produced by plants (also known as phytochemicals) that have antioxidant and other beneficial biological effects possibly contributing to cancer prevention.[6,9,26] Phytochemicals that have received appreciable scientific attention are: carotenoids, flavonoids, phenols, isothiocyanates, allium compounds, and indoles.[6,9,35,140]

International research indicates that antioxidant compounds may protect against many cancer types such as cancer of the lung, mouth and pharynx, esophagus, stomach, colorectum, pancreas, breast, and cervix. [115] Studies incorporating Mediterranean countries also provide evidence on the effects of antioxidant compounds.[88,90,99,105,112,114,124,135,138,139,141-147,149-157]

A recent multicenter case-control study[157] on diet and lung cancer among non-smokers reported minor protective influences for high intakes of all carotenoids, β-carotene, and retinol. In reference to cancers of the oral cavity and pharynx, there is some evidence that β-carotene, vitamin C, and vitamin E may reduce risk 141–143 but the correlation is not always as strong as the correlation determined for fruit intake.[141] A Greek case-control study[124] showed that dietary intake of vitamins A and C were inversely related to the risk for esophageal cancer, while results from a French multi-center case control study[145] supported that vitamin E had an independent protective effect on squamous-cell cancer of the esophagus. Also, two Italian case-control investigations[146,147] reported an appreciable negative association between estimated β-carotene intake and esophageal cancer risk. Several Mediterranean case-control studies have linked vitamin C,[135,138,139,149] vitamin E,[139] β-carotene,[149] and flavonoid intake[150] with the reduction in risk for gastric cancer. Vitamin C[151,152] and carotenoids[112,151,152] were significantly and independently associated with a decreased risk for colorectal cancer. In addition, vitamin E has been shown to reduce colorectal cancer risk.[112] In addition, vitamin C was reported as a protective factor against colorectal adenomas in a Majorcan case-control study.[119] A number of breast cancer studies[88,90,99,105,112,114,153-156] of Mediterranean populations have provided information on the possible role of some antioxidant constituents. In one Greek case-control study,[105] high consumption of total vitamin A was associated with reduction of breast cancer risk, yet, in another Italian case-control investigation,[153] no significant association was identified for retinol. There are studies[88,112,153-156] suggesting that β-carotene may be protective against breast cancer although the observed inverse association is not always as strong as the inverse association related to vegetable consumption.[154] Two breast cancer case-control studies[90,114] did not show a consistent protective pattern for β carotene. Vitamins C[88,99,153,155] and E[88,99,112,153,155] have been shown to protect against breast cancer — but not always.[90,114] Finally, a Greek case-control investigation[84] that assessed diet and prostate cancer provided evidence that vitamin E significantly reduces risk.

Some epidemiological investigations that have evaluated the role of specific antioxidants in reducing cancer risk have not reported a protective effect.[158-161] Also, in some studies,[141,154] it has been pointed out that the reduction of cancer risk evaluated for specific antioxidants was not as pronounced as the risk reduction associated with the respective food intake. It is possible that the Mediterranean Diet, as a whole, is more beneficial than its individual components in preventing free-radical-mediated carcinogenesis, or that unmeasured components of foods may protect against cancer.[32,141,154,162] Ghiselli et al.[162] suggest that the Mediterranean Diet is able to regulate oxidative stress via complex and overlapping mechanisms.[162] The impressive antioxidant potential of the Mediterranean Diet may be attributed to a high intake of combinations of antioxidants but it may also be due to an intrinsic low production of harmful oxidants.[7,162] The characteristics of the Mediterranean Diet that support such a hypothesis are the following:

- A high intake of fresh fruits and vegetables
- A decreased generation of cooking-related oxidants (the oxidative damage and harmful peroxide content is minimized in foods such as meat when cooked in olive-oil-based sauces with onion, garlic, herbs, or wine — a frequent Mediterranean practice
- A decreased usage of antioxidants in the scavenging of small amounts of oxidants leading to lower antioxidant waste[162,164]

Thus, lower catabolism of antioxidants may, in essence, facilitate improved levels of circulating antioxidants.[7,162]

The variability of results reporting on antioxidants suggests how limited our knowledge is in this area of cancer prevention. To better understand the underlying scientific foundation of the cancer-protective benefits of the Mediterranean Diet, it seems important to direct research efforts in specifying the characteristics, functions, and mechanisms involving antioxidants and other potentially beneficial bioactive constituents, found mainly in plant foods and little known at this time.[6]

B. FOODS

1. Fruits and Vegetables

A considerable amount of research supports the beneficial role of fruits and vegetables in cancer prevention.[9,24,26-29,36,164] Anticancer protection due to high consumption of fruits and vegetables may be more pronounced in cancers of the digestive and respiratory tracts than in hormone-related cancers.[24,36,165,166] There is convincing evidence that consumption of fruits and vegetables protects against cancers of the stomach, esophagus, oral cavity and pharynx, and lung.[115] A high consumption of vegetables is likely to protect against colorectal cancer.[115] In a Mediterranean population, it has been estimated that a low consumption of fruits and vegetables may be responsible for 15% to 40% of digestive tract cancers.[24] A high intake of fruits and vegetables may prevent cancer of the endometrium, pancreas, larynx, breast, bladder, cervix, ovary, and thyroid, while intake of vegetables may protect against cancer of the prostate, kidney, and liver. [115] Mediterranean populations consume generous amounts of a wide variety of fruits and vegetables. Dietary studies from the Mediterranean, therefore, present a valuable opportunity to investigate the anticancer potential of fruits and vegetables.[9] About 90% of 65 studies assessing Mediterranean populations report a protective effect of one or more fruits or vegetables in reducing cancer risk.[84-86,88,90,92,94,97,104,106,111,112,114,120,122,124,132,134,135,144-148,157,164-203]

Internationally, a large number of stomach cancer studies have investigated the preventive role of fruits and vegetables.[115] A recent report[167] on the consumption of plant foods and stomach cancer from the Seven Countries Study Research Group concluded that fruits were inversely associated with stomach cancer mortality, but no such association was evident for vegetables. From the Mediterranean, several case-control studies[135,165,166,168-173] support the protective effect of fruit and vegetables in preventing stomach cancer. Among these studies, four[136,168,170,173] reported a reduction in gastric cancer risk with increasing intake of raw vegetables, one study[165] and its recent update[166] found that green vegetables reduce stomach cancer risk substantially, while another study[170] identified tomatoes as a significant protective dietary indicator. Also, seven studies[136,165,166,168-171] reported a protective effect from fresh fruit, and four[168-170,173] identified a specific protective benefit from citrus fruits. Citrus fruits contain high amounts of vitamin C, an antioxidant suspected to reduce gastric cancer risk.[135,138,139,149] Also, fruits and vegetables contain potentially protective bioactive constituents that have not yet been identified or studied adequately.[25]

Seven Mediterranean case-control studies[124,145-148,165,166] that have assessed the effect of fruit and vegetable intake on esophageal cancer risk have reported protective associations, and one case-control study[144] reported a significant protective effect for high consumption of fresh fruits.

Relative to cancers of the oral cavity and pharynx, six Italian case-control studies[86,165,166,174-176] have concluded that frequent fruit and vegetable intake is significant in reducing risk. In three of four of these studies, a beneficial influence was shown for carrots,[174-176] while fresh tomatoes,[174] green peppers,[174] green vegetables,[165,166,175,176] raw and cooked vegetables,[86] fruit,[165,166,175,176] and citrus fruit[86] were inversely related to risk of oral and pharyngeal cancer.

Two Mediterranean case-control studies[177,178] have investigated the etiology of diet in lung cancer. One[177] reported a significant protection against lung cancer due to frequent consumption of carrots, while the other[178] demonstrated a protective effect from a high consumption of fruits.

Eleven Mediterranean case-control studies[120,165,166,179-186] have supported the protective action of vegetables in reducing the risk for colorectal cancer. A study carried out by Manousos et al.[179] in Athens, Greece, identified consumption of vegetables (especially cabbage, beets, spinach, and lettuce) as a statistically significant protective factor against colorectal cancer. A population-based case control study[180] of colorectal cancer in Majorca found that a high intake of cruciferous vegetables reduced risk significantly. Also, two French case-control studies[120,181] reported that vegetables, as a general food group, may prevent colorectal cancer[120], or colon cancer.[181] Furthermore, the results of seven Italian case-control studies [165,166,182-186] exhibited a beneficial role of vegetables in reducing the risk for colorectal cancer. Specifically, three of these studies[165,166,182] showed an inverse association between intake of green vegetables and risk of colorectal cancer, three other studies documented the protective effect of raw and cooked vegetables[184,185], and vegetables[186], while another study[183] showed a significant protection due to frequent consumption of tomatoes and spinach. To quantify the preventive properties of vegetables against colorectal cancer, Franceschi et al.[185] estimated that the consumption of an additional daily serving of vegetables may reduce colorectal cancer risk by more than 20%.

Tomatoes are a common and frequent food choice among Mediterranean populations.[164] A consistent and remarkable anticancer effect of tomatoes has been documented.[24,164,186,187] According to the findings of three Italian case control studies[170,187,188], the protection of tomato intake is notable for reducing the risk of digestive cancers (oral cavity and pharynx, esophagus, stomach, colon, and rectum). The advantage of a high tomato intake against gastrointestinal tract cancers may be superior to that of green vegetables.[187] The fact that tomatoes are a dominant and characteristic food choice among Mediterranean populations, especially in Greece and Italy, may explain in part the identified benefit of this food.[164,187] Actual mechanisms that could interpret the means by which tomatoes confer protection are not well established. Tomatoes, however, contain rather large amounts of lycopene, a carotenoid that does not possess provitamin A activity like β-carotene does. It is hypothesized that lycopene, a compound quite resistant to heat and cooking when compared with β-carotene, may be significant in improving the body's overall antioxidant potential.[187]

The available Mediterranean data on dietary factors and the risks of endometrial, cervical, ovarian, pancreatic, laryngeal, thyroid, bladder, breast, prostate, renal, and hepatic cancer is sparse for each cancer type individually. Four case-control studies, one from Greece[94] and three from Italy[165,166,189], are suggestive that vegetables [94] or green vegetables[165,166] and fruit[189] prevent endometrial cancer. One case control study on cancer of the cervix[190] and three on ovarian cancer[122,165,166] have reported a protective effect for green vegetables[122,165,166,190] and carrots.[122,190] Four Italian case-control investigations[165,166,191,192] showed that fruit consumption may decrease the risk for cancer of the pancreas, while two studies[165,166] have reported the beneficial effect of green vegetables. For laryngeal cancer, five case-control studies[92,165,166,193,194] have reported on the preventive properties of fruits and vegetables. Specifically, a high intake of vegetables[92,194] and frequent consumption of green vegetables[165,166,193] were associated with decreased risk of laryngeal cancer. Citrus fruits,[92,194] orange juice,[92] and fruits in general[165,166,193,194] were also inversely related to laryngeal cancer risk. Case-control studies[165,166,195,196] on diet and thyroid cancer have also identified fruits and vegetables as protective dietary indicators. In more detail, green vegetables,[165,166,195] green salads,[196] carrots,[196] and citrus fruits[196] were shown to protect significantly against thyroid cancer. Five Mediterranean case-control studies[104,165,166,197,198] have examined the role of fruits and vegetables in bladder cancer. Only one study from Spain[104] reported that consumption of fruits and vegetables was not related to the risk of bladder cancer. The other four studies observed inverse risk associations for green vegetables,[165,166,197] spinach,[198] carrots,[197,198] and fruit.[165,166] The Mediterranean evidence on breast cancer and fruits and vegetables is not entirely consistent. A number of Mediterranean investigations[88,90,97,106,132,134,165,166,186] support that intake of vegetables may reduce breast cancer risk. Two Greek breast cancer case control studies[97,106] noted a statistically significant risk reduction due to overall frequent vegetable consumption. Also, raw vegetables,[88,90,186] green vegetables,[132,165,166] cucumber,[106] lettuce,[106] carrots,[106,186] potatoes,[88] garlic, and onions[134] lowered breast cancer risk. Three investigations, though, reported that vegetables[111,114] or cooked vegetables[88] were not related to breast cancer risk. Fruits were reported to decrease risk of breast cancer in some studies[97,106] but not in others.[88,111,165,166] The pattern of association between fruits and vegetables and prostate cancer is also not consistent.[84,85,165,166,199,200] The results of two studies[165,166] support that fruits and green vegetables convey significant protection against prostate cancer. Also, a Greek case-control study[85] on benign prostatic hyperplasia found that fruits were inversely related to risk. However, three other studies were not able to show such an effect for fruits[84,200] or vegetables,[84,199,20], although one of these investigations[84] reported that consumption of tomatoes, especially when cooked, decreased the risk for prostate cancer. It is thought that the antioxidant lycopene in tomatoes, whose availability increases with cooking, may be in part responsible for the observed protection.[164] With respect to renal cancer, one case control study[201] from Italy found no association with fruits and vegetables in general, although carrots alone were inversely related with risk. Two other studies[165,166] found that consumption of fruits and green vegetables decreased the risk for renal cancer. Among four case control studies[165,166,202,203] that considered the role of fruits or vegetables in liver cancer, two[165,166] reported a protective effect of green vegetables, one observed that higher consumption of some vegetables reduced risk[202], another[165] found that fruits decreased risk, while two others[166,203] did not.

Although the Mediterranean data on each cancer type is not extensive, it is in overall agreement with international evidence that a diet rich in fruits and vegetables contributes to cancer prevention.[115] A variety of dietary constituents and mechanisms have been examined or proposed[26,29] to explain the protective action of fruits and vegetables against various cancer types. Some of the possible anticancer components found in fruits and vegetables are dietary fiber, vitamins C and E, folic acid, selenium, carotenoids, flavonoids, isoflavones, indoles, phytosterols, isothiocyanates, coumarins, saponins, protease inhibitors, allium compounds, and D-limonene, to name a few.[26] It has been suggested that these agents act synergistically and that multiple complementary mechanisms are in effect.[26] Proposed anticancer mechanisms include antioxidant activity, ability to modulate cell differentiation, enhanced activity of enzymes that detoxify carcinogens, suppressed production of nitrosamines facilitated primarily by vitamin C, modified hormone metabolism, improved gastrointestinal environment (affecting gastrointestinal bacteria, bile acid composition, pH, fecal bulk, and transit time), maintained integrity of intracellular structures, altered DNA methylation, maintenance of normal DNA repair, elevated degradation of cancer cells, and suppressed cell proliferation.[26,29] Despite the lack of detailed knowledge on responsible anticancer substances and associated mechanisms, the study of fruits and vegetables has provided solid support for their protective effects in cancer prevention. Indeed, in lieu of available scientific evidence, it has been suggested that consumption of fruits and vegetables may be the most salient factor in the dietary etiology of human cancer.[36] From a public health perspective, this implies that special attention ought to be paid to maintaining the high intake of fruits and vegetables in Mediterranean populations, while other populations should be encouraged to improve their fruit and vegetable consumption.

1. Grains

Traditionally, dietary guidelines have recommended that consumption of carbohydrates be emphasized, especially in the form of complex carbohydrates and starches, to reduce chronic disease risk, including some forms of cancer.[73,80] Such broad dietary guidance has been challenged, given the little information on actual positive health outcomes related to high starch diets.[204] Willet[204] and Slavin et al.[205] have claimed that greater attention must be paid to promote, specifically, the intake of whole grains for disease prevention, because epidemiological studies, as limited as they are at this time, demonstrate rather consistently that whole grains decrease chronic disease risk. Recently, the new dietary guidelines were described in the Report of the Dietary Guidelines Advisory Committee on the Dietary Guidelines for Americans, 2000.[206] The guideline that pertains to grains recommends eating "a variety of grains daily, especially whole grains."[206]

Comprehensive reviews of cancer research indicate that whole-grain cereals possibly decrease stomach cancer risk.[115] Also, cereals may decrease the risk of colorectal cancer, while refined cereals and their relative lack of micronutrients, when compared with whole grains, may be responsible for increasing the risk for esophageal cancer.[115] In addition, an expanded review and meta-analysis of case-control evidence[207] on whole-grain consumption and cancer risk supports that intake of whole-grain foods may decrease the risk of various cancer types such as colorectal, gastric, other digestive-tract cancers, pancreatic, and hormonally related neoplasms.

Research investigations have focused primarily on the effects of dietary fiber on chronic disease risk and not major foods such as whole grains. Yet, disease protection conferred by whole grains may be stronger than isolated constituents in these foods. [205] There is increasing interest in studying further the potential contribution of types of grain products and associated constituents, to the prevention of cancer development. Besides dietary fiber, beneficial component candidates of grains include oligosaccharides, antioxidant agents including vitamins, minerals, and phenolic compounds, as well as phytoestrogens and protease inhibitors.[205,208] Plausible interpretations for the cancer-preventive advantage of whole grains include: improvement of the gastrointestinal environment and containment of cell proliferation of abnormal cells, reduction of tumor incidence associated with the presence of specific compounds, like β-sitosterol, induction of detoxification systems, suppression of oxygen radical production, protection against oxidative damage, and prevention of carcinogen production due to antioxidant compounds.[205] It is also hypothesized that phytoestrogens may modulate hormonal metabolism in beneficial ways, e.g., increase in total menstrual cycle length, which may lower the risk of hormonally related neoplasms.[205] Protease inhibitors in whole grains may be involved in inhibition of tumor promotion, while a wide range of phytochemicals may be responsible for stopping initial DNA damage and limiting postinitiation processes.[205] Since beneficial constituents are likely to be found in higher quantities in minimally processed foods, studies have attempted to identify possible differences between whole and refined grains relative to cancer risk.[208] This distinction may be of particular importance because gastrointestinal transit time is shorter for refined grains than it is for whole grains. A preference for refined grains, in consequence, leads to sharper increases in glycemic overload and increases in insulin and insulin-like growth factor I, which enhances growth of tumor cells *in vitro*.[209,210] Grains constitute a dominant staple of the Mediterranean Diet and a number of Mediterranean dietary studies have assessed the potential role of grains in cancer.[86,88,90,94,97,101,106,112,120,122,130,136,146,167-171,173,174,176,179-181,183,184,189,191,195,196,202,203,209,211-214]

With respect to stomach cancer, a follow-up investigation[167] of the Seven Countries Study showed that whole grains did not affect risk. However, refined grains increased stomach cancer risk, a finding that was associated with decreased fruit consumption.[167] The authors acknowledged that high consumption of refined grains may be an indicator of the adverse effects related to a diet poor in fruit.[167] Several Mediterranean case-control studies[136,168-171,173,209,211] have reported on various cereal foods in relation to stomach cancer risk. One Greek study[168] that considered the broad category of cereals or grains, and one Italian study[209] that evaluated the effect of refined grains, found that risk for gastric cancer was positively and significantly associated with elevated intake. An Italian study[169] that assessed pasta and rice together as main contributors of starch in the Italian diet documented a mild positive correlation with gastric cancer risk. On the contrary, two studies[170,173] found that bread and pasta[170] or cereals and rice[173] did not affect gastric cancer risk appreciably, while the results of two other investigations[136,171] supported that increased consumption of bread, pasta, and rice[171] or pasta and rice[136] decreased gastric cancer risk. In another study,[168] pasta as a separate food item was shown to increase significantly and independently the risk for stomach cancer. With respect to consumption of bread, La Vecchia et al.[169] found no significant effect on stomach cancer risk. On the other hand, Trichopoulos et al.,[168] who assessed brown bread separately, observed that consumption of this food item was inversely and significantly associated with gastric cancer risk while white bread did not demonstrate a noteworthy contribution. In agreement with international data,[115] Mediterranean evidence on cereals, as a general food group, and stomach cancer provides diverse observations. Such inconsistency may relate to the fact that degree of grain refinement was not explicitly assessed in all studies. Interestingly, though, Mediterranean studies[168,169,211] that examined whole-grain foods support, uniformly, that higher consumption of whole grains is related to decreased gastric cancer risk.

Dietary Mediterranean studies[130,183,209,211,212] on colorectal cancer risk have frequently differentiated cereals as to whole vs. refined. Three of these studies[183,211,212] have observed a risk reduction in relation to higher whole-grain food intake. A follow-up energy-adjusted analysis[130] of the Seven Countries Study on plant foods and colorectal cancer mortality found that grains, refined and whole, did not influence risk. However, in crude analyses of the same data, i.e., before data was adjusted for energy intake, whole grains were inversely associated with the same risk. Two case-control studies[179,184] were not able to demonstrate a relationship between cereal-based foods and colorectal cancer. Seven case-control investigations[120,180,181,183,209,212] showed increasing colorectal cancer risk with increasing intakes of various cereal foods. One study[120] reported a positive association for pasta and rice but not for bread, yet another report[183] identified bread as a food that increases risk although, as indicated earlier, whole-grain foods specifically were protective in the same study. Also, increased intakes of bread and pasta[112], bread and cereal dishes[212], cereals[180], and refined cereals[181,209] were positively related to elevated colorectal cancer risk. In light of these findings, it appears that degree of grain processing may be an important factor in determining colorectal cancer risk. Almost all Mediterranean studies[130,183,211,212] that reported separately on whole-grain foods support an inverse relationship with colorectal cancer risk, whereas studies[112,120,180,181,183,209,212] that did not specify degree of refinement or distinctly assessed refined cereals documented an increase in risk.

Mediterranean studies[146,209,211,213] on esophageal cancer and grains are few. One study[213] is in agreement with international evidence that dominant consumption of a single grain in a population's diet, as a staple food, e.g. corn, may increase the risk of esophageal cancer.[115] Grains per se may not increase risk for esophageal cancer directly.[115] Rather, their lack of protective dietary constituents may be responsible for the observed elevated risk, as a consequence of deficient diets when there is preference for one type of grain or degree of grain refinement.[115] Indeed, refined cereals were found to increase risk for esophageal cancer,[209] while whole grains decreased risk in one investigation[210] but not significantly in another.[146]

Case control studies[86,174,176,209,211,213] have provided information on grains and cancers of the oral cavity and pharynx. Two studies[175,211] exhibited the beneficial influence of whole-grain foods in reducing risk. A recent study[86] demonstrated that intake of white bread was inversely associated with risk. One the other hand, frequent consumption of pasta or rice and polenta[174], corn[213], or refined foods in general[209] were positively related to risk of cancers of the oral cavity and pharynx.

Relative to hepatic cancer, three Mediterranean analytical epidemiological studies[202,203,211] have examined the contribution of grains. Whole-grain bread and pasta[202] or whole-grain foods as a broad food group [211] were shown to decrease risk. One Greek case-control study on hepatic cancer[202], though, reported that cereals were essentially without influence. Grains in relation to pancreatic cancer risk were assessed in two investigations.[191,211] One reported no association for whole-grain bread or pasta[191], the other showed a nonsignificant decreased risk related to whole-grain foods.[210] In the case of breast cancer, two Greek investigations[97,106] did not identify a notable role of grains, but another study[211] showed that consumption of whole grains significantly reduced risk. Three Italian reports documented a significant increase in breast cancer risk directly associated with consumption of bread[88,90,214], and cereal dishes[88,214], mainly in the form of refined wheat. A possible explanation for this increased risk is that bread and cereal dishes were substantial contributors to energy intake, which was also found to be a risk factor for breast cancer.[88] In two studies,[101,189] the risk of endometrial cancer appeared to be inversely related to frequent intake of whole-grain foods,[189] whole-grain bread and pasta.[101] In two other studies[94,211] of endometrial cancer, intake of cereals in general[94] or whole-grain cereals[211] did not affect risk appreciably. Higher consumptions of whole-meal bread or pasta,[122] and whole-grain foods[211] were inversely associated with risk for ovarian cancer. Interestingly, limited evidence on thyroid cancer shows that whole-grain food intake[211] may not confer a protective benefit, while consumption of foods such as pasta or rice, and bread[195,196] or refined grains[209] may be positively associated with risk. Risk for cancers of the gallbladder, larynx, prostate, bladder, and kidney were significantly reduced by frequent consumption of whole-grain foods in an Italian integrated series of case-control studies.[211] In addition, a significant elevation of risk for cancer of the larynx was noted in relation to refined-grain intake.[209]

Cereals and cereal-based foods constitute an important food category that contributes a sizeable portion of energy to many diets, including the Mediterranean. Nevertheless, present knowledge on the role of grains in the development of different types of human cancer is largely inconclusive. The overall emerging trend is that whole-grain foods may provide a desirable influence in reducing cancer risk. Epidemiological and experimental investigations, including designs of intervention, are warranted to identify beneficial patterns of grain intake, responsible constituents of grains, and associated mechanisms. Finally, there is a need to delineate the differences in cancer risk related to extent of grain refinement and subsequent dietary content.[215]

1. Olive Oil

Olive oil is a central component of the Mediterranean Diet, representing the primary choice of fat among people living in olive-growing areas.[34] In an international comparison, dietary fat data[46] showed that Greece, Italy, and Spain consume, respectively, 71%, 42% and 37% of their estimated total vegetable fat intake from olive oil. A more recent report indicates that, in Greece, about 50% of dietary fat intake is monounsaturated, predominantly contributed by olive oil consumption.[216] Several explanations have been offered for the possible anticancer potential of olive oil: 1) its unique fatty acid profile, with special emphasis on the monounsaturated fatty acid oleic acid, which is more resistant to oxidation than polyunsaturated fats, 2) its antioxidant content such as vitamin E, flavonoids, and polyphenols such as hydroxytyrosol, and 3) its content of other beneficial microconstituents including squalene and β-sitosterol.[6,35,217,218] Besides its own possible cancer-preventive properties, it is important to note that, within the context of the Mediterranean eating pattern, olive oil promotes the plentiful intake of vegetables and legumes as main and accompanying dishes.[35] Consequently, the liberal intake of olive oil can be viewed as a Mediterranean food habit that facilitates and maintains the vegetarian aspects of the Mediterranean Diet.

Although available evidence on cancer and olive oil is not conclusive, a number of Mediterranean studies have supported that olive oil may be either neutral or modestly protective against various malignancies such as cancer of the breast, colon, ovary, endometrium, prostate, pancreas, stomach, esophagus, and lung.[217]

A number of Mediterranean case-control studies[88,96,97,99,100,106,111] have reported on consumption of oils and breast cancer. Of these, one study[106] did not find an association for olive oil, or other fats and oils. The majority of breast cancer studies[88,96,97,99,111] exhibited a minor benefit for olive oil that did not reach statistical significance. Only one Spanish investigation[100] showed that consumption of olive oil lowered the risk of breast cancer significantly.

Case-control studies from Greece,[179] Italy,[87,182,183] Spain,[118] and France[120] have investigated either monounsaturated fat or olive oil with respect to colon cancer. A positive correlation was reported in three of these studies.[179,182,183] The French study[120] found that oils (mainly olive oil) reduced risk, while a recent Italian investigation [87] that controlled for energy, identified a weak beneficial effect for olive oil that was partly confounded by consumption of vegetables. The Spanish study,[118] conducted in Majorca, showed no distinct relationship for consumption of fat, after adjusting data for energy. The authors attributed the absence of association to the overwhelming consumption of olive oil in the studied population, implying a neutral role for olive oil. A genetic study[219] reported a statistically significant inverse association between monounsaturated fat derived mainly from olive oil and risk for a specific colorectal cancer (wild type Ki-*ras* genotype). This finding provides interesting insight for the weak or null associations being reported in epidemiological studies. The authors[219] concluded that, to identify meaningful associations, it may be important, when designing case control investigations, to stratify by tumor genotype.

With respect to ovarian cancer, one case-control study[103] from Greece showed a statistically significant inverse association for monounsaturated fat, mainly from olive oil. Also, an Italian study[122] on ovarian cancer and diet, found no association for consumption of oil. Two case-control studies[94,101] have assessed the role of olive oil or monounsaturated fat chiefly derived from olive oil in relation to endometrial cancer. Both identified an inverse, yet nonsignificant, relationship for frequent consumption of olive oil[101] or monounsaturated fat.[94] Two recently published Greek case-control studies[84,85] have investigated prostate cancer[84] and benign prostatic hyperplasia[85] in relation to olive oil. Both[84,85] documented a lack of association. Interestingly, in the prostate study,[84] monounsaturated fat intake, which was derived from red meat and olive oil combined, increased risk, but without reaching statistical significance. The conflict of findings between the null effect of olive oil and possible adverse influence of monounsaturated fat may be due to the beneficial vitamin E content of olive oil, which was found to significantly reduce prostate cancer risk.[84] No consistent association was noted for monounsaturated fat derived mostly from olive oil in a Greek investigation[102] on cancer of the pancreas. However, a more recent Italian study on pancreatic cancer that evaluated fats in seasonings showed in two analyses[192,220] that intake of oil, primarily olive oil,[220] and olive oil specifically,[192] were inversely and significantly related to risk.

Decreased risk of stomach cancer was correlated with olive oil consumption in an Italian case-control study,[170] and in a recent Spanish ecological study [91] Mediterranean research on esophageal cancer is limited.[124,145] Results suggest that monounsaturated fat increases risk of esophageal adenocarcinoma,[124] while monounsaturated fat,[124] olive oil, or olives[145] may be inversely associated with esophageal squamous-cell carcinoma. Finally, a preliminary presentation of data from a lung cancer case-control study in Italy[221] is suggestive that olive oil used as dressing but not for cooking may be inversely associated with the risk for lung cancer.

It is evident that a small number of Mediterranean studies provide information on the significance of olive oil for each cancer type. Also, a number of these investigations[106,120,122,179,182,183] have not adjusted their data for energy intake, making interpretation of their results challenging. The hint of promise for the cancer-preventive potential of olive oil certainly deserves further scientific research. Lipworth et al.[217] have specifically recommended the need for:

- Prospective randomized intervention trials of moderate to high-risk populations where olive oil will substitute for other fats in the diet
- Major cohort investigations that include Mediterranean populations, such as the European Investigation into Cancer and Nutrition (EPIC) currently in progress
- Assessment of the cancer-preventive properties of monounsaturated fat derived mainly from olive oil, while controlling for other types of fats in typical Western societies such as those in northern Europe and North America
- A multicenter Mediterranean case-control study designed to evaluate the role of olive oil in reducing cancer risk.

1. Red Meat and Fish

High consumption of red meat probably increases the risk of colorectal cancer, and perhaps cancer of the pancreas, breast, prostate, and kidney.[215] It seems that grilled meat and fish possibly increase the risk for stomach cancer, while limited data indicate that cured or smoked meat may also increase the risk for stomach cancer.[115] Diverse or scanty international findings on the relationship between meat consumption and cancers of the mouth and pharynx, larynx, esophagus, lung, gallbladder, liver, ovary, cervix, and bladder preclude a clear comprehensive assessment.[115,222] There is little information suggesting that frequent fish consumption may decrease the risk for breast and ovarian cancer.[215]

The Mediterranean Diet has been described as a traditional dietary pattern that incorporates animal foods in small amounts.[223] The low consumption of red meat, next to the high consumption of fruits and vegetables, is a distinguishing dietary characteristic contributing to the low rates of cancer observed in the Mediterranean.[32,36] Mechanisms by which red meat increases cancer risk have not been elucidated adequately. The fat, protein, or iron content of meat, the production of possible carcinogens, such as heterocyclic amines during the cooking of meat, the lack of fiber and antioxidant agents in meat, the displacement of plant foods in the diet that may be caused by frequent high meat intake could be factors implicated in increasing cancer risk.[32,224]

Fish is consumed in small to moderate amounts in various Mediterranean areas.[223] Fish and fish oils provide n-3 fatty acids shown to inhibit tumors of the colon, breast, and prostate in animal models.[225-227] At the human level, it is not clear whether fish itself is influential enough to reduce cancer risk or consumption of fish is an important substitute for foods like red meat.[215] For example, an ecological study of 24 European countries[95] concluded that fish oil consumption was associated with reducing the promotional effects of animal fat in breast and colorectal cancer.

Several Mediterranean studies[120,121,179-185,212,222] have assessed the role of red meat in colorectal cancer or polyps. Five of these case control studies[179,180,182,183,222] detected positive risk associations for consumption of meat, out of which four[179,180,182,183] observed one or more statistically significant association. Six studies[120,121,181,184,185,212] on the other hand, were not able to demonstrate an appreciable influence of meat. Indeed, in a review of scientific evidence, Hill[228] emphasized that an increasing number of European case-control studies seem to point to a null association between meat and colorectal cancer. With respect to fish consumption and colorectal cancer, six case-control studies[120,180,181,183,184,212] did not identify a meaningful association, yet four other investigations[182,185,212,229] reported a decrease in risk with increased consumption of fish.

In a recent Italian case-control study,[191,222,229] increased intake of red meat was positively related to risk for pancreatic cancer[191,222] and fish consumption was inversely related to risk,[191,229] while another earlier investigation on cancer of the pancreas[190] did not observe a consistent association for meat or fish.

In the case of breast cancer, a Spanish ecological study[65] compared mortality trends and past and current dietary factors. A main conclusion of the study was that past intake of meat is likely to be linked to present rising trends of breast cancer mortality in Spain. Also, elevated breast cancer risk estimates have been reported in relation to consumption of meat or pork or processed meat in several case-control studies.[88,99,132,212,222] Inverse risk associations emerged for fish consumption and breast cancer in some studies[88,90,99] but no relationship was documented in another, more-recent, evaluation.[229] Two studies[122,229] have indicated that consumption of fish may confer protection against ovarian cancer, and three studies[11,122,222] support that increased consumption of meat may be disadvantageous. Moderate elevations in the risk of prostate cancer have been attributed to meat consumption in two Italian case-control studies[199,200] but not in two others.[222,230] Mediterranean data[201,222,229] on red meat or fish intake and kidney cancer do not seem to reveal a noteworthy association. Various case-control studies[169,170,171,172,173] from Italy and Spain are in line with international data, that methods of cooking or processing of meat or fish such as grilling, smoking, pickling, and curing, increase the risk for gastric cancer. The content of nitrites and preformed nitrosamines in processed foods — cured in particular — or the subsequent intragastric formation of nitrosamines from nitrites seem to be important factors that contribute to the unfavorable aspects of processed foods as they relate to gastric cancer.[135] With regard to consumption of meat in general and stomach cancer, one case-control study[222] reported a positive nonsignificant association and another ecological investigation detected no relation.[91] Also, an Italian case-control study[229] documented a consistent benefit for consumption of fish in decreasing stomach cancer risk.

For cancer of the oral cavity and pharynx in relation to meat or fish consumption, findings are equivocal. In one study,[175] interestingly, a significant inverse association emerged for meat consumption. In another,[222] no prominent relationship was identified. Furthermore, in a recent investigation,[86] increased intake of processed meats elevated risk for cancer of the oral cavity and pharynx significantly while fish consumption seemed to be protective. Two case-control studies assessed fish intake: one[229] observed a protective effect on risk for cancer of the oral cavity and pharynx and the other[174] did not find a relation. In terms of cancer of the larynx, three Mediterranean case-control studies[193,194,229] documented a decrease in risk associated with fish consumption. As for the relationship between meat and laryngeal cancer, an increase in risk was noted in two studies[193,194] but in another investigation there was no clear pattern.[222] Fish consumption was significantly associated with risk reduction of esophageal cancer in three investigations.[145,147,229] In one of these studies,[145] further analysis of data demonstrated that lean fish was more beneficial than fatty fish. Also, a nonsignificant increase in risk[147] and a lack of relation[222] was reported for meat consumption and esophageal cancer. A French case-control study[148] of diet and esophageal cancer found that fresh meat decreased risk significantly. It has been postulated[115] that, if diets are deficient, higher meat intake may provide needed micronutrients and may ultimately improve risk for esophageal cancer. Such a positive effect is not likely in populations with more adequate diets.[115] No significant association was detected for gallbladder or liver cancer and intakes of meat or fish.[203,222,229] Also, in the case of cervical cancer, La Vecchia et al.[190] did not find a significant relation for meat or liver consumption, foods that were evaluated separately. Studies that have assessed dietary factors and the risk of endometrial cancer have shown either a protective[189,229] or null[101] effect for fish consumption, and a direct increase[101] or no appreciable variation[189] in risk due to frequent intake of meat. With respect to bladder cancer and diet, Mediterranean data is limited as well.[104,197,222] In two studies,[197,222] meat seemed to elevate bladder cancer risk without reaching statistical significance. In another case-control study,[104] meat intake was associated with a moderate statistically significant decrease in risk, but without demonstrating a dose-related trend in relative risk. In the same study,[104] consumption of saturated fat was shown to be a powerful adverse indicator of risk. The apparent contradiction in findings between the opposite effects of saturated fat and meat was not directly addressed by the authors. No convincing association has been seen between fish consumption and risk for bladder cancer.[229] For thyroid cancer, there are reports showing that fish consumption was significantly protective,[195,196] possibly because it is a good source of iodine.[195] Still, one study did not find a noteworthy association between fish intake and thyroid cancer.[229] Results on meat and thyroid cancer are limited and diverse.[196,222] In one study,[196] raw ham was significantly protective, while cooked ham, salami, and sausages increased risk for thyroid cancer significantly. In another study that evaluated consumption of red meat,[222] thyroid cancer risk was not affected materially.

Although, for every cancer type, Mediterranean or international data are not extensive, the overall evidence seems to indicate that, to minimize cancer risk at the public health scale, it is prudent to limit consumption of red meat, while moderate intakes of fish may be desirable.[222,229] This recommendation is coincidentally in agreement with the inherent traditional eating pattern of Mediterranean people.

5. Wine and Alcohol

Assessment of international research shows that consumption of alcohol has not been related to risk reduction of cancer.[115] In contrast, there is adequate evidence that alcohol increases the risk of the following cancers: mouth and pharynx, larynx, esophagus, and liver.[115] Also, alcohol is likely to increase the risk for cancer of the colon, rectum, and breast, and possibly lung.[115] In the case of breast cancer, even moderate alcohol drinking has been linked to increases in risk.[231] It appears that alcohol does not affect bladder cancer risk, and may not modify appreciably the risk for cancer of the stomach, pancreas, prostate, or kidney.[115]

Traditionally, Mediterranean people have consumed small amounts of alcohol, primarily as wine, and in most occasions during the course of meals.[32,128] In some regions, such as Greece, women used to abstain from alcohol altogether.[32,128] Also, in a Mediterranean population, the quality of a healthy diet in terms of consumption of fruit, vegetables, and fish, did not appear to be linked to the drinking of wine or other alcoholic consumption.[232] Indeed, it has been suggested that wine or alcohol is not necessarily an essential component of the Mediterranean Diet prototype.[32,128] The healthful effect of moderate wine consumption in reducing the risk of coronary heart disease has been adequately established[233] and highly publicized. Yet, numerous cancer investigations and reviews from Mediterranean sources[111,132,142-144,146,147,155,175,176,183,184,193,202,234-253] document an increase in cancer risk associated with increasing alcohol consumption for various types of cancer such as mouth and pharynx, larynx, esophagus, liver, breast.

The lack of relationship between bladder cancer and alcohol suggested by international reviews[115] is also evident in the findings of two Mediterranean case-control studies.[197,254] In contrast, a Spanish case-control study[198] is probably the only report, internationally, that observed a significant positive dose–response relationship between alcohol consumption and bladder cancer risk. However, in the same study,[198] a statistically significant risk estimate emerged only for heavy consumption of alcohol. The majority of Mediterranean studies[91,139,169,173] on stomach cancer does not implicate alcohol or wine consumption as important in risk elevation. A French case-control study,[255] on the other hand, found that red wine significantly increased the risk for stomach cancer, and two other stomach cancer studies[135,168] reported mild risk elevations related to alcoholic beverages. With special reference to cancer of the gastric cardia, there is information suggesting that alcohol intake possibly elevates risk.[115,135] Almost all pertinent pancreatic cancer case-control investigations[192,256,258-261] from the Mediterranean have found no association with alcohol drinking. An exception is a French case-control investigation[257] that observed statistically significant decreases in pancreatic cancer risk due to prolonged alcohol consumption (for at least 10 years) when compared with abstinence. The authors of this study[257] suggested that alcohol per se may not be a protective agent against cancer of the pancreas and that possibly other compounds found in some alcoholic drinks could be responsible for the observed protection due to prolonged drinking. No overall association has been shown for prostate[262,263] or renal cancer[201] and alcohol consumption in Mediterranean studies. Reports[122,264,265] on ovarian cancer and alcohol are limited and diverse. One Italian study[122] reported no association between ovarian cancer and alcohol, another more recent Italian study[265] observed a direct and significant trend in risk related to alcohol intake, primarily as wine, and a Greek investigation[264] found that higher intakes of ethanol (more than two servings of alcohol per day) increased risk but moderate consumption did not.

A study[266] on alcohol and mortality in middle-aged men from eastern France showed that moderate drinking of wine, defined as 2 to 5 servings per day, reduced all-cause mortality by 24–31%. This result is not entirely consistent with the majority of alcohol-related evidence presented thus far, although some case-control studies demonstrate that moderate drinking does not affect cancer risk appreciably for locations such as the liver[202] and esophagus.[240,241] Garidou et al.[241] suggested that intake of alcohol as wine during meals may be an important Mediterranean habit that helps attenuate the undesirable effects of alcohol on the lining of the esophagus. More importantly, the typical generous consumption of fruits and vegetables among Mediterraneans may confound the harmful influence of alcohol on cancer risk.[241,267] Thus, it is important to clarify how diet, especially the Mediterranean Diet, may ameliorate the impact of alcohol on cancer risk. Mechanisms on how alcohol intake could be involved in cancer development are not adequately defined. Alcohol affects the metabolism of steroid hormones, their blood levels, and availability [253] This is a possible mode of action for hormonally related neoplasms such as breast cancer. Additional research is needed to learn more about responsible mechanisms of action, the significance of different types and amounts of alcoholic drinks, and the importance of drinking patterns over time, in relation to cancer outcomes.[253]

Alcohol intake, in any form, even when consumed moderately, may increase some types of cancer, such as breast, oral, or laryngeal cancer.[231,250,268,269] For this, the public health recommendation to "limit consumption of alcoholic beverages, if you drink at all,"[80] is justified and in line with the optional use of alcohol in the Mediterranean Diet.

IV. THE MEDITERRANEAN DIET AS A WHOLE

Our current knowledge of how diet affects cancer risk is incomplete. Nevertheless, evidence from Greece, Italy, Spain, and France, relating dietary factors to cancer risk, shows that integral components of the traditional Mediterranean Diet, namely high consumption of plant foods, conservative intakes of animal foods, and modest to no alcohol drinking, may play a role in the prevention of cancer and the lower cancer rates observed in Mediterranean areas. Diet, though, is probably not the only factor responsible for the health of Mediterranean populations.

Investigations[92,270-272] that assess diet as a whole, dietary quality, and diversity offer promise in better understanding the value of complete dietary patterns in health outcomes. Such studies are quite meaningful because they allow us to quantify, by use of indices, e.g., the Mediterranean Adequacy Index,[272] the deviation of changing dietary habits from the traditional Mediterranean Diet and they facilitate the estimation of effect of total dietary deviation on disease risk. For example, Crosignani et al.[92] projected a 36% survival advantage for laryngeal cancer in those individuals whose eating pattern matches closely the Mediterranean Diet. In terms of intervention research, one report[7] demonstrated the usefulness of the Mediterranean Diet as a successful and appealing means to reduce cancer levels. In this four-year randomized trial,[7] there was a statistically significant 61% reduction in cancer and a comprehensive 56% reduction in deaths and cancer. Such findings are reassuring for the protective efficacy of the Mediterranean Diet and accentuate the necessity for prospective studies that will further elucidate the finer characteristics and underlying mechanisms of the "optimal" diet for maximum health benefit and minimum risk.

Economic growth, industrialization, urbanization, and changes in family structure are powerful factors affecting life-style, including a gradual abandonment of dietary traditions for more "westernized" food choices that favor animal foods. Mediterranean countries are currently undergoing such transition with concurrent increases in noncommunicable diseases such as cancer. No harmful effect has been related to the traditional Mediterranean Diet, so far, and prevention of disease by adopting it long-term is likely. Thus, multiple sources[11,14,16,31] have emphasized the need for coordinated public health efforts to maintain the traditional eating habits among Mediterranean populations and promote, if possible, this healthful eating model in developed societies with worrisome patterns of chronic disease.

REFERENCES

1. Keys, A., Coronary heart disease in seven countries, *Circulation*, 41, 1, 1970.
2. Keys, A., *Seven Countries: a Multivariate Analysis of Death and Coronary Heart Disease*, Harvard University Press, Cambridge, MA, 1980.
3. Blackburn, H., *On the Trail of Heart Attacks in Seven Countries*, University of Minnesota, Minneapolis, MN, 1995.
4. Toshima, H., Koga, Y., and Blackburn, H., Eds., *Lessons for Science from the Seven Countries Study: a 35-year Collaborative Experience in Cardiovascular Disease Epidemiology*, Springer-Verlag, Tokyo, 1994.
5. Kromhout, D., Menotti, A., and Blackburn, H., Eds., *The Seven Countries Study: a Scientific Adventure in Cardiovascular Epidemiology*, Brower Offset, Utrecht, 1994.
6. Hakim, I., Mediterranean diets and cancer prevention, *Arch. Intern. Med.*, 158, 1169, 1998.
7. de Lorgeril, M., Salen, P., Martin, J. L., Monjaud, I., Boucher, P., and Mamelle, N., Mediterranean dietary pattern in a randomized trial: prolonged survival rate and possible reduced cancer rate. *Arch. Intern. Med.*, 158, 1181, 1998.
8. Helsing, E., Traditional diets and disease patterns of the Mediterranean, circa 1960s, *Am. J. Clin. Nutr.*, 61, S1329, 1995.
9. Tavani, A., and La Vecchia, A., Fruit and vegetable consumption and cancer risk in a Mediterranean population, *Am. J. Clin. Nutr.*, 61, S1374, 1995.
10. Filiberti, R., Kubik, A., Reissigova, J., Merlo, F., and Bonassi, S., Cancer, cardiovascular mortality, and diet in Italy and the Czech Republic, *Neoplasma*, 42, 275, 1995.
11. Serra-Majem, L., La Vecchia C., Ribas-Barba, L., Prieto-Ramos, F., Lucchini, F., Ramon, J. M., and Salleras, L., Changes in diet and mortality from selected cancers in southern Mediterranean countries, 1960–1989, *Eur. J. Clin. Nutr.*, 47, S25, 1993.
12. Benito, E. and Cabeza, E., Diet and cancer risk: an overview of Spanish studies, *Eur. J. Cancer Prevent.*, 2, 215, 1993.
13. Giacosa, A. and Visconti, P., The Mediterranean diet, *Eur. J. Cancer Prevent.*, 1, 197, 1992.

14. Hill, M. and Giacosa, A., The Mediterranean diet, *Eur. J. Cancer Prevent.*, 1, 339, 1992.

15. Decarli, A. and La Vecchia, C., Diet and Cancer, in: *The Mediterranean Diets in Health and Disease*, Spiller, G. A., Ed., Van Nostrand Reinhold, New York, 1991, Chap. 15.

16. ECP workshop on the Mediterranean diet, Cosenza, 28–29 June 1991, *Eur. J. Cancer Prevent.*, 1, 79, 1991.

17. La Vecchia, C., Negri, E., Franceschi, S., Parazzini, F., Marubibi, E., and Trichopoulos, D., Diet and cancer risk in northern Italy: an overview from various case-control studies, *Tumori*, 76, 306, 1990s.

18. World Health Organization, *The World Health Report*, World Health Organization, Geneva, 1997.

19. Doll, R. and Peto, R., The causes of cancer: quantitative estimates of avoidable risks in the United States today, *J. Natl. Cancer Inst.*, 66, 1191, 1981.

20. Wynder, E. L. and Gori, G. B., Contribution of the environment to cancer incidence: an epidemiological exercise, *J. Natl. Cancer Inst.*, 58, 825, 1977.

21. Armstrong, B. and Doll, R., Environmental factors and cancer incidence and mortality in different countries, with special reference to dietary practices, *Int. J. Cancer*, 15, 617, 1975.

22. Doll, R., Muir, C., and Waterhouse, J., *Cancer Incidence in Five Continents*, Springer-Verlag, New York, 1970.

23. World Cancer Research Fund, and American Institute for Cancer Research, Food, nutrition, and the prevention of cancer: a global perspective, American Institute for Cancer Research, Washington, D. C., 1997, Chap. 1.

24. La Vecchia, C. and Tavani, A., Fruit and vegetables and human cancer, *Eur. J. Cancer Prevent.*, 7, 3, 1998.

25. Willet, W. C. and Trichopoulos, D., Summary of the evidence: nutrition and cancer, *Cancer Causes Control*, 7, 178, 1996.

26. Steinmetz, K. A. and Potter, J. D., Vegetables, fruit, and cancer prevention: a review, *J. Am. Diet. Assoc.*, 96, 1027, 1996.

27. Block, G., Patterson, B., and Subar, A., Fruit, vegetables, and cancer prevention: a review of the epidemiological evidence, *Nutr. Cancer*, 18, 1, 1992.

28. Negri, E., La Vecchia, C., Franceschi, S., D' Avanzo, B., and Parazzini, F., Vegetable and fruit consumption and cancer risk, *Int. J. Cancer*, 48, 350, 1991.

29. Steinmetz, K. A. and Potter, J. D., A review of vegetables, fruit and cancer epidemiology, *Cancer Causes Control*, 2, 325, 1991.

30. Nestle, M., Traditional models of healthy eating: alternatives to "techno food," *J. Nutr. Educ.*, 26, 241, 1994.

31. Nestle, M., Mediterranean diets: historical and research overview, *Am. J. Clin. Nutr.*, 61, S1313, 1995.

32. Willet, W. C., Sacks, F., Trichopoulou, A., Drescher, G., Ferro-Luzzi, A., Helsing, E., and Trichopoulos, D., Mediterranean diet pyramid: a cultural model for healthy eating, *Am. J. Clin. Nutr.*, 61, S1402, 1995.

33. Trichopoulou, A., Toupadaki, N., Tzonou, A., Katsouyanni, K., Manousos, O., Kada, E., and Trichopoulos, D., The macronutrient composition of the Greek diet: estimates derived from six case-control studies, *Eur. J. Clin. Nutr.*, 47, 549, 1993.

34. Trichopoulou, A. and Lagiou, P., Healthy traditional Mediterranean diet: an expression of culture, history, and lifestyle, *Nutr. Rev.*, 55, 383, 1997.

35. Trichopoulou, A., Lagiou, P., and Papas, A. M., Mediterranean diet: are antioxidants central to its benefits? in: *Antioxidant Status, Diet, Nutrition, and Health*, Papas, A. M., Ed., CRC Press, Boca Raton, Fl, 1998, Chap. 6.
36. Levi, F., Cancer prevention: epidemiology and perspectives, *Eur. J. Cancer*, 35, 1046, 1999.
37. World Health Organization, and Food and Agriculture Organization, Food and health indicators in Europe: nutrition and health, 1961–1990, World Health Organization Regional Office for Europe, Nutrition Unit, Geneva, 1993.
38. World Health Organization, Tobacco or health: a global status report, World Health Organization, Geneva, 1997.
39. World Health Organization Cancer Mortality Databank, http://www-dep.iarc.fr/dataava/globocan/who.htm, 1999.
40. Black, R. J., Bray, F., Ferlay, J., and Parkin, D. M., Cancer incidence and mortality in the European Union: cancer registry data and estimates of national incidence for 1990s, *Eur. J. Cancer*, 33, 1075, 1997.
41. Armstrong, B. and Doll, R., Environmental factors and cancer incidence and mortality in different countries, with special reference to dietary practices, *Int. J. Cancer*, 15, 617, 1975.
41. Doll, R., Muir, C., and Waterhouse, J., *Cancer Incidence in Five Continents*, Springer-Verlag, New York, 1970.
43. Higginson, J., Population studies in cancer, *Acta IUCC*, 16, 1667, 1960.
44. Wynder, E. L., Lemon, F., and Bross, I. J., Cancer and coronary artery disease among Seventh-day Adventists, *Cancer*, 12, 1016, 1959.
45. Benito, E. and Cabeza E., Diet and cancer risk: an overview of Spanish studies, *Eur. J. Cancer Prevent.*, 2, 215, 1993.
46. Rose, D. P., Boyar, A. P., and Wynder, E. L., International comparisons of mortality rates of cancer of the breast, ovary, prostate, and colon, and per capita food consumption, *Cancer*, 58, 2363, 1986.
47. Lagiou, P., Trichopoulou, A., Henderickx, H. K., Kelleher, C., Leonhauser, I. U., Moreiras, O., Nelson, M., Schmitt, A., Sekula, W., Trygg, K., and Zajkas, G., Household budget survey nutritional data in relation to mortality from coronary heart disease, colorectal cancer and female breast cancer in European countries. DAFNE I and II projects of the European Commission. Data Food Networking, *Eur. J. Clin. Nutr.*, 53, 328, 1999.
48. La Vecchia, C., Harris, R., and Wynder, E. L., Comparative epidemiology of cancer between the United States and Italy, *Cancer Res.*, 48, 7285, 1988.
49. Mettlin, C., Global Breast Cancer Mortality Statistics, *CA Cancer J. Clin.*, 49, 138, 1999.
50. Wynder, E. L., personal communication, 1997.
51. World Cancer Research Fund, and American Institute for Cancer Research, Food, Nutrition, and the Prevention of Cancer: a global perspective, American Institute for Cancer Research, Washington, D. C., 1997, introduction.
52. Trichopoulou, A., Lagiou, P., and Gnardellis, C., Traditional Greek diet and coronary heart disease, *J. Cardiovasc. Risk*, 1, 9, 1994.
53. Levi, F., La Vecchia, C., Lucchini, F., and Negri, F., Cancer mortality in Europe, 1990–1992, *Eur. J. Cancer Prevent.*, 3, 109, 1994.
54. Food and Agriculture Organization, FAOSTAT Statistics Database, Nutrition, Food Balance Sheets, http://apps.fao.org/, 1999.

55. Giacco, A. and Riccardi, G., Comparison of Current Eating Habits in Various Mediterranean Countries, in: *The Mediterranean Diets in Health and Disease*, Spiller, G. A., Ed., Avi, Van Nostrand Reinhold, New York, 1991, Chap. 1.

56. Hulshof, K. F., van Erp-Baart, M. A., Anttlainen, M., Becker, W., Church, S. M., Couet, C., Hermann-Kunz, E., Kesteloot, H., Leth, T., Martins, I., Moreiras, O., Moschandreas, J., Pizzoferrato, L., Rimestad, A. H., Thorgeirsdottir, H., van Amelsvoort, J. M., Aro, A., Kafatos, A. G., Lanzmann-Petithory, D., and van Poppel, G., Intake of fatty acids in Western Europe with emphasis on trans fatty acids: the TRANSFAIR Study, *Eur. J. Clin. Nutr.*, 53, 143, 1999.

57. Kromhout, D., Keys, A., Aravanis, C., Buzina, R., Fidanza, F., Giampaoli, S., Jansen, A., Menotti, A., Nedeljkovic, S., Pekkarinen, M., Simic, B. S., and Toshima, H. Food consumption patterns in the 1960s in seven countries, *Am. J. Clin. Nutr.*, 49, 889, 1989.

58. Trichopoulou, A. and Lagiou, P. The DAFNE food data bank as a tool for monitoring food availability in Europe. Data Food Networking, *Pub. Hlth. Rev.*, 26, 65, 1998.

59. Gonzalez, C. A., Dietary patterns in Europe—preliminary results of dietary habits in the EPIC Study. European Prospective Investigation on Cancer and Nutrition, *Eur. J. Cancer Prevent.*, 6, 125, 1997.

60. Trichopoulou, A., Kouris-Blazos, A., Wahlqvist, M. L., Gnardellis, C., Lagiou, P., Polychronopoulos, E., Vassilakou, T., Lipworth, L., and Trichopoulos, D., Diet and overall survival in elderly people, *Br. Med. J.*, 331, 1457, 1995.

61. Gonzalez, C. A., Torrent, M., and Agudo, A., Dietary habits in Spain: an approximation, *Tumori*, 76, 311, 1990.

62. Moreiras-Varela, O., The Mediterranean diet in Spain, *Eur. J. Clin. Nutr.*, 43, Suppl. 2, 83, 1989.

63. Zilidis, C., Trends in nutrition in Greece: use of international data to monitor national developments, *Pub. Hlth.*, 107, 271, 1993.

64. Alberti-Fidanza, A., Paolacci, C. A., Chiuchiu, M. P., Coli, R., Fruttini, D., Verducci, G., and Fidanza, F., Dietary studies on two rural Italian population groups of the Seven Countries Study. 1. Food and nutrient intake at the thirty-first year follow-up in 1991, *Eur. J. Clin. Nutr.*, 48, 85, 1994.

65. Prieto-Ramos, F., Serra-Majem, L., La Vecchia, C., Ramon, J. M., Tresserras, R., and Salleras, L., Mortality trends and past and current dietary factors of breast cancer in Spain, *Eur. J. Epidemiol.*, 12, 141, 1996.

66. World Cancer Research Fund, and American Institute for Cancer Research, Food, Nutrition, and the Prevention of Cancer: a Global Perspective, American Institute for Cancer Research, Washington, D. C., 1997, Chap. 5.

67. Wynder, E. L., Cohen, L. A., Muscat, J. E., Winters, B., Dwyer, J. T., and Blackburn, G., Breast cancer: weighing the evidence for promoting the role of dietary fat, *J. Natl. Cancer Inst.*, 89, 766, 1997.

68. Potter, J. D., Nutrition and colorectal cancer, *Cancer Causes Control*, 7, 127, 1996.

69. Kolonel, L. N., Nutrition and prostate cancer, *Cancer Causes Control*, 7, 83, 1996.

70. Hill, H. A. and Austin, H., Nutrition and endometrial cancer, *Cancer Causes Control*, 7, 19, 1996.

71. Weisburger, J. H. and Wynder, E. L., Dietary fat intake and cancer, *Hematol. Oncol. Clin. North Am.*, 5, 7, 1991.

72. World Health Organization, Diet, Nutrition, and the Prevention of Chronic Diseases, Technical Report 797, World Health Organization, Geneva, 1990.

73. National Research Council, Committee on Diet and Health, Food and Nutrition Board, and Commission on Life Sciences, *Diet and Health, Implications for Reducing Chronic Disease Risk,* National Academy Press, Washington, D. C., 1989, Chap. 22.

74. National Academy of Sciences, *Diet, Nutrition, and Cancer,* National Academy Press, Washington, D. C., 1982.

75. Rose, D. P., Dietary fatty acids and cancer, *Am. J. Clin. Nutr.,* 66, S998, 1997.

76. Grundy, S. M., What is the desirable ratio of saturated, polyunsaturated, and monounsaturated fatty acids in the diet? *Am. J. Clin. Nutr.,* 66, S988, 1997.

77. Prentice, R. L. and Sheppard, L., Dietary fat and cancer: consistency of the epidemiologic data, and disease prevention that may follow from a practical reduction in fat consumption, *Cancer Causes Control,* 1, 81, 1990.

78. Cohen, L. A., Thompson, D. O., Maeura, Y., Choi, K., Blank, M. E., and Rose, D. P., Dietary fat and mammary cancer. I. Promoting effects of different dietary fats on N-nitrosomethylurea-induced rat mammary tumorigenesis, *J. Natl. Cancer Inst.,* 77, 33, 1986.

79. Carroll, K. K., Experimental evidence of dietary factors and hormone-dependent cancers, *Cancer Res.,* 35, 3374, 1975.

80. American Cancer Society Dietary Guidelines Advisory Committee, Guidelines on Diet, Nutrition and Cancer Prevention: Reducing the Risk of Cancer with Healthy Food Choices and Physical Activity, American Cancer Society, Washington, D. C., 1996.

81. Miller, A. B., Berrino, F., Hill, M., Pietnen, P., Riboli, E., and Warendorf, J., European School of Oncology Task Force, Diet in the etiology of cancer: a review, *Eur. J. Cancer,* 30A, 207, 1994.

82. Wynder, E. L., Weisburger, J. H., and Ng, S. K., Nutrition: the need to define "optimal" intake as a basis for public policy decisions, *Am. J. Public Health,* 82, 346, 1992.

83. Byers, T., Dietary trends in the U.S., Relevance to cancer prevention, *Cancer,* 72, 1015, 1993.

84. Tzonou, A., Signorello, L. B., Lagiou, P., Wuu, J., Trichopoulos, D., and Trichopoulou, A. Diet and cancer of the prostate: a case-control study in Greece, *Int. J. Cancer,* 80, 704, 1999.

85. Lagiou, P., Wuu, J., Trichopoulou, A., Hsieh, C. C., Adami, H. O., and Trichopoulos, D., Diet and benign prostatic hyperplasia: a study in Greece, *Urology,* 54, 284, 1999.

86. Franceschi, S., Favero, A., Conti, E., Talamini, R., Volpe, R., Negri, E., Barzan, L., and La Vecchia, C., Food groups, oils and butter, and cancer of the oral cavity and pharynx, *Br. J. Cancer,* 80, 614, 1999.

87. Braga, C., La Vecchia, C., Franceschi, S., Negri, E., Parpinel, M., Decarli, A., Giacosa, A., and Trichopoulos, D., Olive oil, other seasoning fats, and the risk of colorectal carcinoma, *Cancer,* 82, 448, 1998.

88. Favero, A., Parpinel, M., and Franceschi, S., Diet and risk of breast cancer: major findings from an Italian case-control study. *Biomed. & Pharmacother.,* 52, 109, 1998.

89. Trichopoulou, A. and Lagiou, P., Re: Correlating nutrition to recent cancer mortality statistics, *J. Natl. Cancer Inst.,* 89, 1725, 1997.

90. Braga, C., La Vecchia, C., Negri, E., Franceschi, S., and Parpinel, M., Intake of selected foods and nutrients and breast cancer risk: an age- and menopause-specific analysis, *Nutr. Cancer,* 28, 258, 1997.

91. Corella, D., Cortina, P., Guillen, M., and Gonzalez, J. I., Dietary habits and geographic variation in stomach cancer mortality in Spain, *Eur. J. Cancer Prevent.,* 5, 249, 1996.

92. Crosignani, P., Russo, A., Tagliabue, G., and Berrino, F., Tobacco and diet as determinants of survival in male laryngeal cancer patients, *Int. J. Cancer*, 65, 308, 1996.
93. Francheschi, S., Favero, A., Decarli, A., Negri, E., La Vecchia, C., Ferranoni, M., Russo, A., Salvini, S., Amadori, D., Conti, E., Montela, M., and Giacosa, A., Intake of macronutrients and risk of breast cancer, *Lancet*, 347, 1351, 1996.
94. Tzonou, A., Lipworth, L., Kalandidi, A., Trichopoulou, A., Gamatsi, A., Hsieh, C. C., Notara, V., and Trichopoulos, D., Dietary factors and the risk of endometrial cancer: a case-control study in Greece, *Br. J. Cancer*, 73, 1284, 1996.
95. Caygill, C. P., Charlett, A., and Hill, M., Fat, fish, fish oil and cancer, *Br. J. Cancer*, 74, 159, 1996.
96. La Vecchia, C., Negri, E., Franceschi, S., Decarli, A., Giacosa, A., and Lipworth, L. Olive oil, other dietary fats, and the risk of breast cancer (Italy), *Cancer Causes Control*, 6, 545, 1995.
97. Trichopoulou, A., Katsouyanni, K., Stuver, S., Tzala, L., Gnardellis, C., Rimm, E., and Trichopoulos, D., Consumption of olive oil and specific food groups in relation to breast cancer in Greece, *J. Natl. Cancer Inst.*, 87, 110, 1995.
98. Katsouyanni, K., Trichopoulou, A., Stuver, S., Garas, Y., Kritselis, A., Kyriakou, G., Stoikidou, M., Boyle, P., and Trichopoulos, D., The association of fat and other macronutrients with breast cancer: a case-control study from Greece. *Br. J. Cancer*, 70, 537, 1994.
99. Landa, M. C., Frago, N., and Tres, A. Diet and risk of breast cancer in Spain, *Eur. J. Cancer Prevent.*, 3, 313, 1994.
100. Martin-Moreno, J. M., Willet, W. C., Gorgojo, L., Banegas, J. R., Rodriguez-Artalejo, F., Fernandez-Rodriguez, J. C., Maisonneuve, P., and Boyle, P., Dietary fat, olive oil intake and breast cancer risk, *Int. J. Cancer*, 58, 774, 1994.
101. Levi, F., Franceschi, S., Negri, E., and La Vecchia, C., Dietary factors and the risk of endometrial cancer, *Cancer*, 71, 3575, 1993.
102. Kalapothaki, V., Tzonou, A., Hsieh, C. C., Karakatsani, A., Trichopoulou, A., Toupadaki, N., and Trichopoulos, D., Nutrient intake and cancer of the pancreas: a case-control-study in Athens, Greece, *Cancer Causes Control*, 4, 383, 1993.
103. Tzonou, A., Hsieh, C. C., Polychronopoulou, A., Kaprinis, G., Toupadaki, N., Trichopoulou, A., Karakatsani, A., and Trichopoulos, D., Diet and ovarian cancer: a case control study in Greece, *Int. J. Cancer*, 55, 411, 1993.
104. Riboli, E., Gonzalez, C. A., Lopez-Abente, G., Errezola, M., Izarzugaza, I., Escolar, A., Nebot, M., Hemon, B., and Agudo, A., Diet and bladder cancer in Spain: a multi-centre case-control study, *Int. J. Cancer*, 49, 214, 1991.
105. Katsouyanni, K., Willet, W., Trichopoulos, D., Boyle, P., Trichopoulou, A., Vasilaros, S., Papadiamantis, J., and MacMahon, B., Risk of breast cancer among Greek women in relation to nutrient intake, *Cancer*, 61, 181, 1988.
106. Katsouyanni, K., Trichopoulos, D., Boyle, P., Xirouchaki, E., Trichopoulou, A., Lisseos, B., Vasilaros, S., and MacMahon, B., Diet and breast cancer: a case-control study in Greece, *Int. J. Cancer*, 38, 815, 1986.
107. Berrino, F. and Muti, P., Mediterranean diet and cancer, *Eur. J. Clin. Nutr.*, 43, Suppl. 2, 49, 1989.
108. Franceschi, S., Russo, A., and La Vecchia, C., Carbohydrates, fat and cancer of the breast and colon-rectum, *J. Epidemiol. Biostat.*, 3, 217, 1998.
109. Farchi, S., Saba, A., Turrini, A., Forlani, F., Pettinelli, A., and D'Amicis, A., An ecological study of the correlation between diet and tumour mortality rates in Italy, *Eur. J. Cancer Prevent.*, 5, 113, 1996.

110. Taioli, E., Nicolosi, A., and Wynder, E. L., Dietary habits and breast cancer: a comparative study of the United States and Italian data, *Nutr. Cancer*, 166, 259, 1991.
111. Toniolo, P., Riboli, E., Protta, F., Charrel, M., and Cappa, A. P., Calorie-providing nutrients and risk of breast cancer, *J. Natl. Cancer Inst.*, 81, 278, 1989.
112. Franceschi, S. and Favero, A., The role of energy and fat in cancers of the breast and colon-rectum in a southern European population, *Ann. Oncol.*, 10, suppl. 6, 61, 1999.
113. La Vecchia, C., Favero, A., and Franceschi, S., Monounsaturated and other types of fat, and the risk of breast cancer, *Eur. J. Cancer Prevent.*, 7, 461, 1998.
114. Richardson, S., Gerber, M., and Cenee, S., The role of fat, animal protein and some vitamin consumption in breast cancer: a case-control study in southern France, *Int. J. Cancer*, 48, 1, 1991.
115. World Cancer Research Fund, and American Institute for Cancer Research, Food, Nutrition, and the Prevention of Cancer: a Global Perspective, American Institute for Cancer Research, Washington, D. C., 1997, Chap. 4.
116. Trichopoulou, A., Tzonou, A., Hsieh, C. C., Toupadaki, N., Manousos, O., and Trichopoulos, D., High protein, saturated fat and cholesterol diet, and low levels of serum lipids in colorectal cancer, *Int. J. Cancer*, 51, 386, 1992.
117. Franceschi, S., La Vecchia, C., Russo, A., Favero, A., Negri, E., Conti, E., Montella, M., Filiberti, R., Amadori, D., and Decarli, A., Macronutrient intake and risk of colorectal cancer in Italy, *Int. J. Cancer*, 76, 321, 1998.
118. Benito, E., Stiggelbout, A., Bosch, F. X., Obrador, A., Kaldor, J., Mulet, M., and Munoz, N., Nutritional factors in colorectal cancer risk: a case-control study in Majorca, *Int. J. Cancer*, 49, 161, 1991.
119. Benito, E., Cabeza, E., Moreno, V., Obrador, A., and Bosch, F. X., Diet and colorectal adenomas: a case-control study in Majorca, *Int. J. Cancer*, 55, 213, 1993.
120. Macquart-Moulin, G., Riboli, E., Cornee, J., Charnay, B., Berthezene, P., and Day, N., Case-control study on colorectal cancer and diet in Marseilles, *Int. J. Cancer*, 38, 183, 1986.
121. Macquart-Moulin, G., Riboli, E., Cornee, J., Kaaks, R., and Berthezene, P., Colorectal polyps and diet: a case control study in Marseilles, *Int. J. Cancer*, 40, 179, 1987.
122. La Vecchia, C., Decarli, A., Negri, E., Parazzini, F., Gentile, A., Cecchetti, G., Fasoli, M., and Franceschi, S., Dietary factors and the risk of epithelial ovarian cancer, *J. Natl. Cancer Inst.*, 79, 663, 1987.
123. Franceschi, S., Levi, F., Conti, E., Talamini, R., Negri, E., Dal Maso, L., Boyle, P., Decarli, A., and La Vechia, C., Energy intake and dietary pattern in cancer of the oral cavity and pharynx, *Cancer Causes Control*, 10, 439, 1999.
124. Tzonou, A., Lipworth, L., Garidou, A., Signorello, L. B., Lagiou, P., Hsieh, C., and Trichopoulos, D., Diet and risk of esophageal cancer by histologic type in a low-risk population, *Int. J. Cancer*, 68, 300, 1996.
125. Miller, A. B., An overview of hormone-associated cancers, *Cancer Res.*, 38, 3985, 1978.
126. Koumantaki, Y., Tzonou, A., Koumantakis, E., Kaklamani, E., Aravantinos, D., and Trichopoulos, D., A case-control study of cancer of the endometrium in Athens, *Int. J. Cancer*, 43, 795, 1989.
127. La Vecchia, C., Cancers associated with high-fat diets, *J. Natl. Cancer Inst. Inst. Monogr.*, 12, 79, 1992.
128. Kushi, L. H., Lenart, E. B., and Willet, E. C., Health implications of Mediterranean diets in light of contemporary knowledge. 2. Meat, wine, fats, and oils, *Am. J. Clin. Nutr.*, 61, 1416S, 1995.

129. World Cancer Research Fund, and American Institute for Cancer Research, Food, Nutrition, and the Prevention of Cancer: a Global Perspective, American Institute for Cancer Research, Washington, D. C., 1997, Chap. 5.

130. Jansen, M. C., Bueno-de-Mesquita, H. B., Buzina, R., Fidanza, F., Menotti, A., Blackburn, H., Nissinen, A. M., Kok, F. J., and Kromhout, D., Dietary fiber and plant foods in relation to colorectal cancer mortality: the Seven Countries Study, *Int. J. Cancer,* 81, 174, 1999.

131. Negri, E., Franceschi, S., Parpinel, M., and La Vecchia, C., Fiber intake and risk of colorectal cancer, *Cancer Epidemiol. Biomarkers Prevent.,* 7, 667, 1998.

132. La Vecchia, C., Decarli, A., Franceschi, S., Gentile, A., Negri, E., and Parazzini, F., Dietary factors and the risk of breast cancer, *Nutr. Cancer,* 10, 205, 1987.

133. La Vecchia, C., Ferraroni, M., Franceschi, S., Mezzetti, M., Decarli, A., and Negri, E., Fibers and breast cancer risk, *Nutr. Cancer,* 28, 264, 1997.

134. Challier, B., Perarnau, J. M., and Viel, J. F., Garlic, onion and cereal fibre as protective factors for breast cancer: a French case-control study, *Eur. J. Epidemiol.,* 14, 737, 1998.

135. Gonzalez, C. A., Riboli, E., Badosa, J., Batiste, E., Cardona, T., Pita, S., Sanz, J. M., Torrent, M., and Agudo, A., Nutritional factors and gastric cancer in Spain, *Am. J. Epidemiol.,* 139, 466, 1994.

136. Cornee, J., Pobel, D., Riboli, E., Guyader, E., and Hemon, B., A case-control study of gastric cancer and nutritional factors in Marseille, France, *Eur. J. Epidemiol.,* 11, 55, 1995.

137. Slavin, J., Jacobs Jr, D. R., and Marquart, L., Whole-grain consumption and chronic disease: protective mechanisms, *Nutr. Cancer,* 27, 14, 1997.

138. Ramon, J. M., Serra-Majem, L., Cerdo, C., and Oromi, J., Nutrient intake and gastric cancer risk: a case-control study in Spain, *Int. J. Epidemiol.,* 22, 983, 1993.

139. Buiatti, E., Palli, D., Decarli, A., Amadori, D., Avellini, C., Bianchi, S., Bonaguri, C., Cipriani, F., Cocco, P., and Giacosa, A., A case-control study of gastric cancer and diet in Italy: II. Association with nutrients, *Int. J. Cancer,* 45, 896, 1990.

140. Kushi, L., Lenart, E. B., and Willet, W. C., Health implications of Mediterranean diets in light of contemporary knowledge. 1. Plant foods and dairy products, *Am. J. Clin. Nutr.,* 61, S1407, 1995.

141. La Vecchia, C., Franceshi, S., Levi, F., Lucchini, F., and Negri, E., Diet and human oral carcinoma in Europe, *Eur. J. Cancer Oral Oncol.,* 29B, 17, 1993.

142. Negri, E., La Vecchia, C., Franceschi, S., and Tavani, A., Attributable risk for oral cancer in northern Italy, *Cancer Epidemiol. Biomarkers Prevent.,* 2, 189, 1993.

143. Tavani, A., Negri, E., Franceschi, S., Barbone, F., and La Vecchia, C., Attributable risk for laryngeal cancer in nortern Italy, *Cancer Epidemiol. Biomarkers Prevent.,* 3, 121, 1994.

144. Tavani, A., Negri, E., Franceschi, S., and La Vecchia, C., Risk factors for esophageal cancer in women in northern Italy, *Cancer,* 72, 2531, 1993.

145. Launoy, G., Milan, C., Day, N. E., Pienkowski, M. P., Gignoux, M., and Faivre, J., Diet and the squamous-cell cancer of the oesophagus: a French multicentre case-control study, *Int. J. Cancer,* 76, 7, 1998.

146. Decarli, A., Liati, P., Negri, E., Franceschi, S., and La Vecchia, C., Vitamin A and other dietary factors in the etiology of esophageal cancer, *Nutr. Cancer,* 10, 29, 1987.

147. Tavani, A., Negri, E., Franceschi, S., and La Vecchia, C., Risk factors for esophageal cancer in lifelong nonsmokers, *Cancer Epidemiol. Biomarkers Prevent.,* 3, 387, 1994.

148. Tuyns, A. J., Riboli, E., Doornbos, G., and Pequignot, G., Diet and esophageal cancer in Calvados (France), *Nutr. Cancer,* 9, 81, 1987.

149. La Vecchia, C., D'Avanzo, B., Negri, E., Decarli, A., and Benichou, J., Attributable risks for stomach cancer in northern Italy, *Int. J. Cancer*, 60, 748, 1995.
150. Garcia-Closas, R., Gonzalez, C. A., Agudo, A., and Riboli, E., Intake of specific carotenoids and flavonoids and the risk of gastric cancer in Spain, *Cancer Causes Control*, 10, 71, 1999.
151. La Vecchia, C., Braga, C., Negri, E., Franceschi, S., Russo, A., Conti, E., Falcini, F., Giacosa, A., Montella, M., and Decarli, A., Intake of selected micronutrients and risk of colorectal cancer, *Int. J. Cancer*, 73, 525, 1997.
152. Ferranoni, M., La Vecchia, C., D'Avanzo, B., Negri, E., Francesci, S., and Decarli, A., Selected micronutrient intake and the risk of colorectal cancer, *Br. J. Cancer*, 70, 1150, 1994.
153. Negri, E., La Vecchia, C., Franceschi, S., D' Avanzo, B., Talamini, R., Parpinel, M., Ferranoni, M., Filiberti, R., Montella, M., Falcini, F., Conti, E., and Decarli, A., Intake of selected micronutrients and the risk of breast cancer, *Int. J. Cancer*, 65, 140, 1996.
154. Bohlke, K., Spiegelman, D., Trichopoulou, A., Katsouyanni, K., and Trichopoulos, D. Vitamins A, C, and E and the risk of breast cancer: results from a case control study in Greece, *Br. J. Cancer*, 79, 23, 1999.
155. Mezzetti, M., La Vecchia, C., Decarli, A., Boyle, P., Talamini, R., and Franceschi, S., Population attributable risk for breast cancer: diet, nutrition, an physical exercise, *J. Natl. Cancer Inst.*, 90, 389, 1998.
156. La Vecchia, C., Ferraroni, M., Negri, E., and Franceschi, S., Role of various carotenoids in the risk of breast cancer, *Int. J. Cancer*, 75, 482, 1998.
157. Brennan, P., Fortes, C., Butler, J., Agudo, A., Benhamou, S., Darby, S., Gerken, M., Jokel, K. H., Kreuzer, M., Mallone, S., Nyberg, F., Pohlabeln, H., Ferro, G., and Boffetta, P., A multicenter case-control study of diet and lung cancer among non-smokers, *Cancer Causes Control*, 11, 49, 2000.
158. Hertog, M. G., Kromhout, D., Aravanis, C., Blackburn, H., Buzina, R., Fidanza, F., Giampaoli, S., Jansen, A., Menotti, A., Nedeljkovic, S., Pekkarinen, M., Simic B. S., Toshima, H., Feskens, E. J. M., Hollman, P. C. H., and Katan, M. B., Flavonoid intake and long term risk of coronary heart disease and cancer in the seven countries study, *Arch. Int. Med.*, 155, 381, 1995.
159. Ocke, M. C., Kromhout, D., Menotti, A., Aravanis, C., Blackburn, H., Buzina, R., Fidanza, F., Jansen, A., Nedeljkovic, S., Nissinen, A., Pekkarinen, M., and Toshima, H., Average intake of anti-oxidant (pro)vitamins and subsequent cancer mortality in the 16 cohorts of the Seven Countries Study, *Int. J. Cancer*, 61, 480, 1995.
160. Van't Veer, P., Starin, J. J., Fernandez-Crehuet, J., Martin, B. C., Thamm, M., Kardinaal, A. F., Kohlmeier, L., Huttunen, J. K., Martin-Moreno, J. M., and Kok, F. J., Tissue antioxidants and postmenopausal breast cancer: the European Community Multicentre Study on Antioxidants, Myocardial Infarction, and Cancer of the Breast (EURAMIC), *Cancer Epidemiol. Biomarkers Prevent.*, 5, 441, 1996.
161. Garcia-Closas, R., Agudo, A., Gonzalez, C. A., and Riboli, E., Intake of specific carotenoids and flavonoids and the risk of lung cancer in women in Barcelona, Spain, *Nutr. Cancer*, 32, 154, 1998.
162. Ghiselli, A., D'Amicis, A., and Giacosa, A., The antioxidant potential of the Mediterranean diet, *Eur. J. Cancer Prevent.*, 6, S15, 1997.
163. James, W. P. T., Duthie, G. G., and Wahle K. W. J., The Mediterranean diet: protective or simply non-toxic? *Eur. J. Clin. Nutr.*, 43 (suppl. 2), 31, 1989.
164. Weisburger, J. H., Evaluation of the evidence on the role of tomato products in disease prevention, *Proc. Soc. Exp. Biol. Med.*, 218, 140, 1998.

165. Negri, E., La Vecchia, C., Franceschi, S., D'Avanzo, B., and Parazzini, F., Vegetable and fruit consumption and cancer risk, *Int. J. Cancer*, 48, 350, 1991.
166. La Vecchia, C., Chatenoud, L., Franceschi, S., Soler, M., Parazzini, F., and Negri, E., Vegetables and fruit and human cancer: Update of an Italian study, *Int. J. Cancer*, 82, 151, 1999.
167. Jansen, M. C., Bueno-de-Meaquita, H. B., Rasanen, L., Fidanza, F., Menotti, A., Nissinen, A., Feskens, E. J., Kok, F. J., and Kromhout, D., Consumption of plant foods and stomach cancer mortality in the Seven Countries Study. Is grain consumption a risk factor? Seven Countries Study Research Group, *Nutr. Cancer*, 34, 49, 1999.
168. Trichopoulos, D., Ouranos, G., Day, N. E., Tzonou, A., Manousos, O., Papadimitriou, C., and Trichopoulos, A., Diet and cancer of the stomach: a case-control study in Greece, *Int. J. Cancer*, 36, 291, 1985.
169. La Vecchia, C., Negri, E., Decarli, A., D'Avanzo, B., and Franceschi, S., A case-control study of diet and gastric cancer in northern Italy, *Int. J. Cancer*, 40, 484, 1987.
170. Buiatti, E., Palli, D., Decarli, A., Amadori, D., Avellini, C., Bianchi, S., Biserni, R., Cipriani, F., Cocco, P., and Giacosa, A., A case-control study of gastric cancer and diet in Italy, *Int. J. Cancer*, 44, 611, 1989.
171. Gonzalez, C. A., Sanz, M. J. Marcos, G., Pita, S., Brullet, E., Saigi, E., Badia, A., and Riboli, E., Dietary factors and stomach cancer in Spain: a multi-centre case control study, *Int. J. Cancer*, 49, 513, 1991.
172. Sanchez-Diez, A., Hernandez-Mejia, R., and Cueto-Espinar, A., Study of the relation between diet and gastric cancer in a rural area of the Province of Leon, Spain, *Eur. J. Epidemiol.*, 8, 233, 1992.
173. Ramon, J. M., Serra, L., Cerdo, C., and Oromi, J., Dietary factors and gastric cancer risk. A case-control study in Spain, *Cancer*, 71, 1731, 1993.
174. Franceschi, S., Bidoli, E., Baron, A. E., Barra, S., Talamini, R., Serraino, D., and La Vecchia, C., Nutrition and cancer of the oral cavity and pharynx in northeast Italy, *Int. J. Cancer*, 47, 20, 1991.
175. La Vecchia, C., Negri, E., D'Avanzo, B., Boyle, P., and Franceschi, S., Dietary indicators of oral and pharyngeal cancer, *Int. J. Epidemiol.*, 20, 39, 1991.
176. Franceschi, S., Barra, S., La Vecchia, C., Bidoli, E., Negri, E., and Talamini, R., Risk factors for cancer of the tongue and mouth. A case-control study from northern Italy, *Cancer*, 70, 2227, 1992.
177. Pisani, P., Berrino, F., Macaluso, M., Pastorino, U., Crosignani, P., and Baldasseroni, A., Carrots, green vegetables and lung cancer: a case-control study, *Int. J. Epidemiol.*, 15, 463, 1986.
178. Kalandidi, A., Katsouyanni, K., Voropoulou, N., Bastas, G., Saracci, R., and Trichopoulos, D., Passive smoking and diet in the etiology of lung cancer among non-smokers, *Cancer Causes Control*, 1, 15, 1990.
179. Manousos, O., Day, N. E., Trichopoulos, D., Gerovassilis, F., Tzonou, A., and Polychronopoulou, A., Diet and colorectal cancer: a case-control study in Greece, *Int. J. Cancer*, 32, 1, 1983.
180. Benito, E., Obrador, A., Stiggelbout, A., Bosch, F. X., Mulet, M., Munoz, N., and Kaldor, J., A population-based case-control study of colorectal cancer in Majorca. I. Dietary factors, *Int. J. Cancer*, 45, 69, 1990.
181. Boutron-Ruault, M. C., Senesse, P., Faivre, J., Chatelain, N., Belghiti, C., and Meance, S., Foods as risk factors for colorectal cancer: a case-control study in Burgundy (France), *Eur. J. Cancer Prevent.*, 8, 229, 1999.

182. La Vecchia, C., Negri, E., Decarli, A., D'Avanzo, B., Gallotti, L., Gentile, A., and Franceschi, S., A case-control study of diet and colorectal cancer in northern Italy, *Int. J. Cancer*, 41, 492, 1988.

183. Bidoli, E., Franceschi, S., Talamini, R., Barra, S., and La Vecchia, C., Food consumption and cancer of the colon and rectum in northeastern Italy, *Int. J. Cancer*, 50, 223, 1992.

184. Centonze, S., Boeing, H., Leoci, C., Guerra, V., and Misciagna, G., Dietary habits and colorectal cancer in a low-risk area. Results from a population-based case-control study in southern Italy, *Nutr. Cancer*, 21, 233, 1994.

185. Franceschi, S., Favero, A., La Vecchia, C., Negri, E., Conti, E., Montella, M., Giacosa, A., Nanni, O., and Decarli, A., Food groups and risk of colorectal cancer in Italy, *Int. J. Cancer*, 72, 56, 1997.

186. Franceschi, S., Parpinel, M., La Vecchia, C., Favero, A., Talamini, R., and Negri, E., Role of different types of vegetables and fruit in the prevention of cancer of the colon, rectum, and breast, *Epidemiol.*, 9, 338, 1998.

187. Francheschi, S., Bidoli, E., La Vecchia, C., Talamini, R., D'Avanzo, B., and Negri, E. Tomatoes and risk of digestive tract cancers, *Int. J. Cancer*, 59, 181, 1994.

188. La Vecchia, C., Mediterranean epidemiological evidence on tomatoes and the prevention of digestive-tract tumors, *Proc. Soc. Exp. Biol. Med.*, 218, 125, 1998.

189. La Vecchia, C., Decarli, A., Fasoli, M., and Gentile, A., Nutrition and diet in the etiology of endometrial cancer, *Cancer*, 57, 1248, 1986.

190. La Vecchia, C., Decarli, A., Fasoli, M., Parazzini, F., Franceschi, S., Gentile, A., and Negri, E., Dietary vitamin A and the risk of intraepithelial and invasive cervical neoplasia, *Gynecol. Oncology.*, 30, 187, 1988.

191. La Vecchia, C., Negri, E., D'Avanzo, B., Ferraroni, M., Gramenzi, A., Salvoldelli, R., Boyle, P., and Franceschi, S., Medical history, diet, and pancreatic cancer, *Oncology*, 47, 463, 1990.

192. Soler, M., Chatenoud, L., La Vecchia, C., Franceschi, S., and Negri, E., Diet, alcohol, coffee, and pancreatic cancer: final results from an Italian study, *Eur. J. Cancer Prevent.*, 7, 455, 1998.

193. La Vecchia, C., Negri, E., D'Avanzo, B., Franceschi, S., Decarli, A., and Boyle, P., Dietary indicators of laryngeal cancer risk, *Cancer Res.*, 50, 4497, 1990.

194. Esteve, J., Riboli, E., Pequignot, G., Terracini, B., Merletti, F., Crosignani, P., Ascunce, N., Zubiri, L., Blanchet, F., Raymond, L., Repetto, F., and Tuyns, A. J., *Cancer Causes Control*, 7, 240, 1996.

195. Franceschi, S., Fassina, A., Talamini, R., Mazzolini, A., Vianello, S., Bidoli, E., Serraino, D., and La Vecchia, C., Risk factors for thyroid cancer in northern Italy, *Int. J. Epidemiol.*, 18, 578, 1989.

196. Franceschi, S., Levi, F., Negri, E., Fassina, A., and La Vecchia, C., Diet and thyroid cancer: a pooled analysis of four European case-control studies, *Int. J. Cancer*, 48, 395, 1991.

197. La Vecchia, C., Negri, E., Decarli, A., D'Avanzo, B., Liberati, C., and Franceschi, S., Dietary factors in the risk of bladder cancer, *Nutr. Cancer*, 12, 93, 1989.

198. Momas, I., Daures, J. P., Festy, B., Bontoux, J., and Gremy, F., Relative importance of risk factors in bladder carcinogenesis: some new results about Mediterranean habits, *Cancer Causes Control*, 5, 326, 1994.

199. Talamini, R., La Vecchia, C., Negri, E., and Franceschi, S., Nutrition, social factors and prostatic cancer in a Northern Italian population, *Br. J. Cancer*, 53, 817, 1986.

200. Talamini, R., Franceschi, S., La Vecchia, C., Serraino, D., Barra, S., and Negri, E., Diet and prostatic cancer: a case-control study in northern Italy, *Nutr. Cancer*, 18, 277, 1992.

201. Talamini, R., Baron, A. E., Barra, S., Bidoli, E., La Vecchia, C., Negri, E., Serraino, D., and Franceschi, S., A case-control study of risk factor for renal cell cancer in northern Italy, *Cancer Causes Control*, 1, 125, 1990.

202. La Vecchia, C., Negri, E., Decarli, A., D'Avanzo, B., and Franceschi, S., Risk factors for hepatocellular carcinoma in northern Italy, *Int. J. Cancer*, 42, 872, 1988.

203. Hadziyannis, S., Tabor, E., Kaklamani, E., Tzonou, A., Stuver, S., Tassopoulos, N., Mueller, N., and Trichopoulos, D., A case-control study of hepatitis B and C virus infections in the etiology of hepatocellular carcinoma, *Int. J. Cancer*, 60, 627, 1995.

204. Willet, W. C., The dietary pyramid: does the foundation need repair?, *Am. J. Clin. Nutr.*, 68, 218, 1998.

205. Slavin, J. L., Martini, M. C., Jacobs Jr, D. R., and Marquart, L., Plausible mechanisms for the protectiveness of whole grains, *Am. J. Clin. Nutr.*, 70, 459S, 1999.

206. Dietary Guidelines Advisory Committee, Dietary Guidelines for Americans 2000, http://www.ars.usda.gov/dgac/dgacguidexp.htm, 2000.

207. Jacobs, D. R., Jr., Marquart, L., Slavin, J., and Kushi, L. H., Whole-grain intake and cancer: an expanded review and meta-analysis, *Nutr. Cancer*, 30, 85, 1998.

208. Kushi, L. H., Meyer, K. A., and Jacobs Jr, D. R., Cereals, legumes, and chronic disease risk reduction: evidence from epidemiologic studies, *Am. J. Clin. Nutr.*, 70, 451S, 1999.

209. Chatenoud, L., La Vecchia, C., Franceschi, S., Tavani, A., Jacobs Jr, D. R., Parpinel, M. T., Soler, M., and Negri, E., Refined-cereal intake and risk of selected cancers in Italy, *Am. J. Clin. Nutr.*, 70, 1107, 1999.

210. Giovannucci, E., Insulin and colon cancer, *Cancer Causes Control*, 6, 164, 1995.

211. Chatenoud, L., Tavani, A., La Vecchia, C., Jacobs Jr, D. R., Negri, E., Levi, F., and Franceschi, S., Whole-grain food intake and cancer risk, *Int. J. Cancer*, 77, 24, 1998.

212. Franceschi, S., Favero, A., Parpinel, M., Giacosa, A., and La Vecchia, C., Italian study on colorectal cancer with emphasis on influence of cereals, *Eur. J. Cancer Prevent.*, 7, Suppl. 2, 19S, 1998.

213. Franceschi, S., Bidoli, E., Baron, A. E., and La Vecchia, C., Maize and risk of cancers of the oral cavity, pharynx, and esophagus, *J. Natl. Cancer Inst.*, 82, 1407, 1990s.

214. Franceschi, S., Favero, A., La Vecchia, C., Negri, E., Dal Maso, L., Salvini, S., Decarli, A., and Giacosa, A., Influence of food groups and food diversity in breast cancer risk in Italy, *Int. J. Cancer*, 63, 785, 1995.

215. World Cancer Research Fund, and American Institute for Cancer Research, Food, Nutrition, and the Prevention of Cancer: a Global Perspective, American Institute for Cancer Research, Washington, D. C., 1997, Chap. 6.

216. Trichopoulou, A., Katsouyanni, K., and Gnardellis, C., The traditional Greek diet, *Eur. J. Clin. Nutr.*, 43, suppl. 2, 9, 1993.

217. Lipworth, L., Martinez, M. E., Angell, J., Hsieh, C. C., and Trichopoulos, D., Olive oil and human cancer: an assessment of the evidence, *Prev. Med.*, 26, 181, 1997.

218. Newmark, H. L., Squalene, olive oil, and cancer risk: a review and hypothesis, *Cancer Epidemiol. Biomarkers Prevent.*, 6, 1101, 1997.

219. Bautista, D., Obrador, A., Moreno, V., Cabeza, E., Canet, R., Benito, E., Bosch, X., and Costa, J., Kis-*ras* mutation modifies the protective effect of dietary monounsaturated fat and calcium on sporadic colorectal cancer, *Cancer Epidemiol. Biomarkers Prevent.*, 6, 57, 1997.

220. La Vecchia, C. and Negri, E., Fats in seasoning and the relationship to pancreatic cancer, *Eur. J. Cancer Prevent.*, 6, 370, 1997.

221. Fortes, C., Forastiere, F., Anatra, F., and Schmid, G., Re: Consumption of olive oil and specific food groups in relation to breast cancer risk in Greece, *J. Natl. Cancer Inst.*, 87, 1020, 1995.

222. Tavani, A., La Vechia, C., Gallus, S., Lagiou, P., Trichopoulos, D., Levi, F., and Negri, E., Red meat and cancer risk: a study in Italy, *Int. J. Cancer*, 86, 425, 2000.

223. Kromhout, D., Keys, A., Aravanis, C., Buzina, R., Fidanza, F., Giampaoli, S., Jansen, A., Menotti, A., Nedeljkovic, S., and Pekkarinen, M., Food consumption patterns in the 1960s in seven countries, *Am. J. Clin. Nutr.*, 49, 889, 1989.

224. Augustsson, K., Skog, K., Jagerstad, M., Dickman, P. W., and Steineck, G., Dietary heterocyclic amines and cancer of the colon, rectum, bladder, and kidney: a population-based study, *Lancet*, 353, 703, 1999.

225. Takahashi, M., Fukutake, M., Isoi, T., Fukuda, K., Sato, H., Yazawa, K., Sugimura, T., and Wakabayashi, K., Suppression of azoxymethane-induced rat colon carcinoma development by a fish oil component, docosahexaenoic acid (DHA), *Carcinogenesis*, 18, 1337, 1997.

226. Rose, D. P. and Conolly, J. M., Effects of dietary omega-3 fatty acids on human breast cancer growth and metastases in nude mice, *J. Natl. Cancer Inst.*, 85, 1743, 1993.

227. Rose, D. P. and Cohen, L. A., Effects of menhaden oil and retinyl acetate on the growth of DU 145 human prostatic adenocarcinoma cells transplanted into athymic nude mice, *Carcinogenesis*, 9, 603, 1988.

228. Hill, M. J., Meat and colorectal cancer, *Proc. Nutr. Soc.*, 58, 261, 1999.

229. Fernandez, E., Chatenoud, L., La Vecchia, C., Negri, E., and Franceschi, S., Fish consumption and cancer risk, *Am. J. Clin. Nutr.*, 70, 85, 1999.

230. La Vecchia, C., Negri, E., D'Avanzo, B., Franceschi, S., and Boyle, P., Dairy products and the risk of prostatic cancer, *Oncol.*, 48, 406, 1991.

231. Rosenberg, L., Metzger, L. S., and Palmer, J. T., Alcohol consumption and risk of breast cancer: a review of the epidemiologic evidence, *Epidemiol. Rev.*, 15, 133, 1993.

232. Chatenoud, L., Negri, E., La Vecchia, C., Volpato, O., and Franceschi, S., Wine drinking and diet in Italy, *Eur. J. Clin. Nutr.*, 54, 177, 2000.

233. Klatsky, A. L., Armstrong, M. A., and Friedman, G. D., Alcohol and mortality, *Ann. Intern. Med.*, 117, 646, 1992.

234. Brugere, J., Guenel, P., Leclerc, A., and Rodriguez, J., Differential effects of tobacco and alcohol in cancer of the larynx, pharynx, and mouth, *Cancer*, 57, 391, 1986.

235. Tuyns, A. J., Alcohol-related cancers in Mediterranean countries, *Tumori*, 76, 315, 1990.

236. Barra, S., Franceschi, S., Negri, E., Talamini, R., and La Vecchia, C., Type of alcoholic beverage and cancer of the oral cavity, pharynx, and oesophagus in an Italian area with high wine consumption, *Int. J. Cancer*, 46, 1017, 1990.

237. Franceschi, S., Talamini, R., Barra, S., Baron, A. E., Negri, E., Bidoli, E., Serraino, D., and La Vecchia, C., Smoking and drinking in relation to cancers of the oral cavity, pharynx, larynx, and esophagus in northern Italy, *Cancer Res.*, 50, 6502, 1990.

238. Talamini, R., Franceschi, S., Barra, S., and La Vecchia, C., The role of alcohol in oral and pharyngeal cancer in non-smokers, and of tobacco in non-drinkers, *Int. J. Cancer*, 46, 391, 1990.

239. Fioretti, F., Bosetti, C., Tavani, A., Franceschi, S., and La Vecchia, C., Risk factors for oral and pharyngeal cancer in never smokers, *Oral Oncol.*, 35, 375, 1999.

240. Tuyns, A. J., Pequignot, G., and Abbatucci, J. S., Esophageal cancer and alcohol consumption: importance of type of beverage, *Int. J. Cancer*, 23, 443, 1979.

241. La Vecchia, C. and Negri, E., The role of alcohol in esophageal cancer in non-smokers, and of tobacco in non-drinkers, *Int. J. Cancer*, 43, 784, 1989.

242. Garidou, A., Tzonou, A., Lipworth, L., Signorello, L. B., Kalapothaki, V., and Trichopoulos, D., Life-style factors and medical conditions in relation to esophageal cancer by histologic type in a low-risk population, *Int. J. Cancer*, 68, 295, 1996.

243. Zambon, P., Talamini, R., La Vecchia, C., Dal Maso, L., Negri, E., Tognazzo, S., Simonato, L., and Franceschi, S., Smoking, type of alcoholic beverage and squamous-cell esophageal cancer in Northern Italy, *Int. J. Cancer*, 86, 144, 2000.

244. Morales-Suarez-Varela, M., Llopis-Gonzalez, A., Castillo-Collado, A., and Vitoria-Minana, I., Cancer of the rectum in relation to components of the Spanish diet, *J. Environ. Pathol. Toxicol. Oncol.*, 10, 214, 1990.

245. Tavani, A., Ferraroni, M., Mezzetti, M., Franceschi, S., Lo Re, A., and La Vecchia, C., Alcohol intake and risk of cancers of the colon and rectum, *Nutr. Cancer*, 30, 213, 1998.

246. Talamini, R., La Vecchia, C., Decarli, A., Franceschi, S., Grattoni, E., Grigoletto, E., Liberati, A., and Tognoni, G., Social factors, diet and breast cancer in a northern Italian population, *Br. J. Cancer*, 49, 723, 1984.

247. Le, M. G., Hill, C., Kramar, A., and Flamanti, R., Alcoholic beverage consumption and breast cancer in a French case-control study, *Am. J. Epidemiol.*, 120, 350, 1984.

248. La Vecchia, C., Negri, E., Parazzini, F., Boyle, P., Fasoli, M., Gentile, A., and Franceschi, S., Alcohol and breast cancer: update from an Italian case-control study, *Eur. J. Cancer Clin. Oncol.*, 25, 1711, 1989.

249. Richardson, S., de Vincenzi, I., Pujol, H., and Gerber, M., Alcohol consumption in a case-control study of breast cancer in southern France, *Int. J. Cancer*, 44, 84, 1989.

250. Ferraroni, M., Decarli, A., Willet, W. C., and Marubini, E., Alcohol and breast cancer risk: a case-control study from northern Italy, *Int. J. Epidemiol.*, 20, 859, 1991.

251. Martin-Moreno, J. M., Boyle, P., Gorgojo, L., Willett, W. C., Gonzalez, J., Villar, F., and Maisonneuve, P., Alcoholic beverage consumption and risk of breast cancer in Spain, *Cancer Causes Control*, 4, 345, 1993.

252. Viel, J. F., Perarnau, J. M., Challier, B., and Faivre-Nappez, I., Alcoholic calories, red wine consumption and breast cancer among premenopausal women, *Eur. J. Epidemiol.*, 13, 639, 1997.

253. Ferraroni, M., Decarli, A., Franceshi, S., and La Vecchia, C., Alcohol consumption and risk of breast cancer: a multi-centre Italian case-control study, *Eur. J. Cancer*, 34, 1403, 1998.

254. Bravo, M. P., Del Rey Calero, J., and Conde, M., Bladder cancer and the consumption of alcoholic beverages in Spain, *Eur. J. Epidemiol.*, 3, 365, 1987.

255. Hoey, J., Montvernay, C., and Lambert, R., Wine and tobacco: risk factors for gastric cancer in France, *Am. J. Epidemiol.*, 113, 668, 1981.

256. Manousos, O., Trichopoulos, D., Koutselinis, A., Papadimitriou, C., Polychronopoulou, A., and Zavitsanos, X., Epidemiologic characteristics and trace elements in pancreatic cancer in Greece, *Cancer Detect. Prevent.*, 4, 439, 1981.

257. Durbec, J. P., Chevillotte, G., Bidart, J. M., Berthezene, P., and Sarles, H., Diet, alcohol, tobacco and risk of cancer of the pancreas: a case-control study, *Br. J. Cancer*, 47, 463, 1983.

258. Clavel, F., Benhamou, E., Auquier, A., Tarayre, M., and Flamant, R., Coffee, alcohol, smoking and cancer of the pancreas: a case-control study, *Int. J. Cancer*, 43, 17, 1989.

259. Bouchardy, C., Clavel, F., La Vecchia, C., Raymond, L., and Boyle, P., Alcohol, beer and cancer of the pancreas, *Int. J. Cancer.*, 45, 842, 1990.

260. Kalapothaki, V., Tzonou, A., Hsieh, C. C., Toupadaki, N., Karakatsani, A., and Trichopoulos, D., Tobacco, ethanol, coffee, pancreatitis, diabetes mellitus, and cholelithiasis as risk factors for pancreatic carcinoma, *Cancer Causes Control*, 4, 375, 1993.

261. Tavani, A., Pregnolato, A., Negri, E., and La Vecchia, C., Alcohol consumption and risk of pancreatic cancer, *Nutr. Cancer*, 27, 157, 1997.

262. Hsieh, C. C., Thanos, A., Mitropoulos, D., Deliveliotis, C., Mantzoros, C. S., and Trichopoulos, D., Risk factors for prostate cancer: a case-control study in Greece, *Int. J. Cancer*, 80, 699, 1999.

263. Tavani, A., Negri, E., Franceschi, S., Talamini, R., and La Vecchia, C., Alcohol consumption and risk of prostate cancer, *Nutr. Cancer*, 21, 24, 1994.

264. Polychronopoulou, A., Tzonou, A., Hsieh, C. C., Kaprinis, G., Rebelakos, A., Toupadaki, N., and Trichopoulos, D., Reproductive variables, tobacco, ethanol, coffee and somatometry as risk factors for ovarian cancer, *Int. J. Cancer*, 55, 402, 1993.

265. La Vecchia, C., Negri, E., Franceschi, S., Parazzini, F., Gentile, A., and Fasoli, M., Alcohol and epithelial ovarian cancer, *J. Clin. Epidemiol.*, 45, 1025, 1992.

266. Renaud, S. C., Gueguen, R., Schenker, J., and d'Houtaud, A., Alcohol and mortality in middle-aged men from eastern France, *Epidemiol.*, 9, 184, 1998.

267. Rimm, E. B. and Ellison, C., R., Alcohol in the Mediterranean diet, *Am. J. Clin. Nutr.*, 61, 1378S, 1995.

268. Marshall, J. R. and Boyle, P., Nutrition and oral cancer, *Cancer Causes Control*, 7, 101, 1996.

269. Riboli, E., Kaaks, R., and Esteve, J., Nutrition and laryngeal cancer, *Cancer Causes Control*, 7, 147, 1996.

270. Drewnowski, A., Henderson, S. A., Shore, A. B., Fischler, C., Preziosi, P., and Hercberg, S., Diet quality and dietary diversity in France: implications for the French Paradox, *J. Am. Diet. Assoc.*, 96, 663, 1996.

271. La Vecchia, C., Munoz, S. E., Braga, C., Fernandez, E., and Decarli, A., Diet diversity and gastric cancer, *Int. J. Cancer*, 72, 255, 1997.

272. Alberti-Fidanza, A., Fidanza, F., Chiuchiu, M. P., Verducci, G., and Fruttini, D., Dietary studies on two rural Italian population groups of the Seven Countries Study. Trend of food and nutrient intake from 1960s to 1991, *Eur. J. Clin. Nutr.*, 53, 854, 1999.

13 The Cyprus Experience

Michael Tornaritis, Savvas C. Savva,
Maria Shamounki, Yiannis A. Kourides,
and Charalambos Hadjigeorgiou.

CONTENTS

I. INTRODUCTION

The diet consumed by Mediterranean populations, the so-called Mediterranean Diet as established in the Greek island of Crete and in southern Italy, has been proven beneficial in promoting human health, and has been credited for the low cardiovascular disease morbidity and mortality in certain Mediterranean areas such as Crete.[1] Recently, this particular diet has been shown to reduce the secondary complications, recurrence, and even death after a first myocardial infarction,[2] and also to reduce the risk for cancer.[3] The credibility of this diet is evaluated in respect to specific components of the foods, such as the monounsaturated fatty acid (C18:1) and the omega-3 fatty acids. High olive oil consumption, the main source of C18:1 monounsaturated fatty acids,[4] reduces serum LDL cholesterol levels and prevents LDL cholesterol oxidation by its antioxidant substances such as tocopherols, polyphenols, and squalenes.[5] Monounsaturated fatty acids (C18:1) do not reduce serum HDL-cholesterol levels (as polyunsaturated fatty acids do)[6] and they have been reported to prevent lipoprotein particles from oxidation.[7] The dietary supplementation of omega-3 polyunsaturated fatty acids, after a myocardial infarction, has reduced the long-term complications of myocardial infarction significantly.[8]

The island of Cyprus lies on the eastern Mediterranean Sea. For centuries, Cypriots have traditionally been nourished on a diet that resembles very much the Mediterranean Diet model. It was, therefore, a surprise to find out that the majority of children in modern Cyprus have moved away from the traditional pattern and now consume a Western-type diet.

Begun in 1995, a large-scale epidemiological survey is being conducted in Cyprus by the Research and Education Program for Child's Health of Cyprus. This program evaluates all 11,000 elementary-school sixth graders every year (in a total population of about 650,000 on the island). School children have been assessed for the presence of cardiovascular disease and other chronic disease risk factors. The 1995 results of this survey indicated that about a third of Cypriot school children were overweight, almost half had high total cholesterol levels, and almost two thirds were not physically fit. The examination of eating habits showed very poor dietary patterns, with marked consumption of fat-rich substances, and a striking absence of nutritionally rich foods like fruit, vegetables, legumes, and cereals.[9]

These results have raised much concern about the future health of the youngest generations of Cyprus, and the Research and Education Program for Child's Health of Cyprus has commenced a longitudinal effort, with the eventual aim of reversing the situation. The status of Cyprus, unfortunately, is in contrast to other countries' "paradoxes." Albania, for instance, the poorest European country with one of the highest infant mortality rates, has a high adult life expectancy with low coronary heart disease mortality, especially in areas where most olive oil, fruits, and vegetables are produced and consumed.[10]

II. HISTORICAL BACKGROUND

Cyprus is among the eastern Mediterranean countries that have been experiencing an epidemiological transition during the last decades. More and more people are involved in business and tourism professions, and most young mothers have their own careers, thus lacking the opportunity to offer their families healthy home-prepared food. Instead, many families consume precooked and fast-food items. People lack the time for exercise, and children spend much of their leisure time in prep schools, watching television, and playing electronic games.[11] Similar changes have also been observed in the Cretan population and it has been shown that they are associated with an increase in the frequency of heart disease risk factors.[12]

The aging of the population, progressive urbanization, and changes in nutritional habits and life-styles predispose people to cardiovascular diseases. The abandonment of the Mediterranean Diet has already been mentioned. The Cypriot population aged over 65 years has increased from 5.8% in 1881 to 6.4% in 1960 and 11.0% in 1992.[13] The island has also experienced a dramatic transition in respect to where its citizens live. In 1881, only 18.9% of Cypriots were living in urban areas, while by 1960, this figure had increased to 35.9%, reaching 68.9% in 1997.[13] For comparison, the World Health Organization reported that 45% of the world's population lived in urban areas in 1995.[14]

III. TRENDS IN MORBIDITY AND MORTALITY IN CYPRUS

Although per capita income is among the highest, and the medical services are among the most advanced in the region, little epidemiological data is available concerning chronic diseases such as cardiovascular diseases, diabetes mellitus, and cancer. Therefore, it was not surprising that Cyprus was not included in the Task Force Report of the European Society of Cardiology on cardiovascular mortality and morbidity statistics in Europe,[15] nor in the 1999 World Health Report of the World Health Organization.[16]

Mortality data are inadequate in Cyprus because death certificates do not always report the cause of death. In 1996, for example, 45.8% of the death certificates did not provide the cause of death.[17] Therefore, most available information comes from inadequate sources such as hospital admissions or discharges, and some other sparse sources. Hospital discharges rates for certain chronic diseases are presented in Table 1. These data should be viewed with caution, mainly because the private medical section in Cyprus has always absorbed a significant proportion of outpatient visits, and fewer clinic admissions.

TABLE 1
Hospital Discharges in Cyprus General Hospitals in 1980 and 1997 for Certain Chronic Diseases

Disease	Hospital Discharges		% Change
	1980[18,19]	1997[20]	
Ischemic heart disease	1133	1699	50
Cerebrovascular disease	589	625	6
Hypertension	127	142	12
Diabetes mellitus	413	398	−4
All cancers	1330	3082	132
Colon cancer	42	171	307

Note: the population increased by 21% during this period.

A. CORONARY HEART DISEASE

The data presented in Table 1 are indicative of a tremendous increase (50%) in ischemic heart disease discharges over the period 1980–1997,[18-20] while, at the same time, the total population increased by 21%.[13] According to a Pancyprian question-naire-based survey performed in 1989, the prevalence of ischemic heart disease was 167 cases per 10,000 population.[21] Ten new cases of acute myocardial infarction were reported, per 10,000 population per year during the period 1990–1994.[22] The peak age of incidence of acute myocardial infarction is estimated to have occurred at the age of 60–70 years among men and at the age of 70–80 years among women during the late 1980s.[23]

Nevertheless, diseases of the circulatory system rank first as a cause of mortality in Cyprus, with ischemic heart disease being responsible for 11.3% of deaths in 1996.[24] This figure is slightly smaller than the ischemic heart disease mortality rate observed in eastern Mediterranean countries (13.6%) and definitely smaller than what was observed in western Europe (25.5%) and in North America (17.9%) in 1998.[16] It must be assumed, however, that the actual mortality rate from ischemic heart disease is larger than the reported rate, since a significant proportion of the deaths that were not properly recorded could also be due to ischemic heart disease.

Although ischemic heart disease mortality in Cyprus is less common than in western countries, there is rising concern due to increasing incidence of the disease in Cyprus at a time when the mortality from the disease has presented a steady decline during the last two or three decades in most European countries[15] and the United States.[25]

B. STROKE

The incidence of cerebrovascular disease increased slightly during 1980–1997. As shown in Table 1, the increase of cerebrovascular disease hospital discharges was 6% between 1980 and 1997, whereas the prevalence of stroke in the population in 1989 was 47 per 10,000 population.[21] Stroke is, apparently, responsible for the majority of paralysis and hemiplegia cases, which were estimated to be 62 per 10,000 population,[21] and also for the 11.4% of (the properly recorded) deaths that occurred in 1996 in Cyprus.[24] This mortality rate is twice as high as that observed in eastern Mediterranean countries (5.3%) and comparable to that observed in Europe (13.7%) and North America (10.3%).[16]

C. DIABETES MELLITUS

The 1989 questionnaire-based survey estimated the prevalence of diabetes mellitus (both insulin-dependent and non-insulin dependent) in Cyprus to be 2.7% of the total population.[21] A recent study screened a representative sample of the population of Cyprus for fasting capillary glucose values and oral glucose tolerance test when appropriate. This study estimated the prevalence of non-insulin dependent diabetes mellitus to be 14.65% in the population aged over 35 years, whereas another 6.25% of subjects were found to have an impaired glucose tolerance.[26] The figures reported in this study are comparable to figures reported for other Mediterranean countries.[26] The incidence of insulin-dependent diabetes mellitus has been estimated at 10.5 cases per 100,000 children less than 15 years of age, per year, which is comparable to the incidence of most European countries.[27]

The government hospital discharges from diabetes mellitus have decreased by about 4% in 1997 in respect to the 1980 figures (Table 1). This may not be an actual reflection of the disease morbidity trends, since a lot of diabetic patients are treated in the private medical sector.

The rate of complications in non-insulin-dependent diabetic subjects is high. Only 35% of diabetic subjects examined in a cohort were free from complications and those were the subjects who had suffered from the disease for a shorter period of time.[28] The high rate of complications can be attributed mainly to the unsatisfactory control of diabetes. An earlier study indicated that only 31% of diabetics had a fair control of their disease.[29]

Cardiovascular complications (namely hypertension and ischemic heart disease) were present in 29% of the subjects, that is, much higher from the rate of complications reported in many European countries. The reported rate of death from cardiovascular complications was 35% in the 40–60 age group.[28] This may well be an underestimation due to underreporting.

D. CANCER

The 1989 survey estimated the prevalence of cancer at 27 cases per 100,000 population.[21] If one takes into account the fact that patients with cancer in Cypriot society considered their disease a stigma, it is safe to assume that the cancer prevalence was well underestimated.

Nevertheless, a tremendous increase of 132% in hospital discharges (Table 1) was observed in 1997 over 1980. Considering that the private medical sector has absorbed a larger proportion of patients with serious illnesses, we can conclude that there was a significant increase in the incidence and prevalence of cancer in Cyprus during this period.

The causes of cancer still remain unclear in the literature. Nutrition has long been proposed as a major causative factor, colorectal cancer being the type of cancer for which the evidence that diet is involved in its etiology is probably the strongest. It is estimated that 80% of colorectal cancer cases could be prevented by dietary modification.[30] Taking into account the dramatic increase in hospital discharges for colon cancer in 1997 over 1980 (307%, Table 1), a significant increase in the incidence of this nutrition-related (at least partially) form of cancer must have occurred in Cyprus during the last two decades.

Cancer in Cyprus ranks second as a cause of mortality. The reported death rate from all forms of cancer in 1996 was 16.8%.[24] This percentage is almost triple the percentage reported in 1998 for eastern Mediterranean countries (6.4%) and slightly smaller than that reported for Europe (19.2%) and North America (18.9%).[16]

In summary, it is obvious that Cyprus has experienced a dramatic increase in morbidity and mortality from certain chronic diseases such as ischemic heart disease, cancer, and stroke, during the last two decades. This increase should be attributed to the impressive life-style transition that has been observed on the island during the past three or four decades, as mentioned above. Although the data presented are not very precise due to underreporting, they clearly denote an increasing trend in the incidence and prevalence of these chronic diseases to figures similar to those seen in developed countries such as Europe and the United States. It is very disappointing that these increasing figures are observed at a time when these diseases are declining in most developed countries.

IV. CARDIOVASCULAR DISEASE RISK FACTORS IN CYPRUS

The increasing trends in chronic diseases discussed above inevitably lead to the discussion of certain predisposing risk factors for these diseases. Data are lacking for adults, since studies performed in Cyprus are very few. One such study[23] has indicated that 77.2% of patients who had an acute myocardial infarction had 1–4 coronary heart disease risk factors. In particular, 35.8% of patients were smokers, 23.9% were hypertensives, 21.2% were diabetics, and 7% had hyperlipidemia.[23] Another study[22] conducted in the early 1990s gave similar figures, except for hypercholesterolemia, which was reported at much higher figures than the previous study. In particular, hypercholesterolemia was reported to be present in 36% of men and 35% of women with an acute myocardial infarction.

Most of the data presented below come from the screening of children in Cyprus for the presence of cardiovascular disease risk factors. This evaluation has been performed since 1995, and children are evaluated at their schools for obesity, hypertension, hyperlipidemia, physical fitness (with the aid of the Eurofit test), and dietary intake. Generally, there is a clustering of cardiovascular disease risk factors (CVDRF) in children 11–12 years of age. Specifically, 47.1% of 3661 boys and 47.7% of 3393 girls had one CVDRF, 18% and 15% had two factors, 4.8% and 3% had three factors and, finally, four CVDRF were noted in 0.5% and 0.2% of boys and girls respectively.[31] The risk factors evaluated in this study were hypercholesterolemia, obesity, high blood pressure, and low performance in a 20-m shuttle run. These figures could mean that children's coronary arteries are already covered with fatty streaks by 2.5%–11.0% and with fibrous plaques by 0.7%–7.2% of their surface.[32]

A. HYPERLIPIDEMIA

Hyperlipidemia is a well-established risk factor for coronary heart disease.[33] Many studies have proven the relationship between hyperlipidemia and atherosclerosis. The on-going Bogalusa Heart Study,[32,34] for example, has repeatedly shown that atherosclerosis may begin in early childhood and is related to plasma levels of total cholesterol and LDL cholesterol.

In a study performed in the district of Nicosia in the late 1980s, 7% of the patients with acute myocardial infarction had hyperlipidemia,[23] whereas in the early 1990, this figure was reported to be at least 35%. A recent study indicated that 63.8% of middle-aged men and 61.5% of middle-aged women have determined their serum lipids and lipoproteins at least once in their lives, but as many as 77.5% of the subjects with very high levels of total cholesterol (> 265 mg/dl) are not treated optimally.[35]

Many children and adolescents in Cyprus have high or borderline levels of total cholesterol (>200 mg/dl and 170–200 mg/dl respectively) and LDL cholesterol (>130 mg/dl and 110–130 mg/dl respectively) according to the guidelines of the American Academy of Pediatrics.[36] Table 2 presents the results of two different studies in

TABLE 2
Percentage of Children and Adolescents in Cyprus with High and Borderline Levels of Total and LDL Cholesterol

	Children 2–12 years (n = 783)[37]	Adolescents 10–18 years (n = 758)[38]
Total cholesterol-borderline (170-200 mg/dl)	37+	32
Total cholesterol-high (>200 mg/dl)	22	10
LDL cholesterol-borderline (110-130 mg/dl)	23	14
LDL cholesterol-borderline (>130 mg/dl)	30	8

+ Values are expressed as percent.

respect to the pathological values of serum total and LDL cholesterol in children and adolescents.

It is obvious that more than half of the children less than 12 years of age,[37] and about 22% of adolescents,[38] have pathological values of their LDL cholesterol, which is related to atherosclerosis even in youth.[34] There are no existing data concerning children's serum lipids for previous decades for comparison purposes, but the comparison of Cypriot adolescents' lipids with their Greek peers'[39] revealed that the Cypriots' lipids are slightly but statistically significantly higher.[38]

B. SMOKING

Smoking is one of the most important CVDRFs,[33] and a variety of mechanisms have been implicated in the contribution of smoking to the procedure of atherosclerosis.[40] Smoking was the most common CVDRF found in Cypriot patients who had an acute myocardial infarction.[22, 23]

It is known that Cypriots have been smoking for centuries. Smoking was common even among females during the Turkish occupation of Cyprus in the Middle Ages (1571–1878). During the 20th century, the smoking habit has been increasing among Cypriots. In 1950, for instance, the consumption of cigarettes was 1014 per capita and, in 1970, 1560 per capita.[41]

A study conducted in 1987 in the district of Nicosia has indicated that adolescents (mostly 18-year-olds) were smoking at a rate of 21.8% (one third of them frequently). The percentage of male smokers was 40.8% whereas that of females was 11.4%.[42] A recent study[43] has shown that the percentage of children who smoke has increased considerably. This study indicated that about 50% of children aged 15–18 years, 30% of children aged 12–15 years, and almost 4% of elementary-school students are frequent or occasional smokers. Smoking children will probably suffer many health consequences later in their adult lives.

C. OBESITY

Obesity is a positive risk factor for atherosclerosis as measured by the Body Mass Index (BMI), but also the amount of *panniculus adiposus* is positively related to the occupation of the coronary arteries' surface.[33] Intra-abdominal accumulation of adipose tissue is related to the insulin resistance syndrome, serum lipid and lipo-protein perturbations, and hypertension, thus leading to increased risk for ischaemic heart disease.[44]

Data concerning the epidemiology of adult obesity in Cyprus are lacking. A research effort to elucidate the epidemiology of pediatric obesity in Cyprus is currently being carried out by the Research and Education Program for Child's Health. However, existing data for children indicate that there is an increasing rate of childhood obesity in Cyprus. A study[31] performed by the Research and Education Program for Child's Health of Cyprus has indicated that 20.3% of boys and 18.1% of girls aged 11–12 years of age are overweight. In this study, the authors used the BMI 85th percentile cutoff points of the United States NHANES II and III data published recently, which are by 6–7% higher than the previously used BMI values.[45]

In 1990, triceps skin-fold-thickness measurement (TST) in children aged 6–11 from the district of Paphos were compared with those of other countries. It was found that Cypriot children had much thicker TST than British (by 3–6 mm) and Norwegian children (by 4–6 mm).[46] In the same district, as shown in Figure 1, mean TST in children 11–12 years old has increased by 26.4% in boys and by 23.7% in girls during the years 1990–1998.[47] The TST measurement is statistically signifi-cantly higher in urban than in rural areas in children. In urban boys, TST was 19 mm, while in rural areas, it was 16.1mm (p < 0.001). In girls residing in urban areas, mean TST was 19.9 mm, whereas girls from rural areas had a mean value of 18mm (p < 0.001).[47] In general, TST measurement is positively correlated to LDL choles-terol,[47] but when only obese children (BMI>22 kg/m^2) were taken into account, TST was negatively correlated to LDL cholesterol.[48]

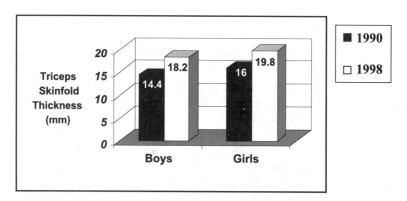

FIGURE 1   Trends in triceps skinfold thickness in 11–12-year-old children between 1990 and 1998.[46]

Leptin is a protein hormone discovered recently. It is derived from the adipose tissue, which is implicated in the pathogenesis of obesity. In a study of Cypriot children aged 10–18, BMI was strongly correlated to serum leptin levels, both in boys (r = 0.704, p < 0.001) and girls (r = 0.741, p < 0.001).[49]

The increasing frequency of obesity raises much concern, since obesity in childhood tends to persist into adulthood,[50] and has been found to be associated with increased risk for all-causes mortality and cardiovascular mortality in adulthood.[51]

D. HYPERTENSION

The prevalence of hypertension in Cyprus is 725 cases per 10,000 population,[21] or about 10.7% of the adult population, a value lower than that observed in other developed countries. However, there was an increase of about 12% in the rate of hospital discharges from 1980 to 1997 (Table 1).[20] Furthermore, among patients with an acute myocardial infarction, 22% to 35% were hypertensives.[22,23]

In children, the actual prevalence of hypertension is unknown, but the authors found that 4.8% of 3661 boys and 6.4% of 3393 girls aged 11–12 had a high blood pressure measurement (> 125 mm Hg).[31] The risk of having high blood pressure was significantly higher among overweight children than in non-obese subjects (odds ratio 7.96 for boys, p < 0.001 and 4.81 for girls, p < 0.001).[52] Both BMI and waist circumference (an index of visceral adiposity in both adults and children) were significant predictors of blood pressure in children in a multivariate analysis.[52]

E. PHYSICAL FITNESS

A sedentary life-style increases the risk for cardiovascular disease, whereas regular exercise prevents it. Three mechanisms have been proposed as mediating the beneficial effects of exercise on human health. In particular, exercise reduces the levels of some cardiovascular disease risk factors (such as the reduction of BMI and serum cholesterol and triglyceride levels, and the increase of serum HDL cholesterol levels),[53,54] has a benefit on metabolism,[55] and decreases the susceptibility of LDL-C to undergo oxidation.[56]

A significant proportion of children in Cyprus (24.2% of boys and 26.4% of girls) were found to have very low cardiorespiratory fitness as measured by the 20-meter shuttle run test.[31] More boys are involved in athletic training than girls (86% and 38%, respectively, p = 0.001). Girls on the other hand, spend more time on sedentary activities (24.6 hours/week for boys and 33.8 hours/week for girls, p = 0.039).[57]

Regular exercise was found to have beneficial effects in children in Cyprus. Thus, athletes were found to have higher mean values of HDL cholesterol than the general population (68.9 mg/dl vs. 59.6 mg/dl, p = 0.02). The time children spend on sedentary activities was found to be positively correlated to LDL cholesterol (r = 0.339, p = 0.02).[57] Finally, children with good performances in the 20-meter shuttle run were found to have lower mean values of LDL cholesterol, both boys (100.8 mg/dl vs. 112.4 mg/dl, p < .0001) and girls (99.1 mg/dl vs. 103.1 mg/dl, p < 0.0001).[58]

V. DIETARY PATTERNS AND FOOD ANALYSIS AND COMPOSITION IN CYPRUS

The role of diet and nutrition in disease has gained special attention since the 1950s, when it was observed that people living in Mediterranean areas such as Crete and south Italy had one of the highest adult life expectancies worldwide, while coronary heart disease, some cancers, and other diet-related chronic diseases were among the lowest.[59]

Cyprus, as an eastern Mediterranean island, had a traditional diet that resembled the Mediterranean Diet as it has been described by Ancel Keys.[60] This diet consisted mainly of grains, greens, all kind of vegetables and legumes mixed with olive oil, cheese (the traditional *challoumi* of Cyprus), and plenty of fruits, and was accompanied with moderate amounts of red wine.

A. DIETARY PATTERNS OF THE MODERN CYPRIOTS

During recent decades, the traditional diet has changed dramatically. The modern diet of Cypriots today very much resembles the diet of North Americans and northern Europeans. Today's diet is based on almost-daily (or even sometimes twice-daily) meat consumption, with regular intake of dairy products and processed meat. The regular consumption of fruits has been replaced, especially in children, by the many available desserts such as cakes, pastries, chocolates, and ice cream. Other alcoholic beverages and soft drinks of the "cola" type have replaced red wine. Most adolescents and even young adults do not meet the family for lunch and dinner, and, instead, visit fast-food shops with friends.

This change in dietary pattern, along with the more sedentary life-style adopted during the past decades by Cypriots, is certainly related to the increasing trends of morbidity and mortality from certain diseases in Cyprus as described above. The beginning of these diseases, such as atherosclerosis, could be in childhood and adolescence, and has been reported to be related to certain "atherogenic" life-styles.[61]

Table 3 presents a typical weekday menu consumed by a modern middle-aged man compared with a farmer's menu of more than 50 years ago. The composition of the foods and beverages (Table 4) was analyzed using the food composition software that was developed in the Department of Social Medicine of the University of Crete and was kindly offered to the Research and Education Program for Child's Health of Cyprus. Although there is a significant daily variation in these meals, especially of the modern man, there are certain striking observations that should be noted. It is very important to note that the total fat contribution to energy is 45% for the modern man, whereas it is only 31% in the older man. Similarly, saturated fat contribution to energy is double in the modern man (16% vs. 8%).

The fat-rich diet of the modern man is at the expense of carbohydrate intake. Thus, the modern man's carbohydrate contribution to energy is 40%, whereas that of the older man was 51%. Another striking observation of these diets is the significant difference in fiber consumption (14 gm for the older man in comparison with only 6 gm in modern man). Finally, we should note the intake of greater amounts of almost all vitamins in the older man, as shown in Table 4.

TABLE 3
Description of the Typical Diet Patterns of a Modern Middle-Aged Man and of a Middle-Aged Farmer More than 50 Years Ago in Cyprus

Meal	Modern Middle-Aged Man	Farmer – 50 Years Ago
Breakfast	Coffee with milk and sugar	A glass of milk (sheep's) with sugar
	Toast with margarine, marmalade, a slice of cheese, and one tomato.	A slice of bread, *anari* (kind of white soft cheese), about 10 olives.
Snack	A cheese pie. Coffee with sugar	A slice of bread, a tomato, and about 10 olives.
Lunch	Roast chicken with fried potatoes, yogurt, village salad, a slice of bread, a glass of Coca-Cola, and an apple.	Beans with olive oil, a slice of bread, tomato, onion, wild greens, vegetables, an apple, and a glass of red wine.
Snack	Apple pie and coffee with sugar.	Grapes
Dinner	Spaghetti with meat sauce and grated cheese.	Same as lunch
Snack	A beer (500 ml) and roasted nuts	—

In comparison with modern Cretan middle-aged men,[62] modern Cypriot men consume more fat as percentage of energy intake. In particular, the percentage of fat contribution to energy was found to be 39.5% in middle-aged Cretan[62] and 45% in middle-aged Cypriots (Table 4). Monounsaturated fatty acid intake as percentage of energy is high in both populations (19.9% in the Cretans, and 18.8% in the Cypriots), whereas the intake of polyunsaturated fatty acids is low in both populations (4.9% in the Cretans and 7% in the Cypriots). Consequently, the carbohydrate intake is greater in the Cretan men, where it confers about 44% of the energy in comparison with 40% in Cypriot men. As in Cyprus though, the Cretans have experienced a significant shift toward higher saturated fat (+ 25%) in the 30 years between 1960 and 1990. This change, along with other life-style changes in the Cretan population, are certainly responsible for the increase of cardiovascular disease risk factors in Crete and possibly also for the increase in coronary heart disease mortality.[12] Therefore, the dietary pattern changes can also be held responsible for the increase in observed morbidity and mortality in Cyprus as reported above.

Modern Cypriot children have abandoned the traditional dietary pattern even more significantly than adults. In a students' congress in 1998, high-school students presented the results of their own questionnaire-based study.[63] These results indicated that modern children's daily menu has "Westernized." Fifteen percent of children have no breakfast at all, and another 35% drink only milk for breakfast. Processed food is consumed very often, since 50% of those children eat processed food for dinner and another 10% for lunch daily. The explanation the students gave for this consumption is lack of time; involvement in prep schools for most of their time does not allow them to join their families for their meals. Thirty five percent of children eat some kind of meat for lunch, whereas only 19% eat some legumes, and even fewer accompany their lunch with salad. These children very seldom consume fruits,

TABLE 4
Nutrient Composition* of the Meals Presented in Table 3

Nutrient	Modern Middle-Aged Man	Farmer – 50 Years Ago
Energy (kcal)	2989	3017
Total fat (gm [% energy])	149 [45]	106 [31]
Saturated fatty acids (gm [% energy])	55 [17]	27 [8]
Monounsaturated fatty acids (gm [% energy])	63 [18]	41 [12]
Polyunsaturated fatty acids (gm [% energy])	18 [6]	7 [2]
Undetermined fatty acids (gm [% energy])	13 [4]	31 [9]
Cholesterol (mg)	392	112
Protein (gm [% energy]	114 [15]	92 [18]
Carbohydrates (gm[% energy])	287 [40]	381 [51]
Fiber (gm)	6	14
Calcium (mg)	1364	1292
Iron (mg)	12	27
Magnesium (mg)	317	375
Phosphorus (mg)	1770	1796
Potassium (mg)	2846	3635
Sodium (mg)	2633	4348
Vitamin A (RE)	735	1964
Thiamin	1.1	2.6
Riboflavin	1.6	3.2
Vitamin B_6 (mg)	1.7	1.2
Vitamin C (mg)	60	105

* The diet analysis was performed with the aid of the food composition software developed in the Department of Social Medicine of the University of Crete, and offered to the Program for Child's Health of Cyprus.

since only about 17% had fruit as an afternoon snack, and even less during the main meals.

The evaluation protocol of the Program for Child's Health of Cyprus includes a 24-hour dietary recall examination, and analysis of the diets consumed by the children using a food composition software. The analysis performed in 8868 children 11–12 years of age in 1999[64] is presented in Table 5, along with the U.S. recommended daily allowances (RDA).[65] The first striking observation from Table 5 is the low energy intake among the children, more pronounced for girls than for boys. This observation, combined with the increased frequency of obesity mentioned previously in this chapter, can be explained only by the sedentary life-style of children, which resulted in a negative energy balance. As described previously, girls in Cyprus are spending more time on sedentary activities than boys, thus expending even less energy than the boys.

The second striking observation is the fact that the intake of total and saturated fat exceeds the RDA by about 30% and 50%, respectively, in both boys and girls. This may well explain, at least to a certain extent, the increased rate of high levels

TABLE 5
Nutrient Analysis of the 24-hour Dietary Recall [Mean Values (± Standard Deviation)] of 8868 Children Aged 11–12 Years During the 1998–99 School Year[6]

Nutrient	Boys (n = 4524)	Girls (n = 4344)	U.S. Recommendations[65] (boys/girls)
Energy (kcal)	1744(389)	1593(361)	2200
Total fat (% energy)	39.0(11.8)	38.6(10.2)	30
Saturated fatty acids (% energy)	15.5(5.5)	15.3(4.1)	10
Monounsaturated fatty acids (% energy)	15.0(5.8)	14.9(5.3)	10
Polyunsaturated fatty acids (% energy)	4.1(2.2)	4.0(2.3)	10
Cholesterol (mg)	227(144)	203(130)	300
Protein (% energy)	14.8(4.8)	14.7(6.4)	15
Carbohydrates (% energy)	46.9(12.4)	47.7(13.0)	55
Fiber (g)	3.7(2.7)	3.6(2.7)	15
Sodium (mg)	2032(746)	1841(739)	500/500
Vitamin A (mg)	622(502)	594(507)	1000/800
Thiamin(mg)	1.00(0.44)	0.88(0.40)	1.3/1.1
Riboflavin (mg)	1.53(0.51)	1.39(0.52)	1.5/1.3
Vitamin B6 (mg)	1.11(0.50)	1.04(0.49)	1.7/1.4
Vitamin C (mg)	97(66)	103(69)	50/50

of serum total and LDL cholesterol mentioned above in this chapter. It is generally believed that dietary cholesterol and saturated fatty acids suppress the LDL hepatic receptors, thus preventing LDL cholesterol clearance.[66] On the other hand, lowering dietary intake of total and saturated fat and increasing monounsaturated and polyunsaturated fat and fiber (that is a diet resembling the traditional Mediterranean Diet) helps to significantly reduce serum total and LDL cholesterol.[67] Even the partial substitution of dietary saturated fat with monounsaturated fatty acids using manufactured foods can achieve significant reductions in serum total and LDL cholesterol.[68] Unfortunately, in this large pediatric sample we have evaluated, the intake of polyunsaturated fatty acids is low, about 8% of energy intake, and the intake of dietary fiber is much lower than optimal, i.e., less than 4 g per day.[64] The increasing trend of colon cancer in Cyprus (Table 1) may be attributed to this lower dietary fiber intake in combination with the regular consumption of "red" meat (e.g., beef and lamb as main dishes) and processed meat (e.g., sausages, hamburgers, smoked, cured and salted meat).[30]

The higher intake of fat as percentage of energy is at the expense of carbohydrates since our sample's carbohydrate intake is almost 10% of energy less than optimal (Table 5).[64] This is, presumably, not only a matter of quantity, but also of quality, since children are consuming foods high in simple sugars. In children, the higher intake of simple carbohydrates is associated with lower serum HDL cholesterol,[69] overeating, and possibly obesity.[70]

The sodium intake of these children is almost four times that of the recommended minimum intake (Table 5). This is certainly a matter of serious concern for the possible harmful consequences, although there is much debate as to what extent salt restriction is appropriate.[71]

Vitamins are essential components of co-factors in a wide range of metabolic reactions. The intake of certain vitamins of Cypriot children, such as vitamin A, thiamine, and B_6, as shown in Table 5, is less than optimal, and this is certainly also a matter for another serious concern. The intake of vitamin C, on the other hand, exceeds the recommended daily allowances, but this is presumably due to the frequent consumption of manufactured orange juice (enriched with sugar and preservatives) instead of the fresh citrus fruits that are plentiful in Cyprus.

B. ANALYSIS AND COMPOSITION OF CERTAIN FOODS IN THE CYPRUS MARKET

The composition of food is an important determinant of its nutritional value. Nutrition, though, receives little attention from the public health sector in Cyprus and there is, as yet, no national nutrition policy.

Fish consumption is inversely related to non-sudden death from myocardial infarction.[72] This benefit is probably mediated through the fatty acid composition of fish, especially of the omega-3 fatty acids. Table 6 presents the fatty acid composition and total fat of six fishes collected from the eastern Mediterranean Sea and two cultured fish at the Institute of Marine Biology in Heraklion, Crete.[73] These fishes are among the most commonly consumed in Cyprus. These data are very interesting in that the amount of omega-3 fatty acids is high in all eight fishes (exceeding the daily requirement of 300 mg), and also in the very low ratio of omega-6/omega-3 fatty acids.

In contrast to fish, the nutritional value of certain snacks purchased from the market of Cyprus is low, since they have a high energy density, which is about 25–30% of the daily energy requirements for some children. The snacks presented (which were unknown in the traditional Mediterranean Diet) provide more than 50% of the energy from fat, even the "light" ones (Table 7).[74] The light snacks (such as light potato chips) contain less saturated fat but much more sodium. The nutritional value of the snacks presented in Table 6 is not optimal. The contribution of proteins is 4–6% in the total energy.

The composition of various traditional Cypriot foods[75-78] (meat and dairy products) is presented in Table 8. As shown, certain dairy products are energy dense. *Challoumi*, for example, the traditional Cyprus cheese, contains more than 50% of its energy as fat, and again, more than 50% of that fat is saturated. The majority of Cypriots consume Challoumi, even nowadays, in most of their meals. Dried *anari* (a type of cheese), which is frequently eaten with pastries, is even more energy dense, and gains more than 60% of its energy from fat. On the contrary, in low-fat Challoumi, most of the fat has been removed, although people seldom consume low-fat dairy products. Nevertheless, most of the dairy products contain about 15 times more saturated than polyunsaturated fat.

TABLE 6
Fatty Acid Composition and Total Fat of Mediterranean Fishes[73]

Fatty Acids	Scomber japonicus (Chub mackerel)[a]	Boopsboops (bogue)[b]	Mullus barbatus (red mullet)[c]	Mullus surmuletus (striped mullet)[d]	Merluccius merluccius (hake)[e]	Pagellus erythrinus (common Pandora)[f]	Pargus pargus (red sea beam)[g]	Sparus aurata (gilthead sea beam)[h]
12:0(mg/100g)	0.1	0.1	0.6	0.4	0.3	0.2	0.1	0.1
14:0(mg/100g)	3.9	5.4	4.2	3.9	4.9	4.0	4.9	5.7
14:1(mg/100g)	0.3	0.5	1.1	0.4	0.6	0.4	0.4	0.4
15:0(mg/100g)	2.7	0.9	1.4	1.9	0.7	0.7	0.4	0.4
16:0(mg/100g)	19.9	19.6	19.8	18.4	18.5	19.8	18.2	19.9
16:1(mg/100g)	2.8	6.0	9.2	8.2	5.5	6.9	6.8	6.8
18:0(mg/100g)	4.6	6.5	6.0	4.6	5.0	7.9	4.0	3.9
18:1(mg/100g)	6.7	20.8	17.5	21.0	19.6	16.4	22.6	25.9
18:2(mg/100g)	1.5	2.3	1.8	3.9	3.0	1.1	6.3	6.5
20:0(mg/100g)	0.6	0.8	0.2	0.8	0.5	0.6	0.3	0.2
20:1(mg/100g)	–	–	1.8	–	–	0.9	–	–
18:3 n-3 (mg/100g)	2.5	2.7	1.9	4.7	2.4	1.8	8.3	7.5
20:2 n-9 (mg/100g)	2.0	0.8	0.7	1.1	0.6	1.1	2.1	1.5
20:2 n-6 (mg/100g)	0.5	0.8	0.7	1.1	0.4	0.4	0.2	0.5
20:3 n-6 (mg/100g)	–	–	0.3	2.2	0.4	0.2	–	0.1
20:4 n-6 (mg/100g)	3.0	1.6	4.1	5.5	2.4	2.5	4.3	3.1
20:5 n-3 (mg/100g)	8.7	5.8	7.0	9.8	4.7	11.4	6.2	2.3
22:4 n-6 (mg/100g)	0.5	1.0	1.7	0.9	0.9	0.6	0.3	0.4
22:5 n-3 (mg/100g)	1.7	2.6	1.7	1.7	3.0	2.7	1.2	1.5
22:6 n-3 (mg/100g)	15.4	10.5	2.0	2.4	11.1	5.6	8.7	7.6
n-6 (%)	5.5	5.7	8.6	13.6	7.1	4.8	11.1	10.6
n-3 (%)	28.3	21.6	12.6	18.6	21.2	21.5	24.4	18.9
n-6/n-3(ratio)	0.2	0.3	0.7	0.7	0.3	0.2	0.5	0.6
Saturated(%)	31.8	33.2	32.1	29.9	29.9	33.2	28.0	30.2
Total Fat(%)	2.2	1.2	3.5	7.0	1.2	2.7	6.2	12.1
n-3 fatty acids (mg/100g)	535	207	390	1207	203	506	1401	2125

– Not detected.
[a]collios, [b]gopa, [c]koutsomoura, [d]barbouni, [e]bakaliaros, [f]lithrini, [g]fagri, [h]tsipoura

TABLE 7
Composition by Chemical Analysis (per 100 g) of Snacks Obtained from the Markets of Cyprus[74]

Food Sample	Energy (kcal)	Fat (g)	Protein (g)	Carbohydrate (g)	SFA[a] (%)	Sodium (mg)	Potassium (mg)
Potato chips "CO" salted	594	41.6	6.8	48.2	40.87	232	801
Potato Crisps "H.A."	552	35.8	8.7	48.8	34.23	386	1603
Potato chips with bacon flavor "M.A"	518	27.9	3.6	63.2	38.79	867	112
"N.S.T." chips	574	38.1	7.8	49.9	18.6	585	241
Light Potato Chips salted	503	27.4	5.3	58.7	15.72	1189	844

[a] Saturated fatty acids

Similarly, some popular traditional items such as smoked sausage and *sheftalia* (type of traditional burger), contain a similar percentage of fat, and are rich in proteins. Items used as appetizers and, frequently, in sandwiches for children, such as *lunza* (a type of deli meat) and smoked ham, are low in fat and, of course, are still rich in proteins.

VI. CONCLUSIONS

This chapter has discussed the increase in chronic disease rates observed in Cyprus during recent decades. It is presumed that this is just an inevitable price that Cyprus is paying for the radical change of its citizens' life-styles, which is thought to have occurred because of the expansion of the economy that Cyprus has experienced during recent years, especially after the Declaration of Independence in 1960.

The life-style changes, mostly the abandonment of the traditional Mediterranean Diet, the adoption of a sedentary way of living, and the increasing frequency of smoking, are certainly directly related to the observed increasing trends of risk factors and morbidity and mortality described in Sections III and IV. Unfortunately, it seems that children in this country are most influenced. Therefore, it is to be expected that, if this status is not reversed, chronic diseases will afflict them as adults.

The evolution of the disease status described in this chapter is certainly not new. It has been observed in both northern European countries such as Finland and in southern Europe in areas such as Crete. In Cyprus, too, certain diet-related risks are apparently increasing at a time when developed countries have succeeded in reducing cardiovascular disease risk factors status, and the morbidity and mortality of related diseases. The experience of those countries should be used and applied to the needs of Cyprus society in order to reverse this status. The effort would be less difficult if the lessons learned in other countries could be adapted properly to this society.

The Research and Education Program for Child's Health of Cyprus has already made a major effort since 1995 by introducing intervention strategies to schoolchil-

TABLE 8
Composition by Chemical Analysis (per 100 gm) of Dairy Products and Meat Products Obtained from the Markets of Cyprus[75-78]

Food	Energy (Kcal)	Proteins (gm)	Carbohydrate (gm)	Fat (gm)	SFA[a] (g/100gm)	MUFA[b] (gm)	PUFA[c] (gm)	Cholesterol (mg)
Challoumi[d]	319	22.4	1.2	25.1	15.1	6.9	1	92
Challoumi low fat	185	26.4	2	8	5.3	2.4	0.3	40
Anari[e] (fresh)	226	10.9	3	21.6	16.6	7.3	1.2	106
Anari (dried)	430	22.2	2.6	39.8	–	–	–	154
Cefalotyri[f]	430	26.6	–	36	–	–	–	–
Yogurt (sheep)	92	6.2	5.8	5.0	–	–	–	–
Yogurt low fat	54.2	6	5.9	0.9	–	–	–	–
Beef sausage	178	19.2	14.3	4.9	–	–	–	–
Traditional smoked sausage	265	21.4	2.1	19	–	–	–	–
Lunza (bacon)	146	26.3	0.5	4.3	–	–	–	–
Smoked salami	292	16.2	8.2	21.9	–	–	–	–
Cooked *sheftalia*[g]	313.5	17.3	12.7	21.5	9	9.5	3.3	53
Smoked ham	106	15.9	4.5	2.8	–	–	–	–
Hamburger	198	16.4	8.9	11.1	–	–	–	–

– Not available
[a] SFA: Saturated fatty acids
[b] MUFA: Monounsaturated fatty acids
[c] PUFA: Polyunsaturated fatty acids
[d] *Challoumi*: Traditional Cyprus cheese
[e] *Anari*: Traditional type of fresh soft cheese
[f] *Cefalotyri*: Type of long-ripened sheep's milk cheese.
[g] *Sheftalia*: Traditional type of burger.

dren and their families. This intervention is a population-based approach, rather than just a high-risk-individual approach. The aim, obviously, is to sensitize the whole population (including the high-risk subjects), where there are many possible candidates for manifesting cardiovascular and related diseases. This approach includes the education of children to change to a healthier way of life. The state strongly supports this effort, and there is encouraging evidence that the public is gradually adopting the appropriate life-style modifications.

REFERENCES

1. Keys A. (Ed.), Seven Countries. *A Multivariate Analysis of Death and Coronary Heart Diseases*. Cambridge: Harvard University Press. 1980.

2. De Lorgeril M., Salen P., Martin J. L., Monjaud I., Delaye J., and Memelle N., Mediterranean Diet, traditional risk factors, and the rate of cardiovascular complications after myocardial infarction. *Circulation*, 99, 779, 1999.

3. De Lorgeril M., Salen P., Martin J. L., Monjaud I., Boucher P., and Mamelle N., Mediterranean dietary pattern in a randomized trial. prolonged survival and possible reduced cancer rate, *Arch. Intern. Med.*, 158, 1181, 1998.

4. Kafatos A.G., Kouroumalis I., Vlachonikolis J., Thedotou C., and Labadarios P., Coronary heart disease risk factors status of the Cretan urban population in the 1980s, *Am. J. Clin. Nutr.*, 54, 83, 1991.

5. Halliwell B., Free radicals and antioxidants: a personal view, *Nutr. Rev.*, 52, 253, 1994.

6. Mensink R.P. and Katan M.B., Effect of a Diet enriched with monounsaturated or polyunsaturated fatty acids on levels of low-density and high-density lipoprotein cholesterol in healthy women and men, *N. Eng. J. Med.*, 321, 436, 1989.

7. Salen P., de Longeril M., Boissonnat P., Monjaud I., Guidolled J., Dureau G., and Renaud S., Effects of a French Mediterranean diet on heart transplant recipients with hypercholesterolemia, *Am. J. Cardiol.*, 73, 825, 1994.

8. GISSI-Prevenzione Investigators. Dietary supplementation with n-3 polyunsaturated fatty acids and vitamin E after myocardial infarction: results of the GISSI-Prevenzione Trial. *Lancet*, 354, 447, 1999.

9. M. Tornaritis. The changing pattern of the Mediterranean diet of the people of Crete and Cyprus, in *Proc. 11th International Ethnological Food Research Conference, Nicosia*, Cyprus, 1996, 60.

10. Gjonca A. and Bobak M., Albanian paradox, another example of protective effect of Mediterranean Life-style? *Lancet*, 350, 1815, 1997.

11. Kourides Y., Tornaritis M., Kourides C., Savvas S., and Hadjigeorgiou C., Relation of excessive television watching and risk of atherosclerosis in children. (In preparation) 1999. (in Greek).

12. Kafatos A., Diacatou A., Voukiklaris G., Nikolakakis N., Vlachonikolis J., Kounali D., Mamalakis G., and Dontas S., Heart disease risk-factors status and dietary changes in the Cretan population over the past 30 y: The Seven Countries Study. *Am. J. Clin. Nutr.*, 65, 1882, 1997.

13. Department of Statistics and Research, Ministry of Finance of Cyprus. *Demographic report 1997*. Printing Office of the Republic of Cyprus, Nicosia, Cyprus, 1998.

14. WHO. Executive Summary. *The World Health Report 1998*. Geneva, World Health Organization, 1, 1998.

15. Sans S., Kesteloot H., and Kromhout D., On behalf of the task force, the burden of cardiovascular diseases mortality in Europe. *Eur. Heart. J.*, 18, 1231, 1997.

16. WHO, *The World Health Report 1999, Making a Difference*. Geneva, World Health Organization, 13, 1999.

17. Department of Statistics and Research, the Ministry of Finance of Cyprus. Personal communication, 1999.

18. Department of Statistics and Research, Ministry of Finance of Cyprus. *Hospital Statistics 1980*. Printing Office of the Republic of Cyprus, Nicosia, 1982.

19. Department of Statistics and Research, Ministry of Finance of Cyprus. Unpublished data, 1980.

20. Department of Statistics and Research, Ministry of Finance of Cyprus. *Health and hospital statistics 1997*. Printing Office of the Republic of Cyprus, Nicosia, Cyprus, 1999.

21. Jefferys M. and Kyriakides D., *Health Status, Utilization and Expenditure on Health Services 1989*. Printing Office of the Republic of Cyprus, Nicosia, Cyprus, 1989.

22. Antoniades L., Simamonian K., Ioannides M., Petrondas D., and Zambartas C., Epidemiology Study of Acute Myocardial Infarction in Nicosia Area Cyprus (AMINA Study Cyprus), *Proc. 11th Annual Meeting of Mediterranean Association of Cardiology and Cardiac Surgery*, Montpelier, France, 1998.
23. Antoniades, L. C., Acute myocardial infarction, Nicosia study — part one, *Cyprus Med. J.*, 10, 23, 1992. (in Greek).
24. Department of Statistics and Research, Ministry of Finance of Cyprus, Unpublished data, 1996.
25. Huston S. L., Lengerich E. J., Conlisk E., and Pessaro K., Trends in ischemic heart disease death rates for blacks and whites — United States, 1981–1995. *Mor. Mor. Wek. Rep.*, 47, 945, 1998.
26. Theophanides C. G., Diabetes epidemiology in Cyprus, *Cyprus Med. J.*, 14, 3, 1996.
27. Skordis N., Kasios J., Toufexis C., Ioannou I., and Hadjiloizou S., Epidemiology of insulin dependent diabetes mellitus in children and adolescents in Cyprus, *Cyprus Med. J.*, 16, 41, 1998 (in Greek).
28. Theophanides C. and G., Beaton M., The epidemiology of diabetic complications in Cyprus, *Cyprus Med. J.*, 16, 17, 1998.
29. Theophanides C. G., Diabetes and its complications in Cyprus, *Cyprus Med. J.*, 4, 5, 1984.
30. Cummings J. H. and Bingham J. A., Diet and the prevention of cancer, *Br. Med. J.*, 317, 1636, 1998.
31. Savvas S., Tornaritis M., Hadjigeorgiou C, Kourides Y., Shamounki M., and Epiphaniou-Savva M., increased frequency of multiple cardiovascular risk factors in children 11-12 years old in Cyprus, *Pediatriki*, 62, 468, 1999, (in Greek).
32. Berenson G. S., Srinivasan S. R., Bao W., Newman III W. P., Tracy R. E., and Wattigney W. A., Association between multiple cardiovascular risk factors and atherosclerosis in children and young adults, *N. Eng. J. Med.*, 338, 1650, 1998.
33. Wissler R. W. and Strong J. P., and the PDAY Research Group, Risk factors and progression of atherosclerosis in youth, *Am. J. Pathol.*, 153, 1023, 1998.
34. Newman W. P. III, Freedman D. S., Voors A. W., Gard P. D., Srinivasan S. R., Cresanta J. L., Williamson G. D., Webber L. S., and Berenson G. S., Relation of serum lipoprotein levels and systolic blood pressure to early atherosclerosis, the Bogalusa Heart study, N. Eng. J. Med., 314, 138, 1986.
35. Hadjigeorgiou C., Tornaritis M., Siamounki M., Savvas S., and Kourides Y., Is Hyperlipidemia Treated Properly in Cyprus? *Proc. 37th Panhellenic Pediatric Conference*, Thessaloniki, Greece, Greek Pediatric Society, Athens, 1999, 168.
36. American Academy of Pediatrics Committee on Nutrition, Cholesterol in childhood, *Pediatrics*, 101, 141, 1998.
37. Moutiris J., Elia A., Eleftheriou O., Eleftheriades A., Sidera M., Agathocleous M., Andreou M., Nikolaides E., and Fessas C., Serum lipids levels in 783 Cypriot children aged 2–12 years old. *Cyprus Med. J.*, 16, 52, 1998 (in Greek).
38. Savvas S., Tornaritis M., Epiphaniou-Savva M., Kourides Y., Hadjigeorgiou C., and Siamounki M., Lipids and lipoproteins levels in Greek-Cypriot adolescents. comparison with Greek data, In preparation, 1999.
39. Schulpis K. and Karikas G. A., Serum cholesterol and triglyceride distribution in 7767 school-aged Greek children. *Pediatrics*, 101, 861, 1998.
40. Parmley W. W., Nonlipoprotein risk factors for coronary heart disease: evaluation and management, *Am. J. Med.*, 102, 7, 1997.
41. Demetriades A. D., Smoking habits in Cyprus, *Cyprus. Med. J.*,4, 23, 1984 (in Greek).

42. Martoudis S. G., The habit of smoking among the undergraduates of the secondary schools in the region of Nicosia, *Cyprus. Med. J.*, 7, 37, 1987.

43. University of Cyprus. Prevalence of smoking habit among children and adolescents in Cyprus. 1999, Personal Communication.

44. Lamarche B., Lemieux S., Dagenais G. R., and Despres J. –P., Visceral obesity and the risk of ischaemic heart disease: insights from the Quebec Cardiovascular Study, *Growth Hormone and IGF Research* 8, 1, 1998.

45. Rosner B., Prineas R., Loggie J., and Daniels S. R., Percentiles for body mass index in U. S. children 5 to 17 years of age, *J. Pediatr.*, 132, 211, 1998.

46. Kourides Y. A.,. Nutritional status of children of Paphos, *Paediatr. N. Gr.*, 9, 190, 1997. (in Greek).

47. Kourides Y., Tornaritis M., Kourides C., Savvas S., Hatzigeorgiou C., and Siamounki M., Obesity in Cyprus in Children 11-12 Years of Age, *Proc. 37th Panhellenic Pediatric Conference*, Thessaloniki, Greece, Greek Pediatric Society, Athens, 1999, 10.

48. Savvas S., Tornaritis M., Hadjigeorgiou C., Kourides Y., Siamounki M., and Epiphaniou-Savva M., Low triceps skinfold thickness is negatively correlated to atherosclerosis indices in overweight children, *Proc. 16th Pancyprian Medical Conference*, Nicosia, Cyprus, 1998.

49. Savvas S., Ierodiakonou M., Tornaritis M., Epiphaniou-Savva M., Georgiou C., Eleftheriou A., and Skordis N., Serum leptin levels in children and adolescents in Cyprus and its relation to sex, puberty stage and obesity. In Preparation 1999.

50. Whitaker R. C., Wright J. A., Pepe M. S., Seidel K. D., and Dietz W. H., Predicting obesity in young adulthood from childhood and parental obesity, *N. Eng. J. Med.*, 337, 869, 1997.

51. Gunnell D. J., Frankel S. J., Nanchahal K., Peters T. J., and Davey Smith G., Childhood obesity and adult cardiovascular mortality: a 57-y follow-up study based on the Boyd Orr Cohort, *Am. J. Clin. Nutr.*, 67, 1111, 1998.

52. Savvas S., Tornaritis M., Epiphaniou-Savva M., Kourides Y., Panagi A., Silikiotou N., Georgiou C., and Kafatos A., Waist circumference and waist-to-height ratio are better predictors of cardiovascular disease risk factors in children than body mass index. Unpublished data.

53. Rodriguez B. L., Curb D., Buchfiel C. M., Abbott R. D., Petrovitch H., Masaki K., and Chiu D., Physical activity and 23-year incidence of coronary heart disease morbidity and mortality among middle-aged men. The Honolulu Heart Program. *Circulation*, 89, 2540, 1994.

54. Hsieh S. D., Yoshinaga H., Muto T., and Sakurai Y., Regular physical activity and coronary risk factors in Japanese men, *Circulation*, 97, 661, 1998.

55. Godsland I. E., Leyva F., Walton C., Worthington M., and Stevenson J. C., Associations of Smoking, alcohol and physical activity with risk factors for coronary heart disease and diabetes in the first follow-up cohort of the heart disease and diabetes risk indicators in a screened cohort study (HDDRISC-1), *J. Intern. Med.*, 244, 33, 1998.

56. Shern-Brewer R., Santanam N., Wetzstein C., White-Welkley J., and Partasarathy S., Exercise and cardiovascular disease. a new perspective, *Arterioscler. Thromb. Vasc. Biol.*, 18, 1181, 1998.

57. Child's Health Program Database of Cyprus. Unpublished data, 1998.

58. Georgiou C., Savvas S., Giangoulli A., Hadjioannou M., Hadjiloizou L., Albanoudes P., and Tornaritis M., The effect of exercise on serum lipids in children, *Proc. 1st Panhellenic Gymnasts Conference*, Nicosia, Cyprus, 1998.

59. Willett W. C., Sacks F., Trichopoulou A., Drescher G., Ferro-Luzzi A., Helsing E., and Trichopoulos D., Mediterranean diet pyramid: a cultural model for healthy eating, *Am. J. Clin. Nutr.*, 61(suppl), 1402S, 1995.
60. Keys A., Mediterranean diet and public health: personal reflections, *Am. J. Clin. Nutr.*, 61(suppl), 1321S, 1995.
61. Boreham C., Twisk J., van Mechelen W., Savage M., Strain J., Cran G., Relationships between the development of biological risk factors for coronary heart disease and life-style parameters during adolescence: the Northern Ireland Young Hearts Project, *Publ. Hlth.*, 113, 7, 1999.
62. Moschandreas J., and Kafatos A., Food and nutrient intakes of Greek (Cretan) adults: recent data for food-based dietary guidelines in Greece, *Br. J. Nutr.*, 81(suppl. 2), S71, 1999.
63. Anonymous, Nutrition, Exercise, and Good Health, *Proc. 3rd Interschool Congress*, Limassol, Cyprus, 1998.
64. Child's Health Program Database of Cyprus, 24-hour Dietary Recall Analysis. Unpublished data, 1999.
65. American Academy of Pediatrics, *Pediatric Nutrition Handbook*, American Academy of Pediatrics, 1993.
66. Dietschy J. M., Dietary fatty acids and the regulation of plasma low density lipoprotein cholesterol concentrations, *J. Nutr.*, 128, 444S, 1998.
67. Mekki N., Dubois C., Charbonnier M., Cara L., Senft M., Pauli A. M., Portugal H., Gassin A. L., Lafont H., and Lairon D., Effects of lowering fat and increasing dietary fiber on fasting and postprandial plasma lipids in hypercholesterolemic subjects consuming a mixed Mediterranean-Western Diet, *Am. J. Clin. Nutr.*, 66, 1443, 1997.
68. Williams C. M., Francis-Knapper J. A., Webb D., Brookes C. A., Zampellas A., Tredger J. A., Wright J., Meijer G., Calder P. C., Yaqoob P., Roche H., and Gibney M. J., Cholesterol reduction using manufactured foods high in monounsaturated fatty acids: a randomized crossover study, *Br. J. Nutr.*, 81, 439, 1999.
69. Starc T. J., Shea S., Cohn S. C., Mosca L., Gersony W. M., and Deckelbaum R. J., Greater dietary intake of simple carbohydrate is associated with lower concentrations of high-density-lipoprotein cholesterol in hypercholesterolemic children, *Am. J. Clin. Nutr.*, 67, 1147, 1998.
70. Ludwig D. S., Majzoub J. A., Al-Zahrani A., Dallal G. E., Blanco I., and Roberts S. B., High glycemic index foods, overeating, and obesity, *Pediatrics*, 103, e26, 1999.
71. de Wardener, Salt reduction and cardiovascular risk: the anatomy of a myth, *J. Hum. Hypertens.*, 13, 1, 1999.
72. Daviglus M. L., Stamler J., Orencia A. J., Dyer A. R., Liu K., Greenland P., Walsh M. K., Morris D., and Shekelle R. B., Fish consumption and the 30-year risk of fatal myocardial infarction, *N. Eng. J. Med.*, 336, 1046, 1997.
73. Tornaritis M., Peraki E., Georgoulli M., Kafatos A., Charalambakis G., Divanack P., Kentouri M., Yiannopoulos S., Frenaritou H., and Argyrides R., Fatty acid composition and total fat of eight species of Mediterranean Fish, *Int. J. Food. Sci. Nutr.*, 45, 135, 1993.
74. Yiannopoulos S., Procopiou E., Tornaritis M., Frenaritou H., Neophytou A., Argyrides R., Akelidou N., and Kafatos A., Nutritional value of snacks purchased from the markets of Crete and Cyprus. In preparation, 1999.
75. Yiannopoulos S.Y., and Argyrides R.S., Composition and Calory Value Determination of Some Cyprus Traditional Food and Food Products, Proc 3rd Cyprus-Greece congress on chemistry and health, 1992.

76. State General Laboratory Cyprus, Preliminary Food Composition Tables of Cyprus Traditional Foods, 1st edition State General Laboratory, Nicosia, Cyprus, 1998.

77. Yiannopoulos S.Y., Frenaritou H., Kokkinofta R, and Argyrides R.S., Halloumi's Traditional Cheese of Cyprus: Composition and Quality, *Proc. 6th Cyprus-Greece Congress on Chemistry and Quality Control in Industrial Products,* Rhodes, Greece, 1999.

78. Yiannopoulos S.Y., Frenaritou H., Kokkinofta R, and Argyrides R.S., Establishing Food Composition Data for Cyprus and Quality Assurance of Analytical Results, *Proc. 6th Cyprus-Greece Congress on Chemistry and Quality Control in Industrial Products*, Rhodes, Greece, 1999.

14 Nutrition Policy Issues and Further Research on the Mediterranean Diet: The Importance of Monounsaturated Fatty Acids

Michael J. Gibney and Helen M. Roche

CONTENTS

I. INTRODUCTION

The Mediterranean Diet is characterized by its level of dietary fat and the composition of that fat. Table 1 illustrates for three southern and three northern EU states.[1-6] The virtues of the Mediterranean Diet have long been espoused by nutrition experts. Most of these virtues have focused on the ability of diets high in monounsaturated fatty acids (MUFA) to lower plasma total and low-density lipoprotein (LDL) cholesterol when substituted for saturated fatty acids (SFA). However, there are other potential beneficial effects of high-MUFA diets that merit further research. Advocates of the Mediterranean Diet immediately enter into direct conflict with the nutrition policies based on the prevailing wisdom, i.e., that lower fat intakes are a universally desirable

TABLE 1
Compositions of Dietary Fat Expressed as a Percentage Of Energy in Typical Southern and Northern EU Member States

	Total Fat	SFA	MUFA	PUFA
Southern				
Spain[1]	38	13	17	5
Greece[2]	40	12	20	5
Portugal[3]	29	9	12	5
Average	36	12	16	5
Northern				
Finland[4]	34	14	11	5
Germany[5]	41	18	15	6
Netherlands[6]	38	15	14	7
Average	38	16	13	6

population goal. A reduction in total fat intake, not a feature of the Mediterranean Diet, will lead to adverse changes in plasma lipids in respect of an increase in plasma triacylglycerol (TAG), a decrease in plasma HDL, and an increase in the proportion of LDL as small, dense LDL. Thus, an objective of this chapter is to examine nutrition policy implications from the promotion of the Mediterranean Diet.

II. POLICY ASPECTS

A. FOOD SUPPLY ISSUES

In the realm of food safety, risk analysis is divided into three separate areas of action: risk assessment, risk management, and risk communication.The first examines the problem to provide a quantitative and sometimes qualitative analysis of the risk. The policy consequences are not considered in this endeavor, but are dealt with by the process of risk management. In effect, having had all aspects or risk teased out, the risk managers decide how society should handle the risk. In the formulation of nutrition policy, risk assessment (e.g., the risk associated with diet-related variation in different fractions of plasma lipids) is usually mixed up with risk management (e.g., to obtain a low risk nutrient intake, a specific set of food targets, such as the food pyramid, are issued). Quite often, these food targets emanating from nutrition "risk-management" are formulated without reference to the wider considerations of the recommendations. As an example, if all (350 million) citizens of the European Union (EU) were to aspire to a Cretan level of olive oil intake (40 g/d), the annual production would have to reach 14,000 metric tons, which is orders of magnitude above present capacity. The land-use implications would be unthinkable, since olive oil production would displace pastures and the production of other crops.

This, then, raises the question of whether olive oil is equivalent in all aspects in relation to nutrition and health to other MUFA-rich oils, such as rapeseed oil, which, in turn, raises a number of research questions that, to date, have not been extensively studied. One such question is whether the non-TAG components of olive oil, particularly virgin olive oil, play any role in the health benefits of this oil source. A second question is whether the positional distribution of fatty acids in the glycerol moiety of TAG differ between olive oil and other high-MUFA oils, and whether this in any way influences the health benefits of olive oil. Even if these issues were to be resolved and all high-MUFA oils were deemed to be equally beneficial, there still remains the issue of how northern-EU diets can be changed. There are basically two options in seeking such change. One is to get people to alter their food choices to those more typical of the Mediterranean Diet. The second is to retain northern-EU food choice patterns but to alter the fat composition of such foods. If the latter strategy were to play a role, further problems would need to be addressed. While it is easy to incorporate MUFA-rich fats into spreadable fats and other such manufactured high-fat foods, it is not so easy to increase the MUFA content of some dry baked foods, e.g., biscuits or of non-processed foods such as dairy products and meats.

B. NUTRIENT-SUPPLY ISSUES

Although the fat contents of the northern-EU and Mediterranean Diets do not differ greatly, the composition of the dietary fat does differ. The northern-EU diet is characterized by higher levels of SFA and lower levels of MUFA. The percent of energy from polyunsaturated fatty acids is fairly constant. A major issue that must be addressed is whether it is more advantageous to leave fat intakes in northern EU at their present high levels while altering the composition of fat, or whether it is best simply to lower fat intakes and replace the fat with carbohydrate. The expression of fatty acid categories as percent of energy can lead to some confusion when examining the question of whether sub-populations who have lower fat intakes actually have altered fat composition. This can be overcome by expressing the intakes of specific fatty acid categories as a percent of the weight of total fat intake. Table 2 compares the intakes of fatty acid categories, using both approaches for sub-populations into the upper or lower tertiles/quartiles (quantiles), for some northern and southern EU countries. Clearly, as percent of energy from total fat falls, so too do the percentages of energy from sub-categories, i.e., SFA, MUFA, and PUFA. However, when expressed as percent of total fat intake, the balance of SFA, MUFA, and PUFA, while differing between the northern and southern parts of the EU, do not differ within either of these regions across quantiles (quartiles or tertiles) of percent of energy from fat. Quite simply, as people within a given region lower their total fat intake, they do not change its composition. This is contrary to the expectation that a reduction in total fat intake will lead to a disproportionate reduction in saturated fat intake. Notwithstanding the difficulties outlined in the preceding section on altering the fat composition of the northern EU diet, nutrition policy must embrace a greater effort to alter the composition of dietary fat, rather than devote itself almost exclusively to extolling the virtues of low-fat diets.

TABLE 2
Dietary Fat Composition Expressed as (a) a Percent of Energy or (b) as Dietary Fatty Acid Categories and a Percent (W/W) in Upper and Lower Quartiles/Tertiles of Percent of Energy from Fat in Typical Southern and Northern EU States

	Low-Fat Diets			High-Fat Diets		
	SFA	MUFA	PUFA	SFA	MUFA	PUFA
(a) Dietary fatty acids as a % of energy						
Southern						
Spain[1]	11	15	4	14	19	10
Greece[2]	8	12	4	15	28	10
Portugal[3]	6	10	4	11	15	11
Northern						
Finland[4]	11	8	4	18	14	12
Germany[5]	14	12	5	21	17	13
Netherlands[6]	12	11	5	17	17	16
(b) Dietary fatty acids as a % of dietary fatty acids						
Southern						
Spain[1]	37	50	13	37	50	9
Greece[2]	34	51	15	30	50	10
Portugal[3]	32	48	20	35	47	11
Northern						
Finland[4]	47	37	17	48	38	12
Germany[5]	45	40	15	46	39	13
Netherlands[6]	41	39	19	40	40	16

C. NUTRIENT RISK-FACTOR ISSUES FOR POLICY

Conventional wisdom argues that high-fat diets predispose to obesity.[7] However, over the last few years, a debate has emerged as to the benefits of maintaining fat intakes at their present level while altering the composition of dietary fat.[8] In effect, that means embracing the dietary fat patterns of the Mediterranean Diet. The hub of the argument in relation to the role of dietary fat composition and the risk of heart disease is twofold. First, the widely held belief that a reduction in fat intake would reduce the incidence of obesity is challenged. Second, it is argued that low-fat, high-carbohydrate diets, while lowering plasma LDL cholesterol levels, lead to elevated levels of plasma TAG, an elevated percent of the LDL fraction as the more atherogenic small, dense LDL, and also a reduction in plasma levels of the cardio-protective HDL fraction. It is totally outside the scope of this chapter to delve into this debate in any depth. It is, however, worthwhile to draw attention to some deficits in the scope of the debate.

It is almost universally accepted that obesity is a major risk factor for hyper-cholesterolemia, hypertriacylglycerolemia, adult-onset diabetes, and hypertension.

However, there is a not insignificant body of research to indicate that these adverse effects can be reduced by physical activity. Several prospective epidemiological studies that have carefully documented baseline cardiovascular fitness have shown that low fitness levels rank about equal, in terms of odds ratios for both all-cause and cardiovascular disease, to conventional risk factors, e.g., hypercholesterolemia, smoking, and hypertension. A recent study has shown that this is true among normal-weight, overweight, and obese subjects.[9]

The case that low-fat, high-carbohydrate diets exert adverse effects on small, dense LDL levels, TAG levels, HDL levels, and even insulin resistance, also needs to be examined. First, these adverse effects are not seen in all studies.[10] Second, these adverse effects of low-fat, high-carbohydrate diets are not seen when the full spectrum of public health nutrition advice is embraced, most notably the consumption of adequate intakes of long-chain n-3 PUFA from fish oil and moderate physical activity.[11,12] The TAG-raising effect of low-fat, high-carbohydrate diets has been shown to be negated by consumption of just 1 g/d of long chain n-3 PUFA.[12]

III. FUTURE RESEARCH AREAS

A. Fat Absorption, Postprandial Lipemia, and Gut Hormone Function: The Role of MUFA

Almost without exception, the many studies that have examined the effects of dietary fat on plasma lipids have focused on fasting blood samples, with almost exclusive attention to cholesterol. In recent years, however, there has been a significant growth in research into the acute, chronic, and acute-on-chronic effects of dietary fats on postprandial TAG metabolism. This arises from the recognition that prolonged and elevated postprandial lipemia is associated with a significant increase in the risk of cardiovascular disease.[13] The most important determinant of the postprandial lipemia response is fasting plasma TAG levels. These can be influenced by a number of dietary factors such as exercise,[14] dietary fat-to-carbohydrate ratio,[15] and intake of long-chain n-3 PUFA. At any given fasting plasma TAG level, the extent of the lipemia response can be influenced by the level of fat ingested and the type of fat ingested.[15] To date, most attention in this regard has been focused on the long chain n-3 PUFA. There is, however, a growing body of evidence to indicate that the main dietary MUFA, oleic acid, plays a key role in linking gut function to postprandial lipemia. A cross-cultural comparison of postprandial lipid metabolism and coagulation factor VII activity in northern and southern European men provided very novel data that showed that southern Europeans metabolized dietary fat very differently from their northern counterparts. As is shown in Figure 1, there was a rapid influx and removal of plasma TAG following the ingestion of the standard test meal by the southern Europeans, whereas plasma TAG concentrations were elevated for a much longer period in the northern European men.[16]

Several *in-vitro* studies using the human gut cell line derived from colon carcinoma, the Caco-2 cell line, have indicated a unique ability of oleic acid (C18:1 n-9) to promote TAG secretion. Van Grevenbroek et al. (1996) found that both C18:1 n-9 and the main dietary polyunsaturated fatty acid, linoleic acid (C18:2 n-6),

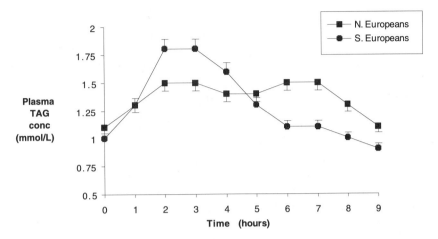

FIGURE 1   Postprandial plasma TAG concentrations following SFA- and MIFA-rich test meals in healthy male volunteers from Northern and Southern Europe (16).

significantly increased basolateral secretion of TAG compared with cells incubated with SFA (palmitic acid C16:0, stearic acid C18:0).[17] Moreover, oleic acid led to a very significant increase in basolateral apo B48 transfer, while none of the fatty acids differed in respect to apo B100 secretion. In a separate comparison of olive oil type and corn oil type fatty acids, the former led to a 50% increase over the latter in basolateral TAG secretion and almost doubled the ratio of TAG to apo B in the secreted chylomicrons.

The transfer of lipids within the enterocyte into nascent chylomicrons is facilitated by an enzyme complex of microsomal transfer protein (MTP) and proteindisulfideisomerase (PDI). The latter is believed to facilitate conformational changes (folding) of apo B to establish a hydrophobic core into which the transfer of lipid is facilitated by the MTP sub-unit of the complex.[18] It remains possible that oleic acid promotes the MTP-mediated lipid transfer into nascent chylomicrons. This hypothesis was tested by Van Greevenbroek et al. (1998) who used a compound (BMS-200150) to inhibit MTP.[19] When cells were incubated with oleic acid, the lipoproteins secreted were predominantly TAG-rich lipoproteins (chylomicrons and VLDL), which were sensitive to inhibition of MTP. Where cells were incubated with palmitic acid, a considerable proportion of the secreted lipoproteins were of the TAG-poor lipoprotein (LDL and IDL). MTP is believed to act early in the synthesis of nascent chylomicrons and it has been suggested that MTP may influence the number of chylomicron particles secreted rather than the lipid composition. Given the observation that oleic acid leads to a significantly greater output of basolateral TAG in Caco-2 cells and the role of MTP in shaping chylomicron synthesis, the interaction of oleic acid and MTP warrants further investigation.

In recent years, several studies have been published indicating a significant effect of dietary fat intake on gut hormone function that may relate to fat absorption and TRL-lipoprotein disposal. Serrano et al. (1997) showed that cholecystectomized patients habituated to high oleic acid or linoleic acid diets for 30 days showed marked differences in gut hormone release in response to an acute-on-chronic fat meal.[20] Whereas linoleic acid led to an acute rise in serum gastrin levels, peaking 30 minutes after fat ingestion, oleic acid in the chronic diet led to no change in serum gastrin with acute fat ingestion. However, the most striking effect was seen with peptide YY (PYY). This hormone tended not to change in concentration with fat ingestion. However, chronic exposure to olive oil led to a very significant rise in serum PYY compared with the linoleic acid diet (i.e., 96 vs. 69 pmol/l). Oleic acid is also established as a potent stimulus to the release of cholecystokinin,[20] which is a highly effective promoter of gall bladder contraction. More recently, Jackson et al. (2000) studied the posptrandial lipid and hormonal response to a test meal in northern Europeans habituated to a diet high in SFA and low in MUFA, and southern Europeans habituated to a high-MUFA diet.[22] Plasma levels of glucose-dependent insulinotrophic polypeptide (GIP) were significantly lower in the northern than the southern Europeans (AUC of 63.2 vs. 116.5 n mol.min). The AUC for plasma insulin was also lower in northern Europeans (105 nmol.min/l) than southern Europeans (229 nmol.min/l). Associated with these profound effects of a high olive-oil diet on the postprandial endocrine response were differences in postprandial lipid response. In southern Europeans, there was an earlier time to apo B-48 peak and a more rapid decline to normal in the southern Europeans. However, there were no differences in lipoporotein lipase activity between subjects from the north and south.

In all of these studies, it is difficult to find a unifying theme to relate the effects of oleic acid on hormones that regulate gastrointestinal function to the effects observed, with more systemically functioning hormones to fat absorption and disposal. Clearly, this is also a very important area for future research. One possible link, albeit an as-yet speculative one, is the observation that exogenous PYY stimulates the synthesis and secretion of intestinal apolipoprotein A IV (apo A-IV) in a dose-dependent fashion.[23] This apolipoprotein is involved in the stimulation of lipoprotein lipase in association with apo C II and is also involved in the induction of postprandial satiety.[24,25] An additive effect of peptide YY and apo A-IV synthesis on chylomicron secretion has recently been suggested.[26] This is supported by the finding that apo A-IV plays a key role in stabilizing chylomicron synthesis.[27]

B. MUFA AND THE IMMUNE SYSTEM

Dietary regulation of the immune and inflammatory processes have been widely studied using *in vitro* cell culture work, animal models, human experiments, and clinical intervention trials. The *in vitro* cell culture studies tend to be somewhat reductionist, since they are necessarily conducted in an environment that cannot link with the many modulators of the immune and inflammatory responses that are sensitive to systemic post-stimulus signals. At the other end of the scale, clinical intervention studies are subject to confounding factors such as degree of severity of the condition under study, stage of the disease, prior surgical treatment, current pharmacotherapies and associated but confounding clinical conditions. Notwithstanding these difficulties, considerable progress has been made in recent years in our understanding of how nutrients influence the immune and inflammatory systems. Without doubt, long chain n-3 PUFA have been shown to have a marked effect on reducing the inflammatory response. However, from the early 1990s, the interest in lipids and the immune system began to be extended to other lipid classes.

Following injection with recombinant human tumour necrosis factor (TNF), protein synthetic rate (PSR %) in the liver and lung is dramatically increased, 88% and 22% respectively, in rats fed maize oil rich in linoleic acid.[28] In contrast, fish oil suppresses PSR percentage in the lung, but stimulates it in the liver. Butter has an entirely opposite effect. Coconut, however, causes a dramatic rise in protein synthetic rate in both the liver (-50%) and the lung (+ 208%). However, when oleic acid was added to the coconut oil diet to a level found in butter, the pattern of response was dramatically altered in both the liver (+ 17%) and the lung (- 22%).

These studies revealed that oleic acid could radically alter the systemic response to TNF injection, TNF being a major mediator of inflammation. Subsequent studies have examined *in vitro* lymphocyte proliferation, stimulated by various mitogens, in cells taken from rats fed various dietary fats.[29] Whereas the stimulation index for animals fed a low-fat diet did not differ from animals fed coconut oil or sunflower oil, there was a very substantial reduction in lymphocyte proliferation in the cells taken from rats fed olive oil, evening primrose oil, or fish oil. Further studies were carried out to compare the same effects between olive oil and high oleic sunflower oil, and no significant differences were observed. Thus, the effect is likely to be the high level of oleic acid and not due to any of the non-saponifiable bioactive lipids found in olive oil. In an evaluation of published data in this area, Jeffrey et al. (1997) showed that the stimulation index was related to the log of the ratio of oleic acid to linoleic acid.[30] In effect, there is a strong response in the suppression of lymphocyte proliferation up to a level of about 36% (w/w) of fatty acids as oleic acid. Thereafter, there is little incremental response. The same authors showed that natural killer (NK) cell activity declines linearly as the level of oleic acid is increased across the range of 20–70 g of oleic acid per 100 g of fatty acids.

More recently, research has begun to focus on the role of dietary fats in adhesion molecule expression in blood mononuclear cells.[31] Such adhesion molecules are an integral part of the binding of lymphocytes and monocytes to tissues. In human endothelial cell lines pre-incubated with different fatty acids and subsequently challenged with TNF alpha, the expression of the vascular cell adhesion molecule-1 (VCAM-1) was significantly reduced compared with controls by oleic and docosahexaenoic acid but not by arachidonic or eicosapentaenoic acids. More recently, in a human feeding study comparing the effects of a high-MUFA or a high-SFA diet for 8 weeks each, the former led to a significant fall in peripheral-blood mononuclear cell expression of ICAM-1 but not Mac-1.[32] The high SFA had no effect on either of these adhesion molecules.

Unraveling the mechanism(s) whereby oleic acid exerts an effect on the inflammatory and immune system will be a challenge. It is likely that the superfamily of peroxisome proliferator-activated receptors (PPARs) transcription factors, the expression of which is regulated by fatty acid, have a role in this process. We already know that these transcription factors, in which there are four mammalian sub-types (α, β, γ, δ), regulate the genes involved in lipid metabolism. A recent study showed that PPARγ pharmacological PPARγ ligands inhibit the inflammatory cytokine response.[33] Northern blot analysis showed that this was a pre-translational event because the PPARγ ligands inhibited monocyte TNFα mRNA expression. Another study demonstrated PPARγ agonists inhibited PMA-induced VCAM-1 expression and monocyte binding to human aortic endothelial cells (HAECs).[34] In Caco-2 cells, it has been demonstrated that pharmacological PPARγ ligands inhibit cytokine gene expression by keeping the pro-inflammatory transcription factor NF-κB in an inactive state. While the entire regulatory sequence up-stream of NF-κB has yet to be resolved, we do know that PPAR ligands, which include fatty acids, alter the phosphorylation status of Iκ-B, which is a prerequisite for NF-κB activation. Since fatty acids are natural PPAR ligands, it is likely that it is through this pathway that oleic acid derived from olive oil has it effects. However, it has yet to be determined whether and how fatty acids and PPARs have a direct effect on 1-κB/NF-κB metabolism. If not, there are intermediates in the signaling cascade, such as protein kinase C, phospholipases, and other kinases, which may transmit the PPAR-induced effects of fatty acids on the inflammatory response. The therapeutic potential and clinical implications of PPARγ ligands and NF-κB inhibition were demonstrated when pharmacological PPARγ ligands significantly reduced colonic inflammation in an animal model of inflammatory bowel disease (IBD).[35] Hence, it remains to be seen if and how fatty acids can attenuate the inflammatory response; this information in turn will have important consequences in relation to chronic inflammatory disease.

REFERENCES

1. Serra-Majem, L., Ribas, L., and Ramon, J.M. Compliance with dietary guidelines in the Spanish populations. Results from the Catalan Nutrition Survey. *Br. J. Nutr.*, 81, S195, 1999.
2. Moschandreas, J. and Kafatos, A. Food and nutrient intakes of Greek (Cretan) adults. Recent data for food-based dietary guidelines in Greece. *Br. J. Nutr.*, 81, S71, 1999.
3. Graca, P., Dietary guidelines and food nutrient intakes in Portugal. *Br. J. Nutr.* 81, S71, 1999.
4. Valsta, L. Food-based dietary guidelines for Finland — a staged approach. *Br. J. Nutr.*, 81, S49, 1999.
5. Herman-Kunz, E. and Thammon, M. Dietary recommendations and prevailing food and nutrient intakes in Germany. *Br. J. Nutr.*, 81, S61, 1999.
6. Lowik, M.R.H., Hulshof, K.F.A.M., and Brussard, J.M. Patterns of food and nutrient intakes of Dutch adults according to intakes of total fat, saturated fatty acids, dietary fibre and of fruit and vegetables. *Br. J. Nutr.*, 81, S91, 1999.
7. Gibney, M.J. Epidemiology of obesity in relation to nutrient intake. *Intl. J. Obesity*, 19, Suppl 5, S1, 1995.
8. Katan, M.B., Grundy, S.M., and Willett, W.C. Beyond low-fat diets. *New Eng. J. Med.*, 337, 563, 1997.
9. Wei, M., Kampert, J.B., Barlow, C.E., Nichaman, M.Z., Gibbons, L.W., Paffenbarger, R.S., and Blair, S.N. Relationship between low cardiorespiratory fitness and mortality in normal-weight, overweight and obese men. *J. Am. Med. Assoc.* 287, 1547, 1999.
10. Turley, E.H.M., Skeaff, C.M., Mann, J.I. and Cox, B. The effect of low-fat, high carbohydrate diets on serum high-density lipoprotein cholesterol and triglyceride. *Eur. J. Clin. Nutr.*, 52, 728, 1998.

11. Wood, P.D., Stefanick, M.L., Williams, P.T. and Haskell, W.L. The effects on plas-malipoproteins of a prudent weight reducing diet with or without exercise, on over-weight men and women. *New Eng. J. Med.* 325, 461, 1991.

12. Roche, H.M. and Gibney, M.J. Postprandial triacylglycerolaemia:the effect of low-fat dietary treatment with and without fish oil supplementation. *Eur. J. Clin. Nutr.* 50, 617, 1996.

13. Roche, H.M. and Gibney, M.J. Postprandial triacylglycerolaemia - nutritional impli-cations. *Prog. Lipid Res.*, 34, 249, 1995.

14. Hardman, A., Interaction of physical activity and diet:implications for lipoprotein metabolism. *Pub. Hlth. Nutr.*, 2, (Suppl 3a) 369, 1999.

15. Mensink, R.P. and Katan, M.B. Effect of monounsaturated fatty acids versus complex carbohydrates on high density lipoproteins in healthy men and women. *Lancet*, i, 122, 1987.

16. Zampelas, A., Roche, H.M., Knapper, J.M.E., Jackson, K.G., Tornaritis, M., Hatzis, C., Gibney, M.J., Kafatos, A., Gould, B.J., Wright, J. and Williams, C.M. Differences in postprandial lipaemic responses between northern and southern Europeans. *Ath-erosclerosis*, 139, 83, 1998.,

17. van Greevenbroek, M.M., van Meer, G., Erkelons, D.W., and de Bruin, T.W.A. Effects of saturated mono- and polyunsaturated fatty acids on the secretion of apo B-con-taining lipoproteins by Caco-2 cells. *Atherosclerosis*, 121, 139, 1996.

18. Gordon, D. Recent advances in elucidating the role of the microsomal triglyceride transfer protein in apolipoprotein B lipoprotein assembly. *Curr.Opin. Lipido.*, 8, 131, 1997.

19. van Greevenbroek, M.M., Robertus-Teunissen, M.G. and de Bruin, T.W. Participation of the microsomal triglyceride transfer protein in lipoprotein assembly in Caco-2 cells:interaction with saturated and unsaturated dietary fatty acids. *J. Lipid. Res.*,39, 173, 1998.

20. Serrano, P., Yago, M., Manas, M., Calpena, R., Mataix, J. and Martinez-Victoria, E. Influence of type of dietary fat (olive and sunflower oil) upon gastric acid secretion and release of gastrin, somatostatin and peptide YY in man. *Dig.Dis.Sci.*, 42, 626, 1997.

21. Konturck, S.J., Tasher, J., and Bilski, J. Physiological role and localization of CCK release in dogs. *Am. J. Physiol.*, 250, G391, 1986.

22. Jackson, K.G., Zampelas, A., Knapper, J.M.E., Roche, H.M., Gibney, M.J., Kafatos, A., Gould, B.J., Wright, J.W. and Williams, C.M. Differences in glucose-dependent insulinotrophic polypeptide hormone and hepatic lipase in subjects of southern and northern Europe. *Am. J. Clin. Nutr.*, 71, 13, 2000.

23. Kalogeris, T.J., Qin, X., Chey, W.Y. and Tso, P. PYY stimulates synthesis and secre-tion of intestinal apolipoprotein A-IV without affecting mRNA expression. *Am. J. Physiol.*, 275, 668, 1998.

24. Goldberg, I.J., Scheraldi, C.A., Yacoub, L.K., Saxena, U., and Bisgaier, C.L. Lipo-protein apo CII activation of lipoprotein lipase. Modulation by apo-lipoprotein A-IV.*J. Biol. Chem.*, 265, 4266, 1990.

25. Fujimoto, K., Cardelli, J.A., and Tso, P. Increased apolipoprotein A-IV in rat mesen-teric lymph after lipid meals acts as a physiological signal for satiation. *Am. J. Physiol.*, 262, 91002, 1992.

26. Tso, P., Liu, M., and Kalogeris, T.J. The role of apolipoprotein A-IV in food intake regulation. *J. Nutr.*, 129, 1503, 1999.

27. Hussain, M.M., Kancha, R.K., Zhou, Z., Luchoomun, J., Zu, H., and Bakillah, A. Chylomicron assembly and catabolism: role of apolipoproteins and receptors. *Biochem. Biophys. Acta*.1300, 151, 1996.

28. Grimble, R.F. Dietary manipulation of the inflammatory response. *Proc. Nutr. Soc.* 51, 285, 1992.

29. Yaqoob, P., Newsholme, E.A., and Calder, P.C. The effects of dietary lipid manipulation on rat lymphocyte subsets and proliferation. *Immunology*, 82, 603, 1994.

30. Jeffrey, N.M., Cortina, A., Newsholme, E.A., and Calder, P.C. Effects of variations in the proportions of saturated, monounsaturated and polyunsaturated fatty acids in the rat diet on spleen lymphocyte function. *Br. J. Nutr.*, 77, 805, 1997.

31. Yaqoob, P. Monounsaturated fatty acids and the immune system. *Proc. Nutr. Soc.*, 57, 511, 1998.

32. Yaqoob, P., Knapper, J.A., Webb, D.H., Williams, C.M., Newsholme, E.A., and Calder, P.C.The effect of olive oil consumption on immune function in middle aged men. *Am. J. Clin. Nutr.*, 67, 129, 1998.

33. Jiang,J., Ting, A.T., and Seed, B. PPAR-γ agonists inhibit production of monocyte inflammatory cytokines. *Nature*, 391, 82, 1998.

34. Jackson, S.M., Parhami, F. Xi, X-P, Berliner, J.A., Hsuceh, W.A., Law, R.E., and Demer, L.L. Perosisome proliferator-activated receptor activators target human endothelial cells to inhibit leucocyte endothelial cell interaction. *Atherioscler. Thromb. Vasc. Biol.*, 19, 2094, 1999.

35. Su, C.G., Wen, X. Bailey, S.T., Jian, W., Rangwala, S.M., Keilbaugh, S.A., Flanigan, A., Murthy, S., Zazar, M.A., and Wu, G.D. A novel therapy for colitis utilizing PPAR-g ligands to inhibit the epithelial inflammatory response. *J. Clin. Invest.*, 104, 383, 1999.

Index

A

a-Aktinin, hydrolysis of, 159
Aaromonas veronii biogroup *sobria*, 215
ACE, see Angiotensin-converting enzyme
Acetic acid, 191
Acinetobacter baumanii, 215
ADA, see American Dietetic Association
Adenocarcinoma, of esophagus, 59
Aegean Sea, 33
Aging
    free radical theory of, 210
    telomeric theory of, 215
AHA, see American Heart Association
Aktin, hydrolysis of, 159
Albania
    adult mortality in, 206
    infant mortality rates of, 342
    milk production in, 130
Alcohol
    cancer risk and, 324
    mood-altering effects of, 181
Alcoholic beverages, 181–201
    availability
        biological factors influencing, 189
        in Muslim countries, 112
        secular trends in for human
            consumption, 183
    beer, 196
    traditional distilled alcoholic beverages
        in Mediterranean region,
        196–197
    trends in alcoholic beverage production
        and availability, 182–189
    wine, 189–195
        composition of wine, 190–193
        wine and health, 195
        wine regions in Mediterranean and
            wine cultivars, 193–195
Alexis of Thurium, 22
Aliphatics, 82
Allium compounds, 315
Almyra, 34
ALP, see Atherogenic lipoprotein phenotype

Amaristeton, 7
American Diabetes Association, 235
American Dietetic Association (ADA), 168
American Heart Association (AHA), 207,
        235, 245
Amino acid(s)
    content, of plant protein sources, 116
    nervous system and, 168
    requirements, 172
    sulfur-containing, 116
    whey protein, 143
Anakatotos, 36
Ancel Keys study, 56
Angiotensin-converting enzyme (ACE), 255
Animal fats, average supply of in selected
        Mediterranean countries and
        U.S., 303
Animal Protein Availability (APA), 164,
        166
Anthocyanidins, 263
Antioxidant(s), 261
    agent, vitamin E as, 89
    anticancer effects of, 311
    excellent source of, 67
    importance of for health-conscious
        public, 118
    intake, emphasis on dietary, 235
    lipophylic, 90
    natural, 89, 90
    waste, 312
APA, see Animal Protein Availability
apoE, see Apolipoprotein E
Apolipoprotein E (apoE), 250, 251
Appetizers, 12
Apple production, in Mediterranean region,
        102
Arachidonic acid, 144
Arginine, 249
Aristotle of Stageira, 16
Artopolides, 8
Artos, 8
Ascorbic acid, 117, 123
Asia Minor, migrants from, 34
Athenaeus, 21, 22

Atherogenesis, process of, 248
Atherogenic life-styles, 350
Atherogenic lipoprotein phenotype (ALP), 269
Atherosclerosis, 192, 347
    benefit of crude fiber against, 59
    characteristics of, 245
    lipid-related risk factor for, 252
    pathogensis of, 246

B

Bacchus, 189
Bacillus cereus, 150
Bananas, availability of in European countries, 109
Barbaralevro, 36
Barley gruel recipe, 13
Beer
    availability, secular trends in for human consumption, 184
    imports, secular trends in proportion of in relation to total availability in Mediterranean countries, 188
    -making, 196
    secular trends of distribution of alcohol availability into, 186
Bellaria, 13
Benzoic acid, 86, 191
Biotin, 139
Bladder cancer, 295, 313, 319, 324
Blended diets, 23
Blood clotting, beneficial role of n-3 fatty acids on, 60
BMI, see Body Mass Index
Body Mass Index (BMI), 233, 347
Bovine spongiform encephalopathy (BSE), 161
Brassicas, 119
Bread
    availability, by degree of urbanization in Greece and Spain, 66
    consumption, pre-World War II Greek, 44
Breast cancer, 295, 314
    case-control studies, 305
    mortality, 303
    olive oil and, 60
    risk, reducing, 304

Breast feeding, importance of emphasized by Soranus, 17
Bronze-Age site, excavation at, 6
Brucella, 149
BSE, see Bovine spongiform encephalopathy

Butter availability, in Mediterranean countries, 135
Butter, 78, 145
    amount of vitamin D in, 86
    contribution of to milk-fat intake, 146
    production of in France, 135
Butyric acid, 144, 146
Byzantine Mediterranean Diet, 23

C

Caffeic acid, 211–212
Cambridge Heart Antioxidant Study (CHAOS), 262
Campylobacter jejuni, 175
Cancer, 293–340, see also specific types
    comparative cancer and dietary patterns of selected Mediterranean countries and U.S., 294–304
    comparison of dietary patterns in early 1960s and 1990s, 297–302
    comparison of total cancer mortality in early 1960s and 1990s, 296–297
    relevant background information, 294–296
    hormone-related, 312
    incidence of in Cyprus, 345
    Mediterranean Diet as whole, 325–326
    mortality, of Seven Countries Study cohorts, 208
    nutritional epidemiology of, 59
    protective effect of vegetables and fruits against, 59
    relationship of Mediterranean Diet to, 56
    risk, fruit and vegetable consumption and, 58
    weighing of evidence, 304–325
        foods, 312–325
        significant nutrient and non-nutrient components, 304–312
Candida albicans, 215